EAT
TO
BEAT
YOUR DIET

EAT

— TO —

BEAT

YOUR DIET

BURN FAT, HEAL YOUR
METABOLISM, AND LIVE LONGER

By

WILLIAM W. LI, MD

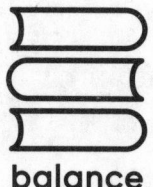

balance

Copyright © 2023 by William W. Li, MD

Cover photographs by Shutterstock
Cover copyright © 2023 by Hachette Book Group, Inc.

Balance
Hachette Book Group
1290 Avenue of the Americas
New York, NY 10104
GCP-Balance.com
Twitter.com/GCPBalance
Instagram.com/GCPBalance

First edition: March 2023

Balance is an imprint of Grand Central Publishing. The Balance name and logo are trademarks of Hachette Book Group, Inc.

The publisher is not responsible for websites (or their content) that are not owned by the publisher.

The Hachette Speakers Bureau provides a wide range of authors for speaking events. To find out more, go to hachettespeakersbureau.com or email HachetteSpeakers@hbgusa.com.

Balance books may be purchased in bulk for business, educational, or promotional use. For information, please contact your local bookseller or the Hachette Book Group Special Markets Department at special.markets@hbgusa.com.

Library of Congress Control Number: 2022949190

ISBNs: 9781538753903 (hardcover), 9781538756539 (large print), 9781538753880 (ebook)

Printed in the United States of America

LSC-H

Printing 1, 2023

This book is dedicated to my parents, who guided me
early in life to harness both the creative and the scientific
as a way to find brighter solutions for the
world around us.

Contents

PART 3
A PLAN FOR LIFE

Introduction

I am not a fan of diets. Never have been. I dislike fad diets, crash diets, pop diets; in fact, any diet that promises massive weight loss "in no time at all!" Most popular diets are not based on science and don't address the true basis for health—which you can't see in the mirror. I am a physician and scientist, and my focus has always been on health, not vanity.

Eat to Beat Your Diet was written to bring you the real science that is missing from all those diet plans. Fighting body fat is vitally important for your health, but not for the reasons you might think. And food is not your enemy. In this book, you will learn through a remarkable set of discoveries backed by validated research studies that the right foods can improve your metabolism and strengthen your body's natural health defenses. By the time you're done, you'll understand how to eat these foods to your advantage, beat back body fat, and optimize your health—all without ever needing to go on a "diet," hence the book's title.

Most diet books preach deprivation and lay out strict rules that take the fun out of your natural way of eating. Instead, I will tell you what foods to *add* to your life and how to enjoy them while healing your metabolism and getting you to your next level of health. Along the way, I'll explain the latest science about how your metabolism really works (it's probably not what you've been told), what your fat does to *support* your health, how shedding even small amounts of weight can have big health benefits, and why, regardless of your age, body type, or size, you do not need to deprive yourself of the joy of food while you are elevating your fitness and ability to resist and fight disease. This book is about mastering your health through metabolism while loving food at the same time. But along the way, you'll also learn how to lose extra weight and shrink your waistline in meaningful and science-backed ways.

* * *

Eat to Beat Your Diet is a sequel to my last book, *Eat to Beat Disease*, in which I discussed how your body resists disease through its five health defense systems—angiogenesis, regeneration, microbiome, DNA protection, and immunity—and how specific foods can support one, two, or even all five of these systems at once. I described the evidence showing how more than two hundred foods can activate these defenses to help us avoid the diseases we fear the most: cancer, heart disease, dementia, diabetes, autoimmune disorders, and more than seventy other conditions, based on the new science of molecular nutrition. By *adding* these beneficial foods to your life, you can raise your health shields against disease. My main message is that some of the most powerful tools for improving your health exist naturally in the foods you eat; you just have to become aware of the complex ways your body responds to what you feed it. This book takes off from there and extends the connections between food and your health defenses to your metabolism and their interplay with body fat.

After *Eat to Beat Disease* was published, I received thousands of emails from readers telling me they felt more fit and had more energy after eating the foods I wrote about. They were happier and more confident about their health once they realized they could embrace food and not fear it. They said they felt empowered to take control of their health using the simple steps I described that they could implement at home. Some even let me know that they were able to stop taking their prescription medications after following the 5 × 5 × 5 plan I proposed in the book.

What caught me completely by surprise was that I also began receiving messages from readers who gleefully told me that they had succeeded in losing weight and slimming down in ways they hadn't experienced before. They were eating the foods I recommended, not starving themselves, and shedding pounds anyway.

Wait, I thought, *they were not reducing their food intake. How could eating food lower their body mass and body fat?*

Drawing on my years of research in medicine and physiology, I did a very deep dive into the science of body fat. I looked at the links between metabolism, fat (also called adipose tissue), and food. What I discovered was mind-opening: most of the ideas we accept as fact about metabolism and fat are not true. Even doctors and nutritionists were getting it wrong!

For instance, you are not born with a slow metabolism that causes you to become fat. It's the other way around. Having too much body fat slows your metabolism. Another common misconception is that you don't need to worry about excess fat unless you are overweight or see unsightly bulges in the mirror. Medical research tells us that slim people can grow dangerous amounts of fat packed inside their bodies.

On the other hand, fat can contribute to good health, because fat is actually an organ. That's right, an organ just like your heart, liver, and lungs. In fact, your fat releases hormones that control the normal function of many of your other organs, even your brain. Fat is also an important heat generator in the body. A layer of it not only provides insulation against the cold; a unique type of fat called "brown fat" can burn away excess amounts of other fat around your middle and elsewhere. By burning fat for energy, brown fat *increases* your metabolism. Of course, fat is also a cushion, but it is so much more. The goal, then, isn't to rid yourself of all your body fat—you just need to tame it.

* * *

There are moments in everyone's life when a light bulb goes off in their head, and they hit on an important new insight that can change their world. These are the moments that scientists live for. For me, that moment came when I realized that the very same food compounds that activate your body's health defenses also trigger cellular actions that improve your metabolism and counter body fat. These compounds are called "bioactives," and I realized that they are key to why my readers were slimming down.

Probing even deeper into the science, I discovered there are multiple ways that bioactives can cause weight loss. Certain foods stop fat cells from expanding; others cause "bad" fat cells to become "good" fat cells; still other foods can redirect a fat stem cell, so it can't create more dangerous fat. Some foods even crank up your brown fat space heater, meaning that you can eat foods to trigger good fat to burn down bad fat. In other words, you can fight fat with fat.

Not all calories are created equal, and my research proves it. Eating the right foods can help you improve and strengthen your metabolism and strip away excess body fat, all while improving your health. In this book, you'll learn about how these discoveries were made and you'll find a unique list of 150 foods I've identified that truly fight fat—all based on evidence from human studies.

* * *

When you look at my list of true Fat-Fighting Foods, it will be clear to you that taming your body fat doesn't require sacrifice and hardship. Quite the opposite: you can enjoy your food while eating to improve your metabolism. This might sound like a paradox, but science says it is not. Taming body fat also doesn't have to be expensive or complicated. Most of the foods on the list are found in your typical grocery store. And when I think about recipes and dishes that can be made with these foods, my mouth begins to water. Healing your metabolism can taste great!

I developed my fondness for tasty food growing up in Pittsburgh, Pennsylvania, a city once known mostly for its steel and glass industry but now recognized as a mecca of medical innovation (and some great restaurants!). Nestled among three rivers and 446 bridges, Pittsburgh is a place of diverse ethnic communities. When I was a kid, there was the annual Pittsburgh Folk Festival that took place in the Civic Arena, a now-defunct sports venue that had a retractable domed roof so unusual-looking that it was featured as a backdrop in multiple movies.*

During the festival, the city's forty-odd nationalities, including Italians, Germans, Hungarians, Slovaks, Poles, Greeks, Chinese, and Filipinos, set up colorful side-by-side food stalls selling small plates of specialties from their homelands to hungry attendees. Enticing smells wafted through the entire venue. I loved sampling tasty bites of traditional cooking while listening to the hosts in the stalls describe the ethnic traditions behind each dish. Through these experiences and a network of family and community, my childhood was filled with flavors and stories of foods from around the world.

Decades later, I still revel in the pleasure of eating. It is something I look forward to every single day, ranking right up there with enjoying good health. What many people don't realize is that those two goals—relishing food and enjoying health—are one and the same; at least, they should be. Based on my more than three decades of scientific research, I know that the right foods can activate the body's power for healing. And contrary to what you might have heard, the foods that are most effective at activating health can also deliver the greatest pleasure. Eating for health can dazzle your taste buds and bring new gustatory delight to your life.

When it comes to eating for both pleasure and health, I look to two parts of the world I have come to know and love: the Mediterranean and Asia. Both regions are, of course, renowned for their delicious and diverse cuisines. The healing power of food is, literally and figuratively, baked into their food cultures. Much of what is known as modern

---

* *The Fish That Saved Pittsburgh* (1979); *Sudden Death* (1995); *Rock Star* (2001); *Zack and Miri Make a Porno* (2008); *She's Out of My League* (2010).

Western medicine had its origins in Italy and Greece. Hippocrates, the father of medicine, was from the Greek island of Kos. His "Hippocratic Oath" is still recited by every medical student on the day they graduate and assume the title of physician. The word "physician," in fact, comes from the Latin *physica*, meaning "natural," while the word "doctor" comes from the Latin *docere*, meaning "teacher."

Nutrition was used for healing when Hippocrates lived in ancient Greece, and the quote "Let food be thy medicine, and medicine be thy food" reflects the thinking of his time.* Ironically, most physicians today are woefully undereducated about modern nutrition. Few are knowledgeable enough to share a proper understanding of food and health with their patients. Medical school education emphasizes the importance of pharmaceuticals for treating disease over natural solutions to maintain health. As a result, generations of doctors have drifted further and further away from medicine's roots, where nutrition was once a key tool in a doctor's toolbox.

Food is also central to health in Asian cultures, which have some of the oldest medical systems in the world. Chinese medicine dates back more than three thousand years and is rooted in the concept that your health is the result of balanced forces known as yin and yang. These balances are influenced by the properties of different foods. One of the earliest-known medical textbooks was assembled by Sun Simiao, who was regarded as China's "King of Medicine." His book *Essential Prescriptions Worth a Thousand Pieces of Gold* was written during the seventh-century Tang dynasty, a golden era of Chinese culture. Simiao devoted an entire section of his textbook to food therapy, including recipes, lists of medicinal herbs, and recommendations for modest eating. Today, medicine in China is a progressive blend of traditional healing approaches mixed with modern biomolecular therapies.

---

* Scholars have determined this is an attribution and not a direct quote from Hippocrates. However, the idea of "food as medicine" was certainly accepted during his time.

The Mediterranean and Asia may seem worlds apart in their traditions, yet two thousand years ago, a remarkable land route called the Silk Road connected these two regions and their foods. This passage served as one of the most influential trading channels in human history, allowing goods, ideas, and ingredients to be exchanged between many different countries and cultures. Established during the Han dynasty, the Silk Road was responsible for the movement of many familiar foods that we eat today from China to Western countries, and vice versa.

I started thinking seriously about these food cultures during a gap year I took before starting medical school. I was interested in learning how food influenced culture, society, and health—so I traveled first to Italy and Greece (this was long before the Mediterranean diet became popular) and then to China to see for myself. Living and eating with locals in Lombardy, Liguria, Veneto, Mount Athos (I embedded myself as a visitor to Greek Orthodox monasteries and even volunteered to help cook Easter feast in one of them!), and the Cyclades and then in Hebei, Shanxi, Sichuan, Hunan, and Jiangsu Provinces planted the seed of an idea in my mind that I later developed into my own style of eating, which I call "MediterAsian." It combines the best of both worlds and uses many of the delicious, metabolism-mending ingredients that you'll learn about in this book.

MediterAsian is how I eat every day, with my food choices inspired by the traditions that span these cultures. I'm going to describe my approach to you and give you some recipes that come from my own kitchen using fat-fighting ingredients that I love to eat. The MediterAsian approach makes it easy to improve your health, inside and out.

* * *

I wrote this book for anyone who can benefit from a better metabolism—and that's everyone, well, everyone who wants to live a longer life filled with greater enjoyment. Whether you are young and fit, in your middle adulthood, or in your senior years, you can apply the new science of body fat, using food to pump up your metabolism and perform at your personal best.

If your doctor has said that you should lose a few pounds, or if you've been struggling to gain better control of your weight, this book will give you a way to achieve your goals while finding (or gaining!) pleasure from your meals. And especially if you have a chronic health condition, fighting excess body fat will help you use your metabolism as a tool to combat diseases, such as cancer, cardiovascular disease, diabetes, auto-immune conditions, dementia, and more. Healing your metabolism heals every part of your body.

Having said all this, it's only fair for me to state who this book is *not* for.

This book is not for a crash dieter, or someone who wants to lose a huge amount of weight in a matter of days, or someone whose only goal is to get a slim beach body, no matter what the cost to their health. If you are looking for a quick and temporary fix that will surely result in a rebound, please look elsewhere. My goal in this book is to help you use your metabolism and body responses to food as a way to lose fat and gain health—with durable benefits.

* * *

Eat to Beat Your Diet has three parts. In Part 1, I tell you about how your body fat is connected to your health defenses and how fat supports your health in absolutely essential ways. You'll learn how fat develops while a fetus is still in the womb, how it sculpts your body as you develop from a baby to child to teenager to young adult and beyond, and how fat behaves differently between men and women in some ways but acts the same in many others. Then, I share new findings about human metabolism that may upend everything you think you know about food, fat, and energy. You'll learn about the power of brown fat as a metabolism healer and how we know that food can activate it to combat fat. *Yes, you really can eat to beat fat!* In fact, I reveal to you the many fat-fighting bioactives found in foods and explain how they tame fat in different, powerful ways.

In Part 2, I take you on a virtual shopping trip to the grocery store to show you how easy it is to find the foods containing these powerful bioactives that improve your metabolism and rightsize fat. We travel to the different sections of the store, from the perimeter to the middle aisles, where you can find many surprising metabolism-boosting ingredients. I highlight the foods that have the greatest scientific evidence for fighting body fat, and I single out the ones I like the most for a delicious MediterAsian approach to eating.

In Part 3, I give you a few coaching tips and a specific plan for how to begin your own MediterAsian program to tune up your metabolism. The plan is both personal and flexible, and I'll show you how to get it started, keep it going, and adapt it to the inevitable changes that you will encounter. It is a plan to establish and maintain a healthy metabolism for your whole life.

* * *

To get the most out of this book, I recommend that you read the chapters in order and not just jump to Part 3 where the MediterAsian plan is. By reading Part 1, you will reframe your entire understanding of body fat and metabolism and how they work together. Before moving on to Part 2, take in all the reasons to respect your body fat and digest the implications of how you can use food to elevate your health. When you read Part 2, you'll learn about all the foods that are beneficial for your metabolism. If this is your own physical copy of the book, use a pen to mark all the foods that you already enjoy or the ones you find interesting and would like to try. If you picked it up at the library, you can snap some photos with your cell phone so you can quickly find the foods you want to remember when you go to the grocery store. Finally, do a quick full read-through of Part 3 to familiarize yourself with the entire plan before you dive in and try it, then go back and read the instructions and tips on how to maximize its benefits.

Once you are familiar with all the steps of the MediterAsian plan, choose a time when you can work it into your life. Use the QR code in Part 3 to get planning guides, practical tips, and updates that I will provide as the science advances.

Get ready for a new life experience. You will transform your metabolism with my sustainable anti-diet approach to food, health, and enjoyment. You will discover it is possible to love your food *and* love your health at the same time—I'm about to show you how. In the spirit of MediterAsian eating, I say to you:

Buon appetito, kalí órexi, and gan bei (干杯)!

PART I

HOW FAT WORKS

Our body is a machine for living. It is organized for that;
it is its nature.
Let life go on in it unhindered and let it defend itself.
—*Leo Tolstoy*, War and Peace

CHAPTER 1

The Surprising Science of Fat, Health, and Disease

If the word "fat" triggers a strong emotion when you hear it, you're not alone. Our language is filled with words like "overweight," "obese," and "heavy" that can bring about judgment, discomfort, disappointment, and even fear. We wince when we see the fat on our frame in the bathroom mirror. It makes us feel less healthy. Even in the grocery store, we feel a negative reaction when we see a rind of fat on a cut of meat in the butcher section. Fat has a bad reputation—but I'm here to tell you that fat is not the villain we've made it out to be.

The truth is, fat is one of the most important tissues in your body. It stores the fuel that your heart needs for pumping, your liver needs to detoxify your blood, and your kidneys need to remove waste and extra fluid from your body. In fact, fat is essential to every organ's functioning. Without any body fat, you would look skeletal and haggard—ultraskinny is a shocking look—and if you stopped eating, you'd run out of life-sustaining energy and die within a couple of months. If you had no food, your body could draw on its fuel reservoir of fat to help you survive—which would be depleted to zero in nine weeks for a woman and seven weeks for a man of average build.*

---

* An "average" adult weighing 70 kilograms (154 pounds) has 30 pounds of fat, which stores 130,600 kilocalories. Women burn, on average, 2,000 kilocalories per day, and men burn 2,500. This means that if all food consumption stopped, fat could theoretically provide fuel for 9.4 and 7.4 weeks, respectively. Practically, however, organ failure would occur long before this point.

Fat insulates you like a sweater when you are exposed to the cold, and it cushions and prevents your internal organs from rupturing if you take a fall. More surprising, science has revealed that fat itself is an actual organ. It releases hormones and chemical signals that control your brain, heart, immune system, and virtually all your body's health systems. Fat is not to be feared but rather respected, although we do need to keep it under control.

The Problem with Excess Fat

Excess body fat *is* a true villain when it comes to your well-being, even in slender people. A common misconception is that you only need to worry about body fat if you are overweight. In reality, even if the number on the scale says "you're healthy," you can have too much fat. Medical research shows that everyone needs to be concerned about the amount of body fat they carry inside their frame.

Whether you have a large body or a small one, excess body fat grows . . . like a cancer. Just like a tumor, fat needs a blood supply to nourish its mass. To grow larger and become dangerous, growing fatty tissue must take on an ever-increasing blood supply by recruiting new blood vessels through a process called angiogenesis—just like a cancer does. Tumors are angiogenesis-dependent, and so is burgeoning fat.

This property of fat has been confirmed using the very tools of cancer research. Scientists at the University of Massachusetts Medical School obtained chunks of belly fat from people undergoing gastric bypass surgery for morbid obesity. They placed tiny pieces of fat in a plastic dish, bathed them with liquid nutrients, and observed what happened. Within four days, new blood vessels began sprouting outward like branches from a tree as the fat attempted to feed itself. This is shown in the two photos from the study (Figure 1.1). The dark mass in the left panel is a piece of fat with a starburst of growing blood vessels radiating

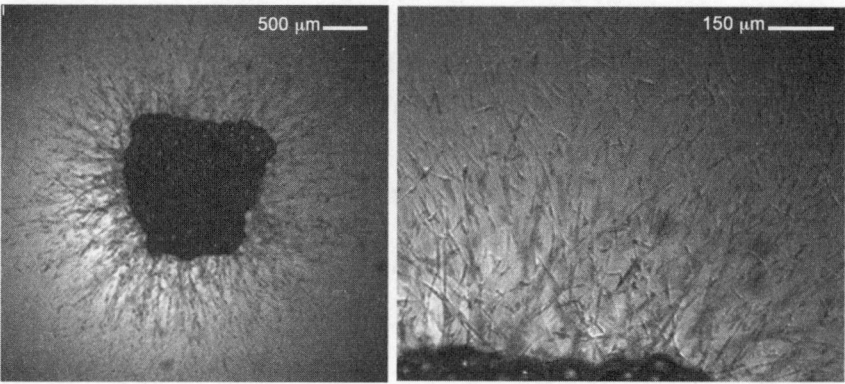

Figure I.I. Fat removed during surgery for morbid obesity in a dish and growing new blood vessels. (Source: Image courtesy of Dr. Silvia Corvera, University of Massachusetts.)

outward. In the right panel is a close-up view: you can see the individual blood vessel cells organizing themselves into tiny tubes.[*]

Once fat improves its blood supply, more oxygen and nutrients flow to feed the cells. But also like a tumor, fat cannot grow if its blood supply is impeded. Researchers have shown in the lab that body fat will actually shrink if angiogenesis is inhibited, and this leads to weight loss.[1] Administering a drug that inhibits angiogenesis can starve fat tissue and cause slimming of the body, even when there is no change in diet.[2] Cutting off the blood supply to tumors is an effective way doctors treat cancer. Now this strategy, called antiangiogenesis, can be applied to controlling body fat.

The best news, however, is that you don't need drugs to cut off fat's blood supply. This approach has been borrowed to study the effects of food because many foods contain natural chemicals that can cut off the blood supply to fat and shrink it. Green tea, for example, contains a bioactive compound called epigallocatechin-3-gallate (EGCG), which is a potent angiogenesis inhibitor.[3] Clinical studies have tested extracts

---

[*] Figure reproduced with permission from O. Gealekman, N. Guseva, et al. "Depot Specific Differences and Insufficient Subcutaneous Adipose Tissue Angiogenesis in Human Obesity," *Circulation* 123, no. 2 (2011): 186–194.

from green tea and shown that people drinking them have reduced abdominal fat and waist circumference.[4] Researchers at Inha University in Korea examined 10,030 subjects in the Korean Genome and Epidemiology Study and found that women who consumed four or more cups of green tea per week had a 44 percent decreased risk of abdominal obesity.[5] All this to say:

You can eat to beat fat.

Eat to Fight Fat

We've known for centuries that eating *less* will help you lose weight, but the unexpected good news is that we've now identified certain foods that when eaten can help burn away excess fat. These foods improve your metabolism, which is vital to your health. You read that correctly: eating the right foods can actively promote fat *loss* and improve your metabolism. Even better, many of the same foods improve your body's health defenses, too. A triple win.

If you are reading this book because you want to lose weight, chances are you have tried dieting before. You may have lost weight temporarily but soon gained it back, since most diets are just too hard to follow for long. You might have felt discouraged by diets that are all about restriction and elimination because you found them onerous and depriving. That's completely understandable. We naturally prefer to enjoy our life and not fear food. So, you may be asking, "Is there a way I can combat fat while embracing and enjoying food?"

The answer is "Yes!" I am going to show you how.

In the chapters ahead, you will learn how you can fight harmful fat, improve your metabolism, and eat for pleasure—all at the same time. And I will show you exactly how to put the latest research to work in your daily menu.

Choosing the right foods can take your health to the next level. In my previous book, *Eat to Beat Disease*, I gave a comprehensive primer on your body's health defense systems. Since then, medical research has greatly expanded our understanding of the many ways our health defenses are linked to our body fat, and vice versa. What this means is that eating to boost your health defenses can also help rein in your body fat. The harm caused by excess body fat also directly hinders the body's health defense systems, making you more vulnerable to disease. In this first chapter, I will lay out, for the first time ever, the fascinating connections among food, fat, and your five health defenses. So let's take a closer look at how each of these systems does its job and how they interact with your body fat.

Heroes of Health: Fat and Your Five Defense Systems

The Angiogenesis System

The prefix "angio-" refers to blood vessels, and "-genesis" refers to growth. Your body is filled with sixty thousand miles of blood vessels that form your circulation—enough to encircle the world twice. These are the highways and byways for blood and everything that's carried within it. Your angiogenesis defense system delivers oxygen and nutrients to every cell in your body. When your blood vessels are healthy, your organs are healthy. This defense system maintains just the right number of blood vessels at all times.

If you are injured and need to heal, or if you are building more muscle, or if you are pregnant and nurturing new life, your angiogenesis system springs into action to grow blood vessels wherever they are needed: just the right amount, not too few and not too many. On the flip side, the system also can adjust itself to prevent too many blood vessels from forming or prune away excess vessels. In short, to maintain good health,

7

you need your angiogenesis system to be operating to groom your circulation.

More than seventy diseases can occur when your angiogenesis system is weakened and there are either excessive or insufficient blood vessels. Some of the most common diseases include obesity, cancer, diabetes, arthritis, and even Alzheimer's disease. Insufficient angiogenesis leads to wounds that do not heal or an oxygen-starved heart and brain and organ failure. Excessive blood vessels, on the other hand, can leak fluid and bleed, causing organ damage. If this should happen in your eyes, leaking vessels can cause vision loss in conditions like age-related macular degeneration and diabetic retinopathy.

Cancer can thwart your angiogenesis defenses by recruiting new blood vessels to bring nutrients and oxygen to cancer cells. This allows tumors to grow and spread (metastasize). A robust, fortified angiogenesis defense prevents this from happening. Without a new blood supply, a tumor cannot expand beyond 2 to 3 millimeters (about 1/10th of an inch) in diameter, roughly the size of the tip of a ballpoint pen. If a cancer does manage to hijack the angiogenesis system, however, new blood vessels sprout into the tumor and nourish cancer cells, fueling the tumor's ability to invade surrounding organs and lethally spread. Cutting off the blood supply to shrink tumors is the basis for cancer treatments called antiangiogenic therapy.

The same principle also applies to fat. The heftier the fat mass, the more blood vessels are needed to keep it nourished. Cut off the blood supply to a mass of fat, and it can't grow larger.

Unlike cancer, however, blood vessels were already baked into your fat from the time you were born. In studies of people with severe obesity, the bigger their waistline, the more blood vessels were present and feeding their fat.[6] The need for blood flow in fat is critical. As I mentioned earlier, a chunk of belly fat removed during surgery and placed in a plastic dish of nutrients will quickly sprout new vessels in an attempt to feed itself.

More than one hundred foods can fortify your body's angiogenesis defenses by either stimulating or inhibiting blood vessel growth. Beyond green tea, foods like turmeric, soybeans, ginseng, and broccoli all prevent unwanted blood vessels from supplying nourishment to cancer cells, and they suppress the growth of fat cells, too.[7] Other foods that support your angiogenesis defenses, such as fruit skins, barley, and even sea bass, can stimulate helpful new circulation for healing. Here's the remarkable part: angiogenesis-inhibiting foods do not starve your organs, and angiogenesis-stimulating foods do not provoke cancer growth. Your body is designed so that when it comes to responding to healthy foods, it takes just what it needs, nothing more, nothing less.[8]

The Regeneration System

Your body contains cells whose job is to constantly regenerate and repair your internal organs. These are your stem cells, also called progenitor cells. They have the amazing ability to morph into any type of cell depending on your body's needs. You were born with 750 million of these progenitors that are stored in your bone marrow, skin, and fat. Throughout life, your stem cells are spurred into action when a damaged organ needs to be repaired or when it grows—like muscle or fat.

The stem cells enter your bloodstream and circulate to the location where they are needed, then they home in to the organ, where they regenerate the tissue. This can occur literally anywhere in your body, such as your intestines, nerves, blood vessels, muscles, bones, liver, lungs, testes, ovaries, and even your heart and brain. Your blood cells and your immune system are constantly replenished by stem cells to keep them fresh and ready for action.

Your fat contains special stem cells called preadipocytes. These cells are essential for health. Preadipocytes create hormone-releasing fat cells—adipocytes—that help your metabolism process blood sugar and blood lipids. The hormones also influence your reproductive system, which in turn communicates with your fat.[9] Your preadipocytes also produce the protective fat padding that safeguards your organs as you jostle through life.

The problem comes when your diet causes your preadipocytes to become overly active and create too many fat cells. Too much fat disrupts your hormones, so your preadipocytes need to be reined in. Foods such as blueberries, goji berries, and turmeric have restraining power over preadipocytes, taming them so that they do not create too many new fat cells.[10]

Another type of stem cell that lives in your fat is called the adipose stromal cell (ASC). These special cells live in the lacework of connective tissue that is embedded within a mound of fat. ASCs have a talent: they are master builders of blood vessels, the ones needed for healthy fat tissue to thrive. When they are overly active, however, ASCs can create an undesirable blood supply that nourishes and expands the fat around your waistline, under your chin, or anywhere in your body.

Medical researchers have tapped into the power of ASCs by pulling them out of a person's fat and injecting them elsewhere in their body in order to tap into their regenerative power. Researchers collect ASCs using liposuction, the same procedure performed by plastic surgeons for body sculpting. The stem cells are harvested and cultivated like seedlings before being reinjected directly into the organ that needs to be healed. This ASC therapy is being tested in clinical trials to regenerate heart muscle in patients with heart failure, to regenerate brain cells in those with Parkinson's disease, and to regrow nerves in people suffering from severe spinal cord injury.[11] Significant clinical improvements have been seen in patients receiving ASCs for all of these conditions.*

In a landmark case, a young man suffered a catastrophic fall that severed his spinal cord at neck level, leading to quadriplegia, a state of paralysis in which he could not move his arms and legs. He received an

---

* To find a clinical trial of adipose stromal cells for a condition of interest, you can go to www.clinicaltrials.gov and type in "adipose stromal cell" and your "[disease]."

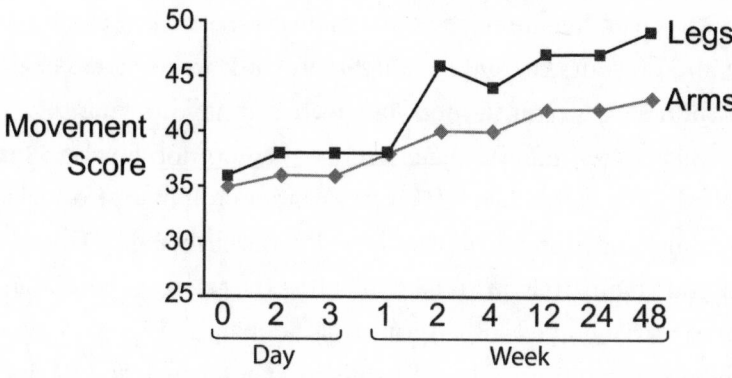

Reversal of Paralysis with Adipose Stromal Cell Therapy

Figure 1.2. Result of ASC injection after spinal cord injury. (Source: Graphic by Diana Saville, adapted from M. Bydon, A. B. Dietz, et al., "CELLTOP Clinical Trial," *Mayo Clinic Proceedings* 95, no. 2 [2020]: 406–414.)

experimental injection of his own ASCs into his spinal cord to see if they could regenerate his nerves.[12] Within months after the treatment, he began regaining movement, the progress of which is shown in Figure 1.2. The vertical axis shows a measure of his ability to move. The horizontal axis shows the time after ASC treatment. The boxed line represents the patient's arms. The diamond line represents his legs. The improvement he experienced over forty-eight months following spinal cord regeneration led to a reversal of his paralysis—an unprecedented feat of medical science!

Remarkably, many foods can trigger regeneration in organs without adding more body fat. In fact, some foods can cause regenerative healing at the same time as they *inhibit* preadipocytes from creating more fat. Mushrooms, barley, cacao, omega-3-containing foods, and coffee and tea have been shown to coax more stem cells to be released into the bloodstream to promote regeneration, but, as you'll soon learn, these are also foods that fight fat.[13]

The Microbiome System

Your microbiome is a health defense made up of 39 trillion bacteria, along with viruses and fungi. These organisms live mostly in your lower gut but also on your skin and in every bodily orifice. Bacteria in particular are surprisingly essential for your well-being. They fine-tune your metabolism, lower blood sugar, reduce cholesterol levels, suppress inflammation, and enhance immunity. Your microbiome also speeds up wound healing and influences your emotional well-being by sending signals to your brain that instruct it to release crucial mood-enhancing hormones such as oxytocin, serotonin, and dopamine.

When your microbiome is disrupted, your physical and mental health can fall apart. A growing body of evidence shows that dysbiosis, the state in which your microbiome is damaged, is associated with an array of diseases including obesity, cardiovascular disease, cancer, autoimmune conditions, irritable bowel syndrome, Alzheimer's disease, depression, schizophrenia, amyotrophic lateral sclerosis, and even autism. Your gut's bacterial makeup can even influence the success of cancer therapy. Whether or not your microbiome is healthy can be a matter of life and death.[14]

Your microbiome is tied to your body fat. Researchers from the Washington University School of Medicine in St. Louis studied fifty-four pairs of twins of different body sizes and checked their microbiomes by collecting fecal samples. They found that twins with lean body types had a different mix of gut bacteria than twins who were obese.[15] Lean subjects also had differences in more than three hundred bacteria genes compared to their obese counterparts.[16]

The diversity of bacteria in your gut is also important. As a general rule, the greater the diversity, the better your health. Lean individuals have a more diverse microbiome than people who are obese. What's important is that you can influence your microbiome directly through the foods you eat. People who consume more plants in their diet have more diverse species of bacteria in their gut than those who shy away from fruits and vegetables.

One particular bacterium, *Akkermansia mucinophila*, is an especially important player among the trillions of bacteria in your body. *Akkermansia* plays a key role in controlling body mass and metabolism, as well as immunity. Researchers have discovered that people who are lean have more *Akkermansia* in their gut than obese people.[17] Even among people who are overweight, those with more *Akkermansia* have a smaller waist-to-hip ratio and their fat cells are smaller in size.[18] Foods like pomegranate, cranberry, turmeric, green tea, and chili pepper help *Akkermansia* grow in the gut because these foods make the intestines secrete more mucous, creating a welcoming environment where this bacterium thrives. Those foods can even help cancer patients respond to immunotherapy treatments because *Akkermansia* plays a role in the immune destruction of cancer cells.[19]

Your microbiome began to develop while you were a fetus in your mother's womb, but it is shaped by your experiences and food choices throughout life. You "pick up" and swallow bacteria without knowing it from touching your pets; from hugging family members and friends; from objects you handle at school, work, restaurants, and shops; and while you are on vacation. What you eat directly influences your gut bacterial health. When you eat plant-based foods, the dietary fiber feeds your microbiome. When they are content and well fed, these bacteria produce three notable metabolites—acetate, butyrate, and propionate—known as short-chain fatty acids. These fatty acids are responsible for many of the health benefits of your microbiome, including streamlining your metabolism and lowering blood cholesterol.

Foods that contain lots of dietary fiber are called "prebiotic" because they nourish your inner biota, your gut bacteria. Leafy green vegetables; fruits like apples, pears, and kiwifruit; mushrooms; whole grains; and nuts like walnuts and macadamia are just some examples of prebiotic foods. "Probiotic" foods are those that contain live bacteria that contribute to the gut ecosystem. They are fermented foods such as kimchi, sauerkraut, pickles, yogurt, kefir, miso, tempeh, and cheese. Fermented foods that contain fiber, such as kimchi and sauerkraut, which are made from pickled cabbage, are both prebiotic *and* probiotic. The products made and released by the bacteria as they grow in the fermented foods are known as "postbiotics," and these aid your metabolism, too.

The DNA Protection System

Your DNA is a six-foot-long folded ribbon of genetic material coiled inside every single one of your 40 trillion cells (very similar to the number of bacteria in your body!). This ribbon contains your genetic code, the instructions for cells to make the proteins your body needs to stay alive. But less than 2 percent of your DNA is used to guide the creation of proteins. Most of your DNA is used to coordinate the inner workings of the two hundred different types of cells in your body to keep them functioning for health.

Your DNA is a defense system that protects your genetic code against the damage that can be wreaked by everyday exposures, including ultraviolet radiation from the sun; radon from the ground; microplastics in your drinking water; and chemicals released by wall paint, carpets, and furniture. These environmental forces create highly reactive atoms known as free radicals. These atoms behave like rogue samurai warriors slashing at your DNA. Left unrepaired, the damaged DNA can create mutations that lead to abnormal cells and, ultimately, to cancer.

Excess body fat also creates free radicals inside your body and increases the risk for cancer-causing mutations.[20] Harmful free radicals are also created by emotional distress; lack of sleep; physical inactivity or extreme physical activity; and eating ultraprocessed food, grilled meats, and chemical preservatives.

Fortunately, damaged DNA is capable of repairing itself. Without this health defense, you would not be here to read this book. You can dial up (or dial down) the strength of the repair mechanisms with the foods you eat. Foods like kiwifruit, carrots, beans, strawberries, and omega-3-rich seafood can boost DNA repair.

Besides repair, parts of your DNA can be switched on or off by your diet, lifestyle, and environment. These are called epigenetic changes. Such changes can protect your health by turning on useful genes or by blocking harmful ones. For example, when parts of your DNA called tumor suppressor genes are turned on, they protect you against prostate, breast, and colon cancer. Foods like soy, cabbage, kale, Brussels sprouts, broccoli sprouts, turmeric, and green tea can switch on these protective genes.[21]

Another type of epigenetic change, called methylation, is associated with lowering body mass. In methylation, the function of a gene is changed by a chemical structure, called a methyl group, which is inserted right into your DNA. The effect is like jamming a screwdriver into a conveyor belt. It halts the manufacturing of certain proteins that cause belly fat to grow and that disrupt your metabolism.

Methylation affects the *function* rather than the structure of your DNA. It is an extra move in the health defense playbook of DNA. A study by scientists at the Norwegian University of Science and Technology compared the DNA of sixty lean and sixty obese women who were between twenty-three and thirty-one years old. They found there were ten specific sites in the DNA that were more methylated—helpfully blocked—in people who are lean compared to those who are obese.[22]

Another link between DNA and fat was discovered by researchers at the Carlos III Health Institute in Madrid, Spain.[23] They tracked the changes in the DNA of 131 obese children, boys and girls between four and nine years old. The children were placed on a personalized version of the Mediterranean diet for one year, along with a supervised physical activity program. Their DNA and physical characteristics were examined at four and twelve months. At both points, the diet and lifestyle interventions led to a decrease in total body fat. When the researchers examined their DNA, they found that those with more DNA methylation had less abdominal fat, smaller body mass, a better metabolism, and more weight loss.

One more way that your DNA defends your health is through structures called telomeres. These are protective caps that prevent your DNA from fraying at its ends. As you age, telomeres shorten like the burning wick of a candle. Anything that slows the shortening process also slows cellular aging. Regular exercise and good-quality sleep, for example, can slow telomere shrinkage, which is why both are important for health.

People with a high body mass have a faster erosion of those crucial telomeres. Children and adolescents who are overweight have shorter telomeres compared to their counterparts who are lean.[24] In adults and the elderly, the impact is even more profound. The Health, Aging and Body Composition Study led by the University of California San Francisco examined 2,721 people in their seventies and measured their body composition and telomere length.[25] Subjects with a lower percentage of body fat and less belly fat had longer telomeres. The good news is that certain foods have been discovered to slow telomere shrinkage. Many of these foods are common in Mediterranean-and-Asian-style eating patterns, and they can also fight body fat, helping your DNA take care of itself—and you.

The Immune System

By far, the most familiar of your body's five defense systems is your immune system. It protects you from external invaders like bacteria and viruses swirling around in your environment. It also protects you from invaders lurking within your body, like cancer cells. Healthy immunity repels disease regardless of its source.

Seventy percent of your immune system is in your intestines, where it communicates with your gut microbiome. Part of your immune system is also embedded in your fat. Like the rest of your body's defenses, your immune system is strongly influenced by the foods you eat.

Your immune system has two main parts: the innate system and the adaptive system. Innate immunity is swift acting and reacts in the same way each time, like a blunt instrument. This part of your immune system causes inflammation, a necessary and brief response when defending your body against invaders. The second part, adaptive immunity, is smarter but slower acting. It is trained to recognize enemies and then develops sophisticated responses to handle each threat. This is where T cells and natural killer cells (also known as large granular lymphocytes) work together to tackle invaders, and where immune B cells learn to produce antibodies. Adaptive immunity is activated inside your body in response to viral infections, a vaccine injection, or a bee sting, or when your immune system is trained by cancer treatments, known as immuno-therapy, to seek out and destroy cancer cells. Together, the elements of these two parts of the immune system function like an army of super soldiers, each with its own special weapons and tactics for detecting, destroying, and clearing out invaders from the fortress of your body.

A healthy immune system can distinguish "friendly forces" (your healthy cells) from "enemies" (everything else). It will ignore your normal cells but immediately spot a threat like a cancer cell. Enemies are swiftly destroyed before they can establish themselves and become dangerous. The microscopic cancers that commonly form in our body do not usually create disease because they are eliminated before they develop into a noticeable tumor.[26] People with a weakened immune system, however, are far more likely to develop dangerous cancers because these microscopic cancer cells remain undetected and are able to grow up and cause harm.[27]

Your immune defenses function like the volume control on a car radio. If the volume is too low, you won't get the right output. This is immune deficiency. If the volume is too high, the noise becomes intolerable. This happens with asthma, severe food allergies, and even hay fever. The volume control on inflammation is especially important to your health. A tiny burst of inflammation is crucial for fighting off infection, but it must be switched off when the battle is won. If inflammation persists and becomes chronic, it can cause damage to your organs. Cancer, heart disease, dementia, diabetes, autoimmune conditions, and obesity are just a few diseases that are tied to the smoldering fire of chronic inflammation.[28] As you will see later, chronic inflammation is caused by excessive body fat.

Here's the thing: normal fat tissue contains immune cells that are a critical part of the response against disease. About 5 percent of all cells in your fat are immune cells called macrophages. They help maintain an adequate blood supply to your fat, and they are also tasked to remove dead fat cells. If your fat expands to an unhealthy size, however, too many macrophages accumulate, and this triggers inflammation.[29]

A study at Columbia University performed fat biopsies of obese as well as lean people to compare their immune cells.[30] They found that, in obese people, macrophages represent a whopping 40 percent of all cells in the fat, eight times above the normal level. The cells also were pumping out inflammatory cytokines, which are chemicals that provoke chronic inflammation.[31] Another study conducted at the Human Research Center on Nutrition in Paris found an even greater, sixteen-fold increase in the number of macrophages in the fat of morbidly obese individuals when compared to lean subjects.[32] After dramatic weight loss from gastric bypass surgery, the macrophages in fat were slashed by half. Controlling body fat lowers inflammation in the body by reducing the number and activity of immune cells that are swarming in the fat.

While excess body fat makes inflammatory cells overactive, it paradoxically dampens other key parts of your immune defenses. The T cells of obese people are less capable of conducting immune surveillance and have difficulty destroying foreign invaders. This translates into more difficulty in avoiding and recovering from infections.[33] Never was this more obvious than during the early days of the coronavirus pandemic in 2020, when obesity was quickly spotted as one of the biggest risk factors for dying from COVID-19.[34]

Food plays an essential role in balancing the impact of fat on your immune system, and vice versa. What you eat can lower inflammation, boost immune defenses, and shrink fat tissue, leading to weight loss. Blueberries, tree nuts, mushrooms, garlic, and broccoli are common foods that support and activate immune cell function yet cause body fat to shrink. Chili peppers increase the number of immune B cells that produce antibodies.[35] Oysters also have immune-boosting and anti-inflammatory properties. Tomatoes, red bell peppers, papayas, citrus fruits, guavas, and strawberries lower inflammation and reduce flares of autoimmune disease. Green tea and chicken soup each have inflammation-quelling benefits.[36] Foods that are high in fiber—leafy greens, apples, pears, and whole grains like whole wheat, oats, and barley—feed your microbiome, which produces the short-chain fatty acids that lower inflammation.

Body Fat and Chronic Illness

With so many connections between your body fat and your health defenses, there are big opportunities and threats when it comes to your health. The opportunity is that you can fortify your defenses and use them to bring excess fat under control. You can even enlist fat as an ally to boost your health defenses. The threat is that too much fat can damage your health defenses, making you more vulnerable to disease. Even if your goal is to see less bulge in the mirror when you step out of the shower, an even more important reason to vanquish excess body fat is to lower the damage it does inside your body, where the destruction is invisible to your naked eye.

The bottom line is that, when it comes to body fat, you can't trust appearances. Fat bulging under the chin, around the torso, over a waistline, and around the thighs is obvious. But slender people can also have unhealthy amounts of body fat packed inside their thin frames like stuffing jammed into a small turkey. You won't be able to see this fat, but the havoc it wreaks can manifest as high blood pressure, high blood cholesterol, and high fasting blood glucose. It's vital that you become aware of your inner health and understand how it is affected by too much body fat.

Blood tests can be revealing. Many people who are not overweight, and even those who are slender, hear from their doctors that they have high blood pressure and their lab tests show high levels of bad LDL cholesterol, high triglycerides, and elevated blood sugar. These are metabolic warning signs that excess fat is lurking somewhere in your body.

The most dangerous type of fat is the kind that is crammed into the crevices inside your abdomen, wrapped around your innards like pastry dough, squeezing your organs in a bear hug. This type of fat is called visceral fat, and it poses a greater health risk than subcutaneous fat—the jiggly stuff that accumulates visibly beneath the skin. Visceral fat encases your kidneys, intestines, and even your heart like a baseball glove. It can infiltrate your breasts if you are a woman and surround the testicles and prostate gland if you're a man. Normal-sized people can walk around with visceral fat billowing deep inside them and never know it until a health disaster strikes.

That is why this book is not simply about slimming down and losing weight. The battle against excess fat goes way beyond vanity. It's a battle for your health—and for some, it may even be a fight for your life. Sure, I want you to feel better by looking good, but my biggest goal is to help you *gain health*, whatever your outward appearance. But first, I'll help you see what I see: the evidence of just how bad excess fat can be when it comes to the diseases you fear the most.

A Double Whammy: Cancer and Diabetes

Too much visceral fat is very dangerous. It releases chemical signals called cytokines that cause inflammation, and it throws your metabolism off-kilter. Excessive amounts of this kind of fat increase your risk for heart disease, stroke, diabetes, Alzheimer's disease, and even cancer. A study out of Weill Cornell Medical College and Memorial Sloan Kettering Cancer Center in New York examined breast tissue removed from women having breast reduction surgery and found that inflammatory fat was present in 35 percent of breasts of normal-sized women.[37] Chronic inflammation from visceral fat raises blood levels of the hormone insulin, a condition known as hyperinsulinemia. This is a sign of metabolic distress.

A high blood insulin level is known to be a risk factor for breast cancer.[38] It's also an ominous sign that predicts cancer death more broadly. A study of almost ten thousand people over a decade by the National Health and Nutrition Examination Survey showed that having high blood insulin *doubled* the risk of dying from cancer, compared to people with normal blood insulin levels. The threat was present even among people who were not obese. When they looked at 6,718 normal-sized subjects, the researchers found that the risk of cancer death was increased by 89 percent in people whose insulin levels were high.[39]

The reason for this is that high blood insulin causes your liver to overproduce a protein called insulin-like growth factor-1 (IGF-1).[40] Too much of this protein can directly spark the growth of cancer cells. IGF-1 can also help cancer cells hijack the body's angiogenesis defense system. High levels of IGF-1 prompt cancer cells to produce a protein called vascular endothelial growth factor (VEGF) that acts as a fertilizer for new blood vessels to grow and feed tumors.[41] You do not want your insulin or IGF-1 levels to be chronically high.

Abnormalities in your body's control of insulin are part of a condition known as metabolic syndrome. The syndrome also includes high blood sugar, high blood pressure, high blood lipids, and too much visceral fat. If you have metabolic syndrome, you are at high risk for diabetes, heart disease, and cancer. Metabolic syndrome doubles the risk of endometrial cancer in women who are obese and increases the risk by 38 percent even in women who are not overweight.[42] Men do not escape the dangers of visceral fat with metabolic syndrome. Inflammatory fat can build up around the prostate gland, and this is associated with more aggressive forms of prostate cancer, even in men who are normal weight.[43]

A massive study was conducted through the Institute for Health Metrics and Evaluation and funded by the Bill and Melinda Gates Foundation to examine the avoidable risk factors of people from 204 countries who were diagnosed with cancer over a decade, from 2010 to 2019. High body mass was one of the top three avoidable risk factors for cancer.[44] The study concluded that a whopping 44 percent of *all* cancer deaths could be avoided if people stopped smoking, reduced alcohol use, and improved their metabolism by lowering body fat and reducing high blood sugar.

The bottom line: no one can afford to have excessive visceral fat—for health reasons. The good news is that eating the right foods can help control this kind of fat. So, what if you don't bring it under control? Well, let's examine more of the consequences.

A Higher Risk of Heart Disease

Most people with obesity have high blood pressure, a condition called hypertension in which the fluid pressure in the arteries is chronically elevated. Hypertension is a major risk factor for all forms of cardiovascular disease, including coronary artery disease, stroke, and heart failure. Too much visceral fat contributes to hypertension. One way it does so is by releasing a hormone called leptin.

Lab studies have shown that leptin stimulates the sympathetic nervous system, leading to a fight-or-flight reaction in your body that increases your blood pressure.[45] You will learn a lot more about leptin in the next chapter. Elevated blood pressure leads to a cascade of events that fells your health like dominoes. It harms your kidneys, which are designed to act as filters to get rid of extra fluid in your body. Once this filtering system is damaged, less fluid is filtered. More fluid accumulates in the body, leading to even higher blood pressure, and this kicks off a destructive cycle. More fluid, higher blood pressure, more kidney damage, even more fluid. Fat also can build up around your kidneys and compress them, further knocking down their filtering ability. Having a fatty kidney doubles your risk for high blood pressure.[46]

Metabolic syndrome results when high blood pressure is combined with high cholesterol, high blood sugar, and excess body fat. You can have this without being obviously overweight. And your risk of cardiovascular disease will skyrocket. A study by scientists at Harvard Medical School, the Medical University of South Carolina, and Boston University examined 1,056 "average-sized individuals" and found that 7 percent of them had metabolic syndrome. These people had a threefold increased risk of heart disease, which manifested as a heart attack, angina, transient ischemic attack, stroke, or poor leg circulation, when compared to people who did not have metabolic syndrome.[47]

When you carry around extra body fat, your heart has to pump harder and faster to not only bring enough blood flow to the rest of your body but also to nourish the fatty tissue itself. Over time, this added strain weakens your heart muscle and can cause heart failure. Excess fat also wreaks havoc on the blood vessels feeding your heart muscle. The cells lining these vessels are called endothelial cells. They are damaged by the inflammatory cytokines released by fat cells, which makes blood flow more difficult to maintain because plaque builds up on the damaged vessel walls and narrows the blood vessels. This causes your blood vessels to become "stiff," and your blood pressure goes up because your circulation has a hard time relaxing.

A study at the Mayo Clinic showed this effect in forty-three young, healthy volunteers who were of normal body weight.[48] They fed the volunteers one thousand extra calories per day to cause them to gain nine pounds, which was about a 5 percent increase in their body weight. The weight gain was primarily due to growing more visceral fat in their belly. This increase led to a 15 percent decrease in the efficiency of their blood flow due to damage to their blood vessel lining. When the volunteers lost the weight they had gained, their blood vessels recovered, and blood flow improved. This shows you how important weight loss can be to reverse the internal damage that you can't see in the mirror.

Your regenerative defenses will normally come to the rescue to repair damaged blood vessels. But the stem cells you need for this fix are themselves damaged by high blood pressure. Researchers from the University Hospital Zurich in Switzerland found that the stem cells in people with high blood pressure were 46 percent less capable of doing their job for regeneration, compared to those from healthy individuals whose blood pressure was normal.[49] High blood cholesterol also cripples the stem cells, so this is another reason people with metabolic syndrome have compromised circulation.[50] These hits to your angiogenesis and regeneration health defenses set you up for heart disease.

Body Fat Causes Lean Diabetes

Type 2 diabetes is closely linked to having too much body fat. The two are so closely related, in fact, that doctors sometimes refer to them together as "diabesity." But how does fat disrupt metabolism? Researchers at Harvard discovered that excess fat stresses out a part of your cell's internal machinery called the endoplasmic reticulum.[51] When this kind of stress occurs, your cells have a hard time responding to insulin, which your cells need to absorb glucose as fuel. When the cells become *insensitive* to insulin, your blood sugar level rises despite the presence of insulin.[52] This is a key connection between obesity and type 2 diabetes.

This link is so profound that an obese individual is eighty times more likely to develop type 2 diabetes than someone of average weight. But the truly surprising fact is that slender people also can develop this form of diabetes if they have too much visceral fat—for the same reason: stressed-out endoplasmic reticulum. As many as 15 percent of people with type 2 diabetes are of a healthy weight. This is known as lean diabetes.[53]

The risks are found in the amount of hidden belly fat. Researchers at the National University of Singapore looked at seventy-six lean and apparently healthy subjects in their early forties and found that those who had early signs of imminent diabetes had more excess visceral fat packed within their abdominal cavities.[54] A special imaging technique known as dual-energy X-ray absorptiometry (DEXA) was used to determine the amount of fat within their bodies. People with lean diabetes can have severe complications from this condition because of damage to the small blood vessels in the retina, kidneys, and nerves.[55] These complications come with a heavy price. A German study showed that people with lean diabetes were more likely to require insulin to treat their diabetes—and, remarkably, they had a 2.5 times *higher* risk of mortality than those people with diabetes who were obese.[56] Now that's an eye-opener.

Body Fat Affects Your Brain

Having too much fat literally messes with your head. A study at University College London examined 9,652 middle-aged people and showed that those who were obese had slightly smaller brains; in fact, 2.4 percent smaller than a person who is of healthy weight.[57] The affected region of the brain was the gray matter, that part that controls movement, memory, speech, emotions, decision-making, and self-control—in other words, the executive functions that are essential for daily life.

When it comes to the brain, once again, it is not just body size that matters. Research led by a team at the Charles E. Schmidt College of Medicine in Florida found that older people who had sarcopenic obesity—low muscle mass but high body fat—had higher rates of cognitive impairment, especially in executive function.[58] A study of 5,186 older adults in Ulster, Northern Ireland, showed that people in their eighties who had high amounts of body fat also had a lower attention span, poorer visual-spatial ability, and immediate as well as delayed memory problems, compared to those with less fat.[59]

An even larger study was conducted in Canada that examined 9,189 subjects across an age span ranging from thirty to seventy-five.[60] The researchers assessed body composition, specifically visceral fat, and assessed brain function using brain imaging and standard cognitive tests. The results showed that having lots of visceral fat is associated with vascular brain injury and reduced cognitive function.[61] The explanation is excess fat provokes chronic inflammation, which disrupts healthy brain function.[62]

Body Fat Affects Your Lungs

Think of your lungs as inflatable lightweight air bags sitting inside your rib cage. When you take a breath, your lungs expand and fill with oxygen, and when you exhale, you blow out carbon dioxide. Typically, we breathe sixteen times in a minute, which means that if you live to be eighty, you will have taken some 673 million breaths. Now consider the consequences of having layers of heavy fat pressing down on your inflatable bags.

How well you can breathe depends on the amount of body fat you have.[63] To inhale, you contract your diaphragm. This pulls down the thick muscle separating your chest from your abdomen and expands your chest cavity like a bellows. A vacuum is created that draws air in from your nose and mouth into your lungs. If there is a large mass of fat sitting inside your bellows, bulging against your diaphragm, it will make it much harder for your diaphragm to pull in air with each breath.

In fact, an obese person can have 30 percent less lung capacity than an average person of normal weight due to excess body fat. Such a dramatic difference reduces the amount of oxygen you take into your body, and this can make even ordinary activities more difficult.[64] The less oxygen your brain, heart, and other organs have, the more likely they are to malfunction. Remember that visceral fat can be invisible—you might not even realize that it's making it harder for you to breathe.

Fat Jams Your Upper Airways

Inhaling is only the beginning of breathing. Air still has to make its way into your lungs, and fat can be an impediment along the way. Excess fat can narrow your airways, the tubes running through your lungs. Worse, it can even make them inflamed. Autopsy studies of overweight people have revealed that the bigger the body mass, the more fat is built up around the airways and the greater the degree of inflammation in them.[65]

Fat can also build up in the back of your throat in an area called the pharynx, where your upper airway begins to descend to your lower airways to your lungs. When you fall asleep, your throat muscles relax and the fat in the pharynx goes flabby. This can partially block your airways, causing the tissues to vibrate when you inhale, leading to loud snoring. Every now and then, the flab can completely obstruct your airway, effectively causing strangulation. As the oxygen levels in your blood plummet, you suddenly awaken, startled. It happens over and over again, all night long. This is called sleep apnea, a serious health problem that affects more than 100 million people worldwide. Sleep apnea results in headaches, daytime exhaustion, irritability, and learning difficulties. The reason? Because you never truly get a good night's sleep. Not only does sleep apnea cause you to be groggy during the day; it also increases your risk of developing diabetes, having a heart attack, winding up with heart failure, or suffering a stroke.[66]

Your Tongue Can Get Fat

A surprising contributor to sleep apnea is tongue fat, a kind of visceral fat. Yes, your tongue can gain weight. Autopsy studies from the San Diego County Medical Examiner's Office measured the amount of fat in the tongues of 121 individuals of varying ages and physical builds who died of natural or accidental causes.[67] The average adult's tongue weighs 99 grams in men, about the same as a bar of soap, and slightly less in women. The entire tongue is made of muscle that can perform acrobatic feats, especially the tip, but it also contains more fat than other muscles in your body. The tip and front are 11 percent fat. The rear third of the tongue—the part that helps you swallow food—is 30 percent fat. The fat there is spread through your tongue muscle like marbling in a ribeye steak. Compare this with your neck muscle or thigh muscle, each of which is only 3 percent fat. In this autopsy study, the bigger the body mass, the greater the amount of tongue fat.

When fat builds up in the rear part of your tongue, it can cause breathing problems during sleep. A study by a group at the University of Pennsylvania examined 121 people and found that those with sleep apnea had 140 percent more tongue fat compared to those who did not have apnea.[68] Loud snoring occurred in the apneic people because their oxygen levels periodically plummeted to critical levels due in part to their floppy tongue fat.

Fatigue and brain fog are only the beginning of the problems caused by sleep apnea. The lack of oxygen also promotes high blood pressure, diabetes, liver disease, dangerous rhythm disturbances in the heart such as atrial fibrillation, and even heart failure.[69] An eighteen-year study of 1,522 people in the Wisconsin Sleep Cohort Study found that people with sleep apnea had a threefold higher rate of mortality.[70] Fatal cardiovascular disease was seen twice as often in people with sleep apnea compared to those who did not have the condition.

Once again, body size can fool you. Even lean people can have fat tongues that cause sleep apnea. Up to 23 percent of young slender people between eighteen and thirty were found to have mild sleep apnea in one clinical study.[71] Besides fatigue, the subjects with sleep apnea also suffered metabolic abnormalities, including a 27 percent reduced insulin sensitivity, so their bodies were forced to produce 37 percent more insulin than people without apnea.

A Swedish study of four hundred women ranging from twenty to seventy found that 50 percent of women had some form of sleep apnea. Eighty-four percent of obese women had the condition, which would be expected. But what was surprising is that slender women also suffered from it.[72] In slim women under forty-five, 20 percent were found to have sleep apnea. In women over fifty-five, 70 percent were apneic—even if they were not overweight. Excess body fat in the belly, the airways, and the back of the tongue is responsible for these dangerous conditions.[73] If you know someone who is slender in build but snores at night, they probably have extra tongue fat.

Research on people with sleep apnea who underwent bariatric surgery or intensive lifestyle modifications to help them lose weight[74] found that those subjects with the greatest improvement in their quality of sleep also lost the most tongue fat as part of their weight loss.

All doctors know that prescribing weight loss is one of the most effective ways to treat sleep apnea. But I'm willing to bet you've never thought of your tongue as being fat, or the importance of slimming it down.

Fat Makes COVID-19 Worse

It was during the COVID-19 pandemic that my attention was drawn to new aspects of body fat. I've always worried about obesity in my patients primarily because of the way it contributes to chronic diseases. But during the first months of 2020, when the coronavirus pandemic was just escalating around the world, obesity was quickly spotted as a major risk factor for being felled by COVID-19. Of course, I knew that obesity hinders the body's immune defenses, but the lethality of COVID-19 on the overweight and obese seemed way out of proportion: these conditions *doubled* the risk of being hospitalized or dying according to an analysis of 3.5 million patients across thirty-two countries during the early months of the pandemic.[75] Why was body fat so harmful, I wondered—and what could we do about it?

One reason that obesity increased the risk of death from COVID-19 is because of the high baseline level of inflammation caused by excess fat raging throughout the body. Infection by the coronavirus made the inflammation even worse. We also knew that the dampened immunity caused by obesity made the coronavirus more difficult to eliminate. Then came the discovery that the coronavirus directly attacks fat cells, and that their destruction ignites even more inflammation.[76] Hormones like leptin released by fat cells in the body of the obese also reduced the number of immune B cells that produce antibodies to fight the coronavirus.[77] The decreased lung capacity of obesity also compromises normal breathing, which increases the danger of any virus that infects the lungs.

But the obesity-related risk goes far beyond the immune system. In the spring of 2020, I was part of an international research team that discovered that COVID-19 causes severe damage to tiny blood vessels everywhere in the body, a serious problem called endotheliopathy. Our discovery changed the treatment of patients with severe COVID-19 by calling for blood thinners to prevent life-threatening blood clots due to the blood vessel damage.[78] Because blood vessels are already compromised in people with obesity, we realized that further vascular injury from the coronavirus infection would cause even greater damage to the kidneys, heart, brain, and even testicles.[79]

Later in the pandemic, I began to research "long COVID"—the prolonged and strange symptoms that arise and persist, sometimes for months or years after one recovers from the initial infection.* This chronic condition is also worse in people who are overweight or obese. The hallmarks of long COVID are persistent blood vessel damage (microvascular injury), chronic inflammation (with autoimmunity), and nerve damage (neuropathy). When there is excess body fat, this can further trigger autoimmune reactions where your body produces antibodies that attack your healthy organs, including blood vessels and nerves.[80] A study of 5,750 healthcare workers in Bari, Italy, who had COVID-19 revealed that having a larger body mass increased the risk of

---

* Long COVID is also known as Post-Acute Sequelae of SARS-CoV-2 infection, or PASC.

long-term effects from the infection that lasted more than one month, making excess body fat a risk factor for long COVID as well.[81]

Lose a Little, Gain a Lot

Although the consequences of excess body fat can be dangerous and devastating, I do have good news: you don't need to lose much weight to score big wins for your health. Unlike the huge amounts of weight loss that fad diets often promise, healthy weight-loss goals are realistic, achievable, and sustainable for almost anyone—and you don't need to get rid of all your fat. You just need to rightsize it, so your body fat can do its job to support your health.

It is important to distinguish intentional weight loss, which is purposeful, from unintentional weight loss, which often is the result of diseases that cause malnutrition or wasting. One study from the Royal Free and University College London Medical School showed that unintentional weight loss is associated with a 71 percent *higher risk* of mortality, while intentional weight loss has a 41 percent *reduction* in mortality.[82]

When you lose weight intentionally, you'll receive the most significant benefits by losing anywhere from one to twenty pounds, for most people. The range of benefits does vary based on how much weight you lose, but those benefits don't add up the way you might expect. Medical researchers have discovered that losing more weight isn't always better.

Let's start at the lower end.

The Surprising Benefits of Losing One to Four Pounds

Losing even a little weight is good for your heart and brain. Researchers from Wageningen University in the Netherlands analyzed twenty-five clinical studies, involving a total of 4,874 individuals, looking at weight reduction and blood pressure. These studies took place over thirty-six years, between 1966 and 2002.[83] Their analysis found that for every two pounds of weight lost, there was a one-point reduction in the subjects' systolic blood pressure, (the top number). Normal blood pressure is 120/70, for example, so 120 is the systolic blood pressure. High blood pressure (hypertension), which begins when your blood pressure is 130/80 or higher, increases the risk of heart disease, stroke, kidney failure, and, later in life, dementia.

Lowering your blood pressure matters in a big way. An analysis of six hundred thousand people involved in clinical trials of blood pressure reduction showed that for every ten-point drop in systolic blood pressure, participants had a 28 percent reduction in risk of heart failure. Thus, losing a mere two pounds lowers the risk of heart failure by 2.8 percent, and losing four pounds reduces the risk by 5.6 percent.[84]

The Benefits of Losing Five Pounds

The sliding scale of benefits really kicks in when you lose five pounds or more. Every bit of weight that is shed unloads your metabolism and helps to reverse the damage that excess fat inflicts on your health defenses. Five pounds of weight loss hits a sweet spot when it comes to reducing cancer risk.

A study supported by the American Cancer Society examined weight change over ten years in 180,885 women from the United States, Australia, and Asia.[85] The women were in their fifties at the start of the study, all were overweight and not taking hormone replacement therapies, and they either had a stable weight (no change) or they had lost varying amounts of weight over the past decade.* The researchers correlated the amount of weight loss to the diagnosis of breast cancer. The results showed that women who lost five pounds or more—and sustained it—had an 18 percent decrease in the risk of developing breast cancer. The benefit increased as more weight was shed. At ten pounds lost, there was a 25 percent lower risk of breast cancer. At twenty pounds,

---

* Their average BMI was 25.1.

the risk declined even further to 32 percent. But even a very achievable five-pound weight loss delivered significant benefits.

The Benefits of Losing Ten to Twelve Pounds

Let's raise the bar on weight loss and look at the benefits of losing ten pounds. This also is an attainable amount of weight for most people to lose and maintain. The benefits include reducing the risk of another deadly disease: endometrial cancer. This cancer develops from the lining of the uterus (the endometrium) in postmenopausal women. There is strong evidence that excess body fat heightens the risk of developing this cancer.[86]

A fourteen-year study led by researchers at Indiana University examined intentional weight loss and endometrial cancer.[87] They enrolled 36,794 women between fifty and seventy-nine, all of whom were overweight and participating in the Women's Health Study.[*] This age bracket is the window of highest risk for endometrial cancer. The researchers monitored these women for weight gain, loss, or stability (no change) over a three-year period. Then they followed their health for the next eleven years.

The study found that those women who lost ten pounds or more during the initial three years had a 39 percent *reduced risk* of endometrial cancer over the next decade.[88] By contrast, women who gained ten pounds or more in those same years had an increased risk of endometrial cancer. The conclusion: even moderate weight loss can have a long-term effect of reducing the risk of a deadly cancer in women.[**]

---

[*] Their BMIs were between 25 and 30, which is classified as "overweight." Their average weight was about two hundred pounds.

[**] I learned a very important tip from one of my medical school professors, Dr. Wayne Christopherson, a gynecological surgeon, that every woman should know. One evening, while making rounds on patients in the cancer ward, he told me, "No woman should ever die of endometrial cancer." He recommended that every woman, after having all the children they want, have a hysterectomy: "If you do not have a uterus, you'll never have endometrial cancer."

In addition to reduced cancer risk, moderate weight loss lowers blood pressure, which, as you've seen, is one of the most beneficial steps you can take for heart health. A Harvard study called TOHP (Trials of Hypertension Prevention) investigated whether intentional weight loss affected mortality over sixteen years, from 1987 to 2013.[89] The researchers enrolled 2,182 men and women between ages thirty and fifty-four. They were overweight, weighing anywhere from 184 to 219 pounds. Those who lost 5 percent or more of their starting body weight (or an average of eleven pounds) had an 18 percent lower risk of death from any cause. Compared to people who gained eleven pounds, those who lost the same amount of weight had a 36 percent reduced death risk. In fact, there was a 14 percent *increase* in mortality risk for every 5 percent weight gain in this study.

The evidence for the lifesaving benefits of losing a modest amount of weight was seen in a meta-analysis by researchers at Wake Forest School of Medicine and Tufts University. They analyzed fifteen well-designed, randomized clinical trials of intentional weight loss, where the effort took place over at least eighteen months and where the subjects started out being obese, meaning they had a lot of weight to lose before they could attain an average weight range.[90] A total of 17,186 middle-aged male and female participants were enrolled in the studies, which ranged in duration from 18 months to 12.6 years. The interventions all involved dietary behavior change, and five of the studies also included some exercise. The results showed that losing a mere twelve pounds was associated with a *15 percent reduction* in all-cause mortality.

Even More Benefit Losing Up to Twenty Pounds

Losing larger amounts of weight brings even more benefits. Twenty pounds is a sizeable amount of weight to lose, though, and it takes a concerted effort to achieve this safely and without resorting to extreme (and usually unsustainable) measures. In general, it's advisable to lose only around one to two pounds a week so you don't lose muscle mass. This means that hitting a twenty-pound weight-loss goal should take place no faster than over two and a half months.

Losing twenty pounds reduces your risk of dying from diabetes. A study by scientists from the US Centers for Disease Control and Prevention, the American Cancer Society, Emory University, and the University of Colorado analyzed data from 49,337 men who were overweight but not obese and were between forty and sixty-four years old. The researchers studied the risks of dying associated with intentional weight loss over thirteen years. The most common causes of death from diabetes include heart attack, stroke, kidney disease, cancer, and vascular disease.[91]

For people with diabetes but no other health conditions, the researchers found those who intentionally lost up to nineteen pounds had a *22 percent* reduced risk of mortality caused by a diabetes-associated condition. In men with diabetes and other health conditions, such as documented heart disease, stroke, and high blood pressure—but no cancer—their diabetes-associated mortality was reduced by an even greater *36 percent*. (See Table 1.1.)

TABLE 1.1. THE HEALTH BENEFITS OF INTENTIONALLY LOSING SMALL TO LARGER AMOUNTS OF WEIGHT

Amount of Weight Loss	Results
1–4 pounds	Lower systolic blood pressure Up to 6% reduced risk of heart failure
5 pounds	18% lower risk of breast cancer
10 pounds	25% lower risk of breast cancer 39% lower risk of endometrial cancer
11 pounds	36% reduced risk of all-cause mortality
12 pounds	15% reduction in all-cause mortality
19 pounds	22% reduced risk of mortality from diabetes
20 pounds	33% reduced risk of breast cancer

Overall, then, losing weight is good for you—but there's a lot more to the story. Losing weight generally means losing fat and, as you've seen, fat has multiple identities and varied roles in the body, both helpful and harmful. To really understand the relationship between food and health, we're going to need to learn how fat really works, from the inside out.

CHAPTER 2

Rethinking Body Fat

All babies have that same adorable look. Like Hershey's Kisses candies coming off the assembly line, they have bulging rolls of fat on their arms and legs, around their cheeks, and under their chin. A plump baby makes you smile, and your instincts are correct: fattiness at this stage of life is absolutely a sign of good health. If you saw a svelte infant with thin arms and legs, a tiny waist, and a chiseled face, you would assume that something was seriously wrong—and you'd be right. In babies, fat is fabulous.

Body size isn't a dead giveaway about adult health, though. Consider Olympic athletes. They train intensely and are at the top of their game every four years. Perfection for them comes in different proportions—the tiny gymnast, the beefy weightlifter, the stocky shot-putter, the svelte figure skater. Excellence is not packaged into a single shape or weight. Professional boxing is another prime example. The sport has seventeen weight classes! They start with minimumweight (yes, that's the correct spelling) at 105 pounds, ascend to featherweight at 126 pounds, then middleweight at 160 pounds, and finally heavyweight at 200 pounds and up. Each boxer fits into one of these categories, and there's a world champion in every weight class. Then there are sumo wrestlers. These legendary Japanese sports figures are behemoths, each weighing in at somewhere between 300 and 400 pounds when they are ready for the *dohyō*, or competition ring. Despite their massive size, sumo wrestlers are highly fit and do not suffer from high rates of the diseases classically associated with obesity, such as heart disease, diabetes, stroke, and cancer.[1] Clearly, large size does not necessarily equate to bad health.

Being thin is not necessarily healthier either. Being underweight carries health risks, as was seen in a study of 1,035,727 patients who underwent a common heart procedure called a cardiac catheterization. In this procedure, dye is injected into the coronary arteries supplying blood to the heart to pinpoint areas of narrowing or blockage that can cause a heart attack. Although the test is routinely performed by cardiologists, it is invasive and can sometimes lead to complications. The researchers wanted to see if the patients' body mass correlated with mortality after the test.[2] Remarkably, they found that patients who were underweight were *three times* more likely to die from complications of the procedure than normal-weight people.

Becoming very lean by losing fat does not necessarily achieve good health. Sports medicine doctors and fitness trainers know this all too well. Some bodybuilders, for example, go on extreme diets during training for competition to lower their body fat levels as far as possible so that their sinewy muscles pop out during flexing to wow the crowd and judges. Bodybuilders often lower their body fat from a safe 10 to 15 percent down to a meager 5 percent. Dropping down to 5 percent body fat can slow your heart rate by 50 percent, bringing it down to dangerous levels.[3] Testosterone levels can plummet by as much as 75 percent. Below 5 percent body fat, people start to lose not only muscle mass but bone mass, too.[4] In young women, ultralow levels of body fat can stop the menstrual cycle and cause infertility.

Researchers at the Li Ka Shing Knowledge Institute and St. Michael's Hospital in Toronto examined fifty-one clinical studies that correlated body weight with death from any cause and found that being underweight is even more risky than being overweight when it comes to mortality. Underweight adults had a 38 percent higher chance of dying from any cause over a five-year period, compared to adults who were severely obese.[5]

So thin is not always better, and big is not always bad. It is time to look more deeply at the science and rethink everything you know about fat.

* * *

Let's start with its proper name: adipose tissue. The term "adipose" comes from the Latin *adipem*, meaning "lard"—the rendered fat of a pig.* Perhaps not the most attractive definition, for sure, but it is historically accurate, since humans have been domesticating pigs for food and handling their fat for more than ten thousand years.[6]

Contrary to popular belief, fat is neither an amorphous blob nor the enemy of health that it's been made out to be. Far from it. Fat is essential to life itself. As I explained earlier, fat is actually an organ that serves you well when it is functioning properly. Mother Nature has cleverly engineered body fat to support your health, and she's organized it in ways so that it can perform its job with great efficiency. Thus, fat is one of your health's greatest allies.

Let me be clear: fat can be diverted from its original health-supporting role to become a real danger to your well-being. Harmful chemicals, poor food choices, lack of exercise, and even insufficient sleep can throw your biology off-kilter, causing fat to accumulate in overly abundant amounts and in all the wrong places. Bad habits can lead to an imbalance between different types of fat, some more harmful than others. You see, fat is not just a single entity. Because fat comes in multiple forms, it can be good for you or bad for you—and you have the power to control which way it goes.

Most biological systems operate within a zone. Whether fat is good or bad for you is all about balance within that zone. Like the tale of Goldilocks and the three bears, the important thing when it comes to

---

* Lard is the fat from a pig, whereas fat from cattle, such as you'd see on a steak, is called tallow.

fat is not having too much or too little—but just the right amount. And just like you need your heart, lungs, brain, and kidneys in order to be alive, you also need your fat to survive.

Forget the mirror and the bathroom scale for one moment. The time has come to develop a new, respectful attitude toward body fat. Fat is critical to maintaining your health. Once you understand how, you'll think about your body, your metabolism, and your approach to weight management very differently.

Meet Your Fat

You are carrying around two kinds of adipose tissue, one of which is called subcutaneous adipose tissue. As its name suggests, it's located under the skin (*sub* is "below"; *cutis* is "skin" in Latin). This is the kind of fat you can pinch with your fingers. Your love handles, the jiggly part under your arms, the mound under your chin, the bulge on your thighs, the curve of your buttocks—all are made of subcutaneous adipose tissue. This makes up 90 percent of the fat in your body.

The other type of fat you have is "visceral" adipose tissue. This makes up 10 percent of the fat of a healthy person. Visceral fat is not usually visible to the naked eye, so you're probably not aware it is there. This type of fat is packed deep inside your body cavities. Visceral fat releases hormones that affect your entire bodily system, filling up the space that exists inside your belly and between organs like your liver, intestines, and stomach as a protective cushion.

You even have a special organ made of visceral fat. It's called the omentum, a fatty apron that has two parts draped across your stomach and intestines and tethered by ligaments to the inner wall of your abdomen.[7] The apron varies in size among individuals. On the small end, it can be 300 grams, about the weight of a can of soup. On the larger end, the omentum can be as much as 1,500 grams, as heavy as a full two-liter bottle of soda.

This apron of fat has a big job to do—it processes energy for your metabolism, regulates your appetite, controls inflammation, and stimulates your health defenses, including regeneration. The omentum is also a vigilant guard on the lookout for serious trouble in your belly. Surgeons call it the "policeman of the abdomen" because it protects you from an infection in case there is ever a perforation in your intestines or if you have a burst appendix. When this happens, your omentum whips into action and wraps itself like an octopus around the area of perforation to seal it off and keep any infection from spreading, which otherwise could be lethal.

When I say fat is an organ, I mean it performs specific vital functions to keep you alive. Visceral fat contains hormones that instruct other organs on what to do, including your brain. The other kind of fat, subcutaneous fat, gives your body its shape and stores fuel for your metabolism. Both kinds of fat act as padding to cushion your muscles, bones, and soft organs, protecting them from rupture due to blunt trauma. If your fat is not performing all of these jobs competently, your health will fail. So, the next time you feel inclined to curse your fat, just remember that without it, you would not survive.

Now let's take a closer look at the specific life-sustaining duties that fat performs for us.

Fat Is Your Fuel Tank

Your fat stores energy that comes from the food you eat. In times of plenty, when food is abundant, any spare energy—extra calories—from your meals and snacks is loaded up into adipocytes. In this way, your body builds up energy reserves, like filling up the gas tank of a car. Adipocytes store the fuel from food by making substances called triglycerides, which are the form of currency for fat-based energy. The process that creates triglycerides in adipocytes is called "lipogenesis." This is essential to a healthy metabolism.

Between meals, when your body needs energy, your adipocytes convert the stored triglycerides back into usable fuel that is released into your bloodstream. This is the fuel that powers up your muscle, supplies your liver, and feeds your brain and other organs. The process that releases this fuel from adipocytes is called "lipolysis." It is similar to drawing gasoline from your gas tank when you are driving a car. The fuel in your bloodstream is used to keep your organs working, but more is needed when you are physically active or exercising. Your flexing muscles and pumping heart need energy, so your adipose tissue releases fuel to sustain them, too. The fuel job of body fat is straightforward. The stored fuel can be released to give the body the energy it needs to run bodily functions. Just like the gas tank of a vehicle, the fat fuel tank can regularly be filled by eating.

However, there's a difference between filling up at the gas station and sitting down at the dinner table: the gas pump at the filling station has a safety cutoff mechanism to prevent you from overfilling your car's gas tank, which would be extremely hazardous if it spilled down the sides of your car and became a spreading pool on the ground. When it comes to eating, people were not so thoughtfully designed. There is no automatic cutoff. Your body's fuel tank can easily be overfilled if you eat too many calories. In a vehicle, extra fuel can be stored in jerricans that are placed in the trunk. In your body, the fuel overload from food fills up your fat, which then has to expand into the trunk space of your body. This is why, if you care about body fat, weight control, and staying healthy, it's imperative to eat in moderation.

Fat Is an Endocrine Organ

Less well known, your fat is a gland that releases hormones. Just like the hormones released by your pituitary, thyroid, adrenal gland, pancreas, and ovaries or testes, your fat hormones control many body functions.

You might be surprised to learn that fat is the largest gland in your body. Fat hormones are made by adipocytes, which release the hormones into the lacy network of blood vessels that penetrate and feed fat tissue. Your circulation then carries the fat hormones to other parts of your body.

When the hormones flow into organs, they deliver instructions on what the organ should do next. Most hormones act like a volume switch to turn up or turn down an organ's level of activity. When your body needs an organ to do more, a larger amount of hormone is released by your fat, and the volume is turned up. When there is enough activity, your fat releases less hormone. There are at least fifteen different kinds of hormones that are released by your fat. These influence the health of your brain, immune system, gut, circulation, muscles, reproductive system, and, especially, your metabolism.* Some fat hormones turn up your metabolism, while others slow it down. Collectively, your fat hormones are called "adipokines." Let's take a look at the ones that have the biggest influence on your health.

Leptin, adiponectin, and resistin are three of the most important hormones released by your fat cells. They not only influence your metabolism, but they also interact with your five health defense systems—angiogenesis, regeneration, microbiome, DNA protection, and immunity. Let's get familiar with the specific functions of each one.

Leptin is known as the satiety hormone. It is an appetite suppressant that tells you to slow down and stop eating. Leptin's influence on appetite is due to a direct chemical connection between your body fat and your brain. Under normal circumstances, when leptin is released into your bloodstream, it travels to the command center of your brain, the hypothalamus. There, the hormone acts on the circuitry of nerves in your brain's hunger center, the orexigenic neurons. These are the

---

* Adiponectin, apelin, chimerin, fibroblast growth factor-21 (FGF21), hepcidin, interleukin-6, leptin, monocyte chemoattractant protein-1, omentin, plasminogen activator inhibitor-1, resistin, transforming growth factor-beta, tumor necrosis factor-alpha, vaspin, visfatin.

neurons responsible for turning on your appetite. Leptin lowers the activity of these neurons, so you feel less hungry. To reinforce this effect, leptin also triggers your brain to produce special proteins that are anorexigenic, which actively shuts off your appetite. By turning down your appetite's on switch and then hitting the off switch, leptin ensures that you will lose the urge to eat for several hours.

When you are not eating—which is technically "fasting"—your body senses it is between mealtimes, so it releases fuel for the energy to keep operations running. Your metabolism revs up and moves the fuel in your fat out of storage mode and sends it into the bloodstream as energy for your organs. As your fat burns down its fuel, it releases less leptin, so your brain's appetite center swings back up, and you start to feel like eating again.

At healthy levels, leptin also activates your immune defenses. When your body cannot make sufficient amounts of leptin, you are more susceptible to infection. The hormone helps your immune cells spring into action to fight bacteria and viruses. Leptin guides your immune system when it needs to mount a proper inflammatory response after an injury. At the same time, leptin helps your immune system unleash T cells against infection. Your T cells release chemicals called cytokines that destroy any invaders that have penetrated your body.[8] In yet another useful immunity role, leptin instructs your immune system to produce protective antibodies.[9]

Leptin protects your heart and cardiovascular system. The hormone tells your blood vessels to dilate in order to improve blood flow to your organs. It activates your angiogenesis defense system to grow new blood vessels and improves your circulation.[10] Leptin also protects the cellular lining of your blood vessels, the vascular endothelium, and it even helps your heart muscle to stay in shape, literally. As you age and the heart muscle weakens, your heart starts to lose its shape and become floppy and wider in diameter. In a study of 432 subjects, researchers from the Framingham Heart Study, Boston University, and Tufts University found that people with higher blood levels of leptin continued to preserve more normal dimensions of their heart as they aged.[11]

Adiponectin is the primary fat hormone that shapes your metabolism. Its job is to make sure things run smoothly in the fuel uptake department. Adiponectin is so important for a healthy metabolism that this hormone is found in your bloodstream at levels one thousand times higher than any other hormone in your body.[12] A sufficient amount of it in your blood is a marker of health. Adiponectin works by helping your body maintain the right amount of glucose (blood sugar) needed for energy. There is always some in your bloodstream providing the fuel to keep the lights on in your organs all day long. This baseline amount of glucose is known as fasting blood sugar, and it's what your doctor measures during a routine checkup for health. Your blood is drawn first thing in the morning before breakfast (you are instructed to fast overnight) to determine how your metabolism performs at its baseline. If your fasting blood glucose is higher than what is considered normal, which is between 70 to 100 milligrams per deciliter, it means there is more energy in your bloodstream than necessary, and your metabolism is not functioning efficiently.

Adiponectin's job is to ensure your blood glucose is always at normal levels. It controls the effects of insulin, the metabolic hormone made by your pancreas. Whenever you eat food, your pancreas releases more insulin. Insulin's job in your blood is to help your cells absorb blood glucose and store the energy. Adiponectin makes your cells more responsive to insulin, so blood glucose can be taken up more quickly and efficiently. This is called insulin sensitivity, and it is crucial for maintaining a healthy metabolism.

When your cells lose their responsiveness to insulin, your blood glucose levels begin to rise to abnormally high levels because your cells cannot suck up the fuel. This is a major problem because without insulin or proper insulin sensitivity, your muscles weaken, your brain becomes sluggish, and your other organs swiftly falter due to lack of energy. All of these symptoms herald the beginnings of metabolic syndrome and foretell the dreaded arrival of diabetes.

Adiponectin is also anti-inflammatory.[13] At the high levels normally found in your bloodstream, this fat hormone protects your entire body from inflammation, and this shields the lining of your blood vessels from being scalded by inflammation. Healthy blood vessels without inflammation are less likely to develop atherosclerosis and suffer the blockages seen in coronary artery disease.[14]

In addition to its effects on insulin sensitivity, adiponectin also stimulates angiogenesis to ensure there are enough blood vessels to deliver insulin to all your cells.[15] Body fat is the factory for adiponectin, so you need to have enough fat around to maintain a healthy metabolism. People who are obese have plenty of body fat, but malfunctions caused by excess fat can make normal levels of adiponectin drop. In obesity, we are more likely to see *low levels* of adiponectin and higher levels of inflammation throughout the body, which poses a danger because many of the worst chronic diseases are caused by inflammation.[16]

Resistin, the third major fat hormone, helps fine-tune the effects of adiponectin by countering its effects. This allows your metabolism to be fine-tuned and slowed, like shifting to a lower gear in a sports car—a vital function, since revving your metabolism at high speeds continuously would wear down your engine. Resistin also helps the body "resist" (hence its name) the effects of insulin, allowing blood glucose to enter cells at a slower, controlled pace, like regulating the flow of hot water in a shower.

This fat hormone helps your body to spark inflammation, which is a completely normal and vital part of your immune defenses. By countering the superpowers of adiponectin, which reduces inflammation, resistin helps to make sure your body can mount an inflammatory response to fight an infection or after an injury. This role in tissue repair is very important. Resistin also promotes angiogenesis so new blood vessels will grow to repair damaged tissues.[17] It also recruits stem cells to help repair heart muscle and other damaged organs. Like many hormones, resistin wears multiple hats when called on to support your health defenses.[18]

These three hormones—leptin, adiponectin, and resistin—are the most important players when it comes to your fat's tremendous influence on your health defenses, which elevates their importance beyond metabolism. These essential fat hormones must be manufactured by adipocytes and released in the right amounts at the right time. When we carry too much body fat, the factory and mission control centers for these hormones are thrown into chaos. Hormonal signals are scrambled, or the hormones are released at the wrong time or in the wrong amounts. The mixed signals confuse your brain, heart, and other organs as well as your circulation and immune system. The consequence of too much body fat is metabolic pandemonium—which is why you need to mind your body fat regardless of your body size.

I'm not going to review the dozen or so other hormones produced by fat, but suffice it to say that healthy amounts of fat are absolutely critical to your ability to store and use fuel and to keep your metabolism running like the finely tuned engine it is designed to be.

Fat Is a Space Heater

Your fat has a third important function: it's your body's space heater. Everyone knows what it is like to step shivering out of the water after a dip in a swimming pool. Shivering occurs when our muscles involuntarily contract to generate heat. This response warms us up. Fat can generate heat, too—only without the need to shiver—and it does so by using a truly remarkable system that is linked to what you eat as well as to the temperature of your environment.

The way fat generates heat is called adaptive thermogenesis. There is one specific type of fat cell, called the brown adipocyte, or brown fat, whose job is to "turn up the heat." Heat generation by brown fat has huge health implications. For one thing, turning on adaptive thermogenesis consumes the fuel from excess fat, which burns away harmful fat and can result in weight loss. Many factors have been discovered that can trigger this process. Cold temperatures can activate brown fat to start thermogenesis. Emotional and physical stress can also ignite brown fat and call it into action. Starvation also causes thermogenesis, but to an unhealthy extreme. Deliberate fasting can encourage thermogenesis in a more controlled way.

In addition to burning down harmful fat, when your adaptive thermogenesis system is turned on, it activates all of your health defense systems: angiogenesis, stem cells, your gut microbiome, DNA protection, and your immune system. Remarkably, this entire set of reactions can be triggered by certain foods—like chili peppers! Your brown fat is the secret to this activation, which we will discuss further in Chapter 3.

The Discovery of Brown Fat

The history of brown fat is fascinating because it was first discovered not in humans but in the Alpine marmot, a large ground-dwelling rodent that resembles a groundhog. In 1551, a Swiss naturalist named Conrad Gessner was dissecting a marmot when he found an odd mass sitting between its shoulder blades.[19] Marmots live in the mountains of central Europe. During frigid winters, marmots hunker down in their burrows to hibernate, and their heart rate and breathing drop to barely perceptible levels.[20] Their bodies generate heat and use stored fat for energy. When spring arrives, they emerge from the burrow lean and ready to load back up on food in order to mate.

Gessner didn't realize that the tissue he found was composed of brown fat. In fact, he described it as "neither fat nor flesh." But soon other scientists began noticing that a similar brown mass was present in the bodies of other hibernating animals, like bats, hamsters, and mice. The lump became known as the hibernating gland.[21] It wasn't until 1961 that an observant physiologist named Robert E. Smith, working at the University of California at Los Angeles, examined the tissue more closely and recognized that the hibernating gland was actually made of fat.* Smith discovered that this unusual brown fat could generate heat, especially when it was exposed to cold temperatures.[22]

Brown fat wasn't discovered in humans until 1964.[23] Just like in the Alpine marmots, the purpose of brown fat in newborn humans is to generate heat and keep them warm. When brown fat is turned on later in life, as you'll learn a lot more about in the next chapter, it can burn away excess fat while increasing metabolism and causing weight loss.

If you find all these features of body fat surprising and a bit overwhelming, don't worry; you are in good company. Medical researchers are astonished at what they discover as they peel back the mysteries of body fat at a furious pace. In the year 2021 alone, there were more than 11,000 scientific articles published on adipose tissue, with more than 2,000 on leptin, 1,500 on adiponectin, and more than 1,000 about brown fat. Now you can see what I mean when I say you need to reconsider your assumptions about fat.

There's just a little more I want to share with you before we take a deep dive into how food influences fat. We all recognize the idealized form of the human figure: the sculpted physique of Michelangelo's statue of David and the curves on the Venus de Milo—these, of course, are not the only beautiful body types. Indeed, the shape of everyone's body and physical identity are sculpted by fat. It's valuable to understand how all the useful, healthy fat in your body is distributed over the course of your lifetime.

From Baby to Babe

Your fat started forming when you were in your mother's womb, before you even had a face and long before your first bite of food. When your father's

---

* The first time I ever heard of brown fat, someone told me it was found in hibernating bears. It turns out, however, that bears don't truly hibernate; they undergo a deep sleep called torpor (another myth busted). And they don't use brown fat to generate heat to keep themselves warm.

sperm met your mother's egg, this activated a blueprint for fat in your future body. For about two weeks, you were just a ball of cells. Then, the stem cells that formed you began to create parts of your head, chest, and abdomen. True, you looked more like a tadpole than a human, with short limbs and a stubby tail, for the first couple of months. Your organs, including fat, took shape inside your nascent body when you were just a few inches long. At around fourteen weeks (three and a half months) after conception, the genetic instructions that create fat cells kicked in, about a third of the way into a full-term, forty-week pregnancy. At this point, you were the size of a lemon and ready to have a face. Fat first formed your cheeks and under your chin, and then it filled in the hollows of your eye sockets.

The story is the same for every developing fetus regardless of your body type as an adult. Before fat forms, a small amount of connective tissue marks the spot the fat cells will call home. Next, blood vessels grow in that area through the process of angiogenesis, laying the groundwork so that oxygen and nutrients will be available to support the tissue that will soon form. This connection between fat and your angiogenesis health defense system starts early in life. Think of it as a home builder marking the construction area, then laying out where the foundation and plumbing will be placed.

Next, preadipocyte stem cells begin to cluster around the new blood vessels.[24] These clusters are called fat lobules, and they resemble a bunch of grapes. About two weeks later, at four months into the pregnancy, the preadipocytes will have morphed, as stem cells do, into true adipocytes. These brand-new fat cells then rapidly fill up with liquid fat until they resemble golden orbs. By roughly six months into the pregnancy, the chubby cheeks of a fetus are clearly seen on a prenatal ultrasound. It's fat that creates the recognizable shapes that wow and delight parents seeing the first images of their baby.*

---

* The timing and formation of human adipose tissue in the fetus were determined in a landmark research study conducted by the University of Michigan and the Hôpital Port-Royal in Paris in 1982. Researchers performed careful studies using microscopic techniques in 805

Over the next two months, no new fat cells are made, but the existing ones get bigger and bigger as they fill up with more liquid fat. Soon after, mounds of fat (now called adipose tissue) form throughout the rest of the body. Subcutaneous fat forms under the skin, while visceral fat forms inside the abdomen—all in the proper amounts needed for health.

These fundamentals are the same for every individual, although the details of this process can play out in very different ways. Our paths begin diverging long before we are born. External factors like what mom eats, the quality and quantity of her food, whether she is prescribed an antibiotic or other medications, environmental toxins she is exposed to, her stress levels, whether she drinks alcohol, smokes, or lives with a smoker—all can affect how much adipose tissue grows during pregnancy and childhood. The link between diet and fat development is one major reason why expectant moms should avoid or limit eating heavily processed foods during pregnancy.

The packaging of foods can cause trouble, too. Phthalates, also known as plasticizers, are commonly used in bottles, plastic wrap, and other food and beverage containers to make them flexible and more elastic. Studies have shown that phthalates can be transferred from the plastic package into prepared or frozen foods like pizza, burritos, hamburgers, french fries, chicken nuggets, and other snacks.[25] Plastics also can be transferred to food products from the gloves worn by food workers in fast-food restaurants.[26]

Moms need to be careful because phthalates are found in bottled water after they leach out from the plastic container.[27] Phthalates belong to a category of compounds called obesogens. The name comes from studies showing a link to obesity markers in children whose mothers

---

human embryos and fetuses at different stages of development and recorded their findings. They found that facial fat was one of the first types of fat to form, and it did so in five stages. Remarkably, until then, very little was known about how and when fat forms in humans.

were exposed to these compounds while pregnant, which puts their offspring at a higher risk of developing obesity.[28]

At the moment of birth, roughly 10 percent of a baby's total body weight is healthy fat. Most of that is subcutaneous white adipose tissue. But there is also brown fat that fills in the interscapular space between its shoulder blades—just like the Alpine marmot. Brown fat isn't what makes babies adorably chubby; that is subcutaneous white fat, the pinchable fat that sits right underneath the skin. In the first six months of human life, there is a steep increase in this kind of baby fat.[29]

Let's take a look at how our fat grows.

Fatty tissue gets bigger in two ways. One way is for existing fat cells to fill up with more liquid fuel. This is called hypertrophy, which means a mass of tissue enlarges by increasing the size of the cells. The second way it grows is for more fat cells to develop from fat stem cells. This is called hyperplasia, in which the mass expands by simply adding more cells. Either way, adipose tissue in babies has plenty of blood vessels for oxygen and nutrients to support it, and there is very little inflammation. The burgeoning amount of fat in babies is picture perfect—and perfectly healthy.

By the time a baby turns one, their fat cells are five times larger than when they were born. Studies have examined what happens to fat from infancy to adolescence and beyond. From age two to five, kids start getting taller and lankier, and body fat declines in both boys and girls. Boys shed roughly 25 percent of their body fat, while girls shed about 20 percent.[30] There's not much difference, which is why young girls and boys are shaped so similarly. It's in the years that follow, during adolescence and adulthood, that the differences in body fat become more dramatic.

Differences in Fat Distribution

The body fat differences between males and females from prepuberty to early adulthood were profiled by researchers at the University of Otago in New Zealand. This is the period when natural body sculpting by fat creates the youthful curves and angles that many have come to see as the ideal of fitness and health. The scientists used the dual energy X-ray absorptiometry, or DEXA, scan to look at areas of the body where fat development in boys and girls might differ the most: the trunk (which is the neck, chest, and abdomen), the waist, and the hip area. The DEXA scan is a classic way to measure body composition in great detail because it can precisely measure total percent body fat, fat mass, visceral adipose tissue, muscle mass, and bone density.

The New Zealand team examined 1,009 healthy children and young adults between the ages of five and twenty-nine, all of whom were of normal weight. They looked for patterns of how and where body fat developed in boys and girls. Males, they found, experienced a burst of fat growth in early puberty, which leveled off as they reached adulthood. Females had a steady gain in fat throughout their maturation. The location where the body fat grew also varied between females and males.

Let's look at the main trunk of the body, the region between the neck and the pelvis. This would be the silhouette between the shoulders and hips. During adolescence, females steadily lost fat in this area, compared to males. In late puberty, they were 17 percent slimmer around their torso, and by young adulthood, they had 34 percent less fat in this region, compared to men.

Next comes the waist. This is where the hourglass-like shape of females emerges as the waist narrows and the hips spread. Indeed, girls almost always have less waist fat than boys, as their waistline shrinks during puberty. In the early stages of puberty, females already have 15 percent less waist fat, but by the end of puberty, they have 35 percent less than males of the same age. By the time women reach their twenties, the differences between women and men are even greater. Women have 48 percent less waist fat.

On to the hips. Females have larger hips than males, and it's not just because of the shape of their pelvis bone—it is partly due to their body fat. The shaping starts before puberty, when the researchers measured 6 percent more hip fat in girls than boys. As they enter puberty, girls have 16 percent more, and by late puberty, they have 47 percent more hip fat than boys. By early adulthood, young women have an average 66 percent more hip fat than young men. Remember, this study was done to profile adipose tissue in a group considered to be of normal weight, where fat performs its duties in the healthy zone.

During adulthood, body fat continues to grow differently between men and women. A landmark study was conducted by researchers from Columbia University, the Technical University of Lisbon in Portugal, and the University of Alabama.[31] They set out to identify how fat is distributed in a healthy body across the entire human life span. They looked at 499 people, of which 147 were children between the ages of five and seventeen, and 352 were adults from eighteen to eighty-eight. All were considered to be of healthy weight. The subjects were from New York and were diverse, including white people, Black people, Hispanic people, and Asian people, including Chinese, Indian, Korean, and Japanese ethnicities.

The researchers performed whole-body scans using magnetic resonance imaging (MRI) to obtain two hundred images of each subject's body fat. This allowed them to calculate total body fat, including the amount of subcutaneous and visceral adipose tissue. They then correlated the amounts of fat with gender and age to look for patterns and then organized the patterns into ten-year increments of life. They asked the question, How does fat change over time between healthy males and females?

The results: With the hormonal changes of puberty, fat patterns started to change. Adult males older than eighteen had 50 percent *more* visceral fat than adult females. But the amount of visceral fat in boys had started increasing at age twelve, and it always exceeded the amount found in girls. In women, visceral fat is slow to start growing, but it starts accumulating at a faster pace after age twenty-six and builds throughout their life. Between the ages of forty and fifty, women gained a little over two cups of visceral fat. In the decade following that, they gain another two cups. So, between the fourth and sixth decades, women gained the equivalent of half of a large soda bottle's worth of visceral fat, the kind you can't see inside the abdomen.

Subcutaneous fat in women, however, accumulated quickly between puberty and age thirty-five—then its growth slowed down. After the age of fifty, the study found women grew very little subcutaneous fat but instead added mostly visceral fat. This is the same time frame in which women undergo menopause. Interestingly, the researchers found no connection between menopause and accumulation of fat in women of a healthy weight range. This means the hormonal changes of menopause, contrary to popular thinking, do not automatically lead to more body fat.

In boys, subcutaneous fat accumulated rapidly until age seventeen. After that, fat growth slowed. By adulthood, men have 20 to 30 percent *less* of this type of fat than women. After age fifty, male subcutaneous fat accumulation dramatically slowed. Healthy women always have more subcutaneous fat than healthy men. And men always have more visceral fat, the harmful stuff, than women.

Where Brown Fat Lives

The fat deposits that we have been talking about so far are mostly white fat. What about brown fat—where is it distributed in your body?

The world's first "atlas" of human brown fat was developed by the US National Institutes of Health.[32] To create this map, researchers studied twenty-eight young, healthy individuals under temperature-controlled conditions. They compared men who were lean versus those who were obese to see if there were any significant differences in the amount or location of brown fat between the two groups. The researchers used computed tomography (CT) and positron emission tomography (PET) scans to identify the locations of brown adipose tissue. They performed the scans in people under a range of ambient temperatures ranging from 60 to 87.8 degrees Fahrenheit because they knew that brown fat is more active and more visible at cooler temperatures, making it easier to spot because of its fluctuating behavior.

The results were eye-opening. Not everyone had the same amount of brown fat. The amounts detected ranged from 500 milliliters to as much as 2,000 milliliters (2 liters) of brown fat in each subject. If you compared that to the size of a large chicken egg, which contains about 50 milliliters of liquid, the amount of human brown fat ranges from the equivalent of ten to forty chicken eggs—which is a lot more than was previously thought existed!

The study showed that brown fat accounts for only a tiny fraction, 1.5 percent, of your total body mass and only 4 percent of your total fat mass. Researchers also discovered that human brown fat is not found in the form of lumps, as was previously described by Conrad Gessner in Alpine marmots, but rather in wafer-thin sheets layered next to bone, muscle, and organs across six anatomical locations: along the sides of the neck, around the collarbone, flanking the armpits, around the spine, behind the breastbone, and inside the abdomen.

The greatest proportion, about 66 percent of the brown fat, was found around the neck, collarbone, and armpit regions. These locations were also responsible for 70 percent of the total brown fat activity in the human body.

There were important differences in brown fat among people who were lean versus those who were obese. Lean subjects had 2.5 times *more* brown fat on average than obese subjects. Also, the brown fat in lean subjects was found to be 4 times more active than the brown fat found in people who are obese. This suggests that brown fat is not fully activated in people who have more overall body fat, so there is an opportunity to fire it up. We will talk more about this opportunity in the next chapter.

How White Fat Changes from Friend to Foe

Many factors cause people to pack on pounds—as white fat—beyond healthy levels. Genetics, environment, diet, and behavior all come into play when it comes to fat becoming too much of a good thing.

There are more than four hundred genes linked to the predisposition of becoming overweight. One of them is particularly common in modern humans: a fat-mass- and obesity-associated gene called the FTO gene, which is found in 43 percent of people![33] The FTO gene is linked to larger waist circumference, faster rate of fat accumulation, bigger hips, and more food consumption—and notably (but perhaps not surprisingly), FTO is also linked to cancer.[34] Having this gene does not guarantee you will become overweight or develop cancer—but it does predispose you to weight gain by the way it influences the amount of food you eat and your food choices. Brain scans of people with the FTO gene show that their frontal cortex, the part of the brain involved with executive decision-making, lit up much more strongly when they were shown an image of a "fattening food," compared to other objects.[35]

A study of 38,759 people by eighteen research centers in the United Kingdom found that those who had the FTO gene were 67 percent more likely to become obese, and not just as an adult. The increased risk started at age seven.[36] But lifestyle can also make a big difference and help to counter the harmful effects of the FTO gene. A major international research project involving ninety-seven medical institutions and 237,434 children and adults showed that overall physical activity, ranging from walking to working out, can lower the obesity risk by 27 percent, even if you have the FTO gene.[37] And a meta-analysis of studies involving 9,563 subjects showed that diet and lifestyle interventions were effective for weight loss in people who carried the FTO gene.[38] So when it comes to this obesity gene, your fate is not set—you can take action to change your destiny.

There are other, less common gene mutations that increase the like-lihood of becoming obese. One gene mutation interferes with the body's ability to manufacture the fat hormone leptin, which, as you've learned, lowers your appetite. With this mutation, the feeling of hunger never goes away, and this results in overeating. This genetic defect is rare and found in only about 7 percent of children with morbid obesity.[39] Other genetic mutations influence the regions of the brain that control appe-tite. The brain disturbances go beyond eating and also interfere with cognition, so affected individuals deteriorate in both mental and physi-cal health.[40]

You might think that eating fried food—which is tasty but unhealthy— is completely voluntary, but the research shows that your genetics can be directing your actions. Your genes can influence what you choose to eat based on what's available in your environment. Consistently making poor choices can cause you to build up body fat beyond the healthy levels.[41] For example, eating fried food is associated with increasing body fat, weight gain, and becoming obese.[42] A Harvard-based study of 37,423 people found that subjects with a genetic predisposition for weight gain were more likely to eat more fried foods, as frequently as four or more times per week.[43] A similar genetic inclination was seen for drinking fat-promoting sodas and sugar-sweetened fruit drinks.[44] With discipline and education, of course, you can learn to make better decisions by recognizing the conse-quences of those choices.

Any time you overeat, you are forcing excessive energy into your body, which is to say you're overloading on fuel. This happens from time to time in everyone's life. Eating for pleasure, which is called "hedonic" eating, can have a wide range of underlying motivations, from being a food connoisseur who enjoys culinary experiences to having a compul-sive eating disorder, despite the body having sufficient energy.

The links among body, brain, and behavior can be measured using a tool called the Power of Food Scale.[45] The higher you score on this scale, the more you are compelled to eat regardless of how much energy your

Fat begets fat.

body needs. Some individuals overeat in response to psychological stress, while others do it when they are distracted, such as while watching a device while eating. Still others eat too much because they eat too quickly and shovel the food into their stomach before their brain can send the signal to stop.[46]

The quality of food also influences whether you gain weight. Foods containing fiber help you reduce body fat by improving your metabolism. Your gut microbiome digests the fiber and produces short-chain fatty acids that not only lower inflammation but also help to quell your appetite and rein in the growth of adipose tissue.[47] The gut bacteria in people who eat less fiber produce fewer short-chain fatty acids and the ones that are made are less potent for lowering appetite.[48] Fewer short-chain fatty acids also means that the unhealthy foods you eat will cause more inflammation, making you even more susceptible to developing a chronic disease.

Crossed Signals

Routine overeating causes your adipocytes to get bigger and bigger until they are filled to their brim with fuel. When your existing fat cells are filled to capacity, more fat cells need to develop to store more excess fuel. Fat begets fat, and the rate at which people with obesity can make new adipocytes can be 2.6 times faster than in normal-weight adults. Rapidly expanding fat causes another serious problem—it can outgrow its blood supply.

Remember that your blood vessels are lifelines for all your tissues, and your angiogenesis defense system stands ready to grow new vessels when you need them. But when fat grows too quickly, angiogenesis can't keep up. The expanding fat cells become oxygen-deprived, and a condition called hypoxia occurs, leading to metabolic mayhem.

Just like a swimmer in the ocean panics when they feel like they might drown, hypoxic fat tissue begins to flail biologically. The hormonal function of fat goes haywire. Adipocytes begin making and releasing adipokines in an uncoordinated and uncontrolled fashion, as fat cells frantically try to recruit more blood vessels by releasing cytokines and growth factors. Lack of oxygen causes inflammation all by itself, but the cytokines trigger even more inflammation, like gasoline being poured onto a fire. This can be clearly seen under a microscope in biopsies of abdominal fat from adolescents who are obese.[49] The combination of it all—malfunctioning hormones, wildly released cytokines, hypoxia, and inflammation—wreaks havoc on your health.

Let's take an even closer look at this metabolic mayhem. The finely tuned functions of adipocytes you learned about earlier are disrupted. Instead of carefully controlling your appetite in coordination with your brain, storing and releasing fuel to power the body, reducing inflammation, and supporting your immune system, your adipocytes spin out of control. Excess fat also means too many triglycerides for the adipocytes to handle. They leak out of adipocytes and backwash into the bloodstream. These leaked fats build up in your organs, especially your liver, where accumulated leaked fat is poisonous. This is called "lipotoxicity," and it can cause liver damage and a condition called nonalcoholic fatty liver disease, which is a major risk factor for liver cancer.[50]

You can eat foods that calm the inflammation caused by excess fat, and this helps to calm the pandemonium in your body. And by simply reducing your caloric intake, you can reduce inflammation by 40 percent. A study out of Louisiana State University placed ten obese subjects on a program of caloric restriction and achieved a 7 percent reduction in body weight. The subjects had their fat biopsied before the study and one year later. By comparing the before and after appearance of the fat under the microscope, the researchers found that calorie restriction not only reduced the size of the fat cells; it also substantially lowered inflammation.[51] After calorie restriction, the subjects' adipocytes also showed greater responsiveness to insulin, meaning there was a reversal of the metabolic defect caused by excess fat, helping the adipocytes go back toward their more normal function.

Another crossed signal that comes with chaos in your body fat involves leptin, the satiety hormone. People with excess fat can develop leptin resistance, a malfunction of the brain's ability to respond to the satiety hormone.[52] With leptin resistance, your adipocytes continue making leptin in an effort to shut down your appetite, but your brain does not respond in the way that it should. Recall that the hormone leptin normally works as a signal that tells the brain's command center, "There's enough energy now, let's put the fork down." With leptin resistance, the brain keeps revving up and tells your body, "You are still hungry, so keep eating." Eating with a brain that is unresponsive to leptin is like trying to call a cell phone that has run out of battery charge. You can dial the number as many times as you want, but no one is going to answer the phone. People with leptin resistance crave food all the time.

When you eat more food, your fat cells release more leptin, but since there is no feedback from the brain, even more leptin is released. This vicious cycle causes levels of leptin to soar in your bloodstream. As with any hormone, too much leptin can be disastrous to your health. Excessive leptin interferes with your immune system and cripples your ability to produce infection-fighting antibodies. When antibody-producing immune B cells were collected from young, healthy, lean people and exposed to high levels of leptin, they could barely muster an antibody's response to the influenza vaccine.[53]

The exact cause of leptin resistance is unclear, but you need to know there is a connection to one common food ingredient: high-fructose additives. Fructose is a form of sugar that is naturally found in many fruits and vegetables, but it shows up in a concentrated, processed form—high-fructose corn syrup—in hard candies, candy bars, sodas, factory-made desserts, and other snacks associated with obesity. When researchers fed lab rats a high-fat diet along with high concentrations of fructose, the rats could no longer respond to leptin and ate food ravenously.[54] But when the high-fructose corn syrup was removed, the high-fat diet alone did not cause leptin resistance.

Fight Fat with Food

Regardless of your genetics or environment, your ultimate goal is to get any excess fat you have under control. This will bring your body back to its natural state of balance when it comes to your metabolism. And this is where the true health benefit of weight loss lies. But conventional wisdom says that to lose weight and body fat, you have to give up enjoyable eating. Sacrifice is the name of the game when it comes to fighting body fat, right? Wrong.

Science says you should actually *feed your metabolism* with the right kinds of foods to direct your body to burn down excess fat and rein it in to healthier levels. There's no need for harsh deprivation, and you also do not have to clear-cut your fat with surgery, suck it out of your body, or freeze it to death. With a food-based approach, you can keep the crucial energy-generating, hormonal, and thermal properties of your fat running properly—the way it should be, so you can optimize your metabolism and your health. Eating to fight fat means you don't have to resort to strict diets and makes it possible for you to live a pleasurable life.

It's a rather startling concept the first time you encounter it: fight fat with food? Yes! In the next chapter, I am going to tell you exactly how this works—and how you can use food to flip the switch and burn away unwanted fat. Eating the right way will help you rightsize your metabolism, reduce your waistline, and lose pounds. Regardless of whether your body size is small, medium, or large, this is a science-based way to achieve your next level of health. Let's take a look at how all of this helps your metabolism.

Yo-Yo Dieting Can Be Beneficial

Many people find they cannot stay on a diet, especially the more extreme ones, so even if a diet leads to weight loss, they soon regain what they lost. The temptation to eat unhealthy foods or unhealthy amounts of food can be too hard to resist after a period of intense

deprivation. You may have experienced this yourself. The typical solution? You get back on the same or another diet and try to lose the weight
all over again. This pattern is called weight cycling and is more popu-
larly known as "yo-yo dieting"—your weight goes down and up and
down again like a toy yo-yo.[55] Conventional wisdom says this is terrible
for your health, and common sense might lead you to believe this could
be true.

You might be surprised to learn that, provided you are not stuffing
yourself with junk food, multiple attempts at weight loss can be beneficial, even though I don't recommend highly restrictive dieting. Yo-yo
dieting is only unhealthy when the food you eat on the rebound involves
sodas, ultraprocessed snacks, fried foods, and red and processed meats,
all of which can grow dangerous visceral fat. This was shown in a study
from the University of Nottingham, Kings College, and the University
of East Anglia in England.[56] The researchers examined the dietary habits of 2,218 twins and found that those who ate mostly red and processed
(deli) meat, eggs, and fast and fried foods had much more visceral fat
than those who ate fruits and foods made with whole grains.*

Yo-yo dieting has been found to lower the risk of cancer. Researchers
from the National Cancer Institute, the University of North Carolina,
and the University of Regensburg in Germany studied 161,738 men and
women in the AARP Diet and Health Study. They looked at the number
of times each person had tried to lose at least *five pounds* over a twenty-
year period and compared this with the risk of death from any cause.[57]
What they found was that making one or two attempts at dieting and
then giving up led to only a modest 6 percent reduced risk of death from
any cause. But there was a 9 percent reduction from seven to eight

---

* Interestingly, the high visceral fat in these people was associated with one gut bacteria,
Eubacterium dolichum, and high blood levels of chemicals found in red and processed meats.
The chemicals were alpha-hydroxyisovalerate and butyrylcarnitine, found in blood as
metabolites after eating red and processed meat and eggs. *Eubacterium dolichum* is the first
bacterium to be associated specifically with visceral fat gain.

TABLE 2.1. REDUCED MORTALITY RISK BASED ON NUMBER OF ATTEMPTS TO LOSE AT LEAST FIVE POUNDS AT MIDLIFE

# of Attempts	Reduction in Death from Any Cause
1–2	6%
3–4	4%
5–6	9%
7–8	9%
9–10	13%
>11	12% (22% for cancer)

attempts, and those who made eleven or more attempts to lose weight experienced an even greater 12 percent reduced risk of death—a doubling of the benefit from trying only once or twice. When researchers looked at specific diseases, they found that more than eleven attempts at intentional weight loss of at least five pounds reduced the risk of dying from cancer by 22 percent (see Table 2.1).

This eye-opening result tells us that being persistent in losing small amounts, even five pounds, through weight cycling is actually beneficial, not harmful. Obviously, it's much better to keep off any weight you lose and not have to yo-yo diet at all. But anyone can lose five pounds, gain it back, and lose it again without detriment. The key is not to load up on junk food between cycles.

Putting It All Together

When it comes to weight loss, shedding even small amounts is attainable and worth it because it can reduce the risk of a whole host of threatening health conditions. Dropping just five pounds can make you live longer (and lighter). As you continue to lose more weight, you gain even more advantages. Weight loss is a sliding scale of health benefits.

And if you regain the initial weight you lost, don't despair. Go back to the basics and shed it again. And again. Repeated weight loss is not the "yo-yo of death" as it was once thought to be—and it doesn't ruin your metabolism either, so long as you do not load up on unhealthy food between cycles. As you will learn in Part 2, it is very possible to eat food that is delicious and lose weight, so you never feel the need to go back to extreme diets. Eating to beat your diet means eating better, enjoying your food, losing weight a little at a time, and repeating your efforts if needed.

All of this is connected to your metabolism. In the next chapter, I will share the scientific secrets of how your metabolism really works. Get ready to challenge a lot of your preconceptions—and a lot of what you might have learned from books, online, and even from your doctor.

CHAPTER 3

Heal Your Metabolism

Now that you've learned about the science of body fat, it's time to understand your metabolism—and how to eat to beat the need for a diet. Chances are you know that a strong metabolism is vital for good health, but it's also likely that much of what you believe to be true about metabolism and body fat is wrong.

For decades, conventional wisdom has said that some people are "doomed to get fat" because they were born with a genetically slow metabolism, so nothing can be done about it. Another popular belief is that as you reach middle age, your metabolism slows down, making it hard to lose weight. Eating small, frequent meals and consuming various drinks and supplements are popular metabolism hacks, but new discoveries tell us we haven't heard the whole story about metabolism—and how it really works.

It turns out that every human is born with . . . the exact same metabolism! And it is hardwired to operate in only four patterns over the course of your life. It is not a slow metabolism that causes you to gain body fat; rather, it is your body fat that slows your metabolism. The accumulation of excess fat forces your metabolism to slacken like a heavy load placed on the roof of a race car. The good news is that this means you *can* control your metabolism by shedding fat. Not only can weight loss help restore a slowed metabolism, you can also fire up your metabolism by activating your brown fat.

Metabolism is not destiny, and it's also much more than simply burning calories.

Your metabolism is a system that controls every single function in your body; it is the basis for life itself. The term comes from the Greek *metabole*, meaning "change." Your body is in a continuous state of change: moving, growing, digesting, thinking, breathing, healing, and simply functioning. Just as a car has many connected parts—from the gas tank to the engine to the wheels and everything in between—all working together to keep the vehicle road-ready, so, too, is your metabolism working as the sum of thousands of interconnected biochemical and cellular reactions that operate collectively to keep you alive and well. When you get sick, a robust metabolism helps you recover and rebound to your usual self. A damaged metabolism is guaranteed to result in illness and a longer recovery from any encounter with disease.

How does your metabolism interact with body fat? Their connection is fuel, the biochemical energy coming from the food you eat. Your fat (adipose) tissue stores the fuel. Your metabolism draws energy from fat tissue's fuel reservoir to power the rest of your body. Again, similar to a vehicle, the higher the quality of fuel you feed your engine, the better it will function and the longer it will run. Placing low-quality fuel in your body will eventually wear down your metabolism and wreck your health.

Metabolism Revealed

The concept of metabolism dates back to at least the thirteenth century and is inextricably linked to nutrition. An Egyptian physician named Ibn al-Nafis wrote the first documented description in 1260 CE: "Both the body and its parts are in a continuous state of dissolution and nourishment, so they are inevitably undergoing permanent change."[1] In 1614, a Venetian physician named Santorio Sanctorius tried to measure his own metabolism. He weighed his meal before eating and compared it to the weight of his feces later to determine what his body had extracted from the foods he ate.[2] Famously, these measurements were

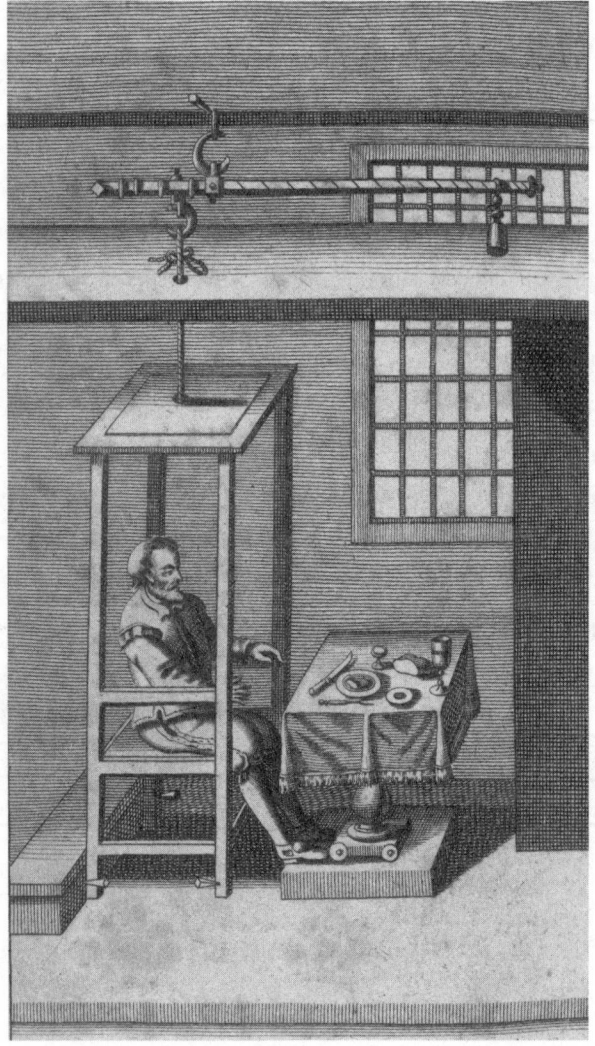

Figure 3.1. Engraving of Santorio Sanctorius sitting on his weighing chair.

taken using his own invention: Sanctorius sat in a chair device that was suspended like a swing set and connected to a weight scale (see Figure 3.1). While eating, working, defecating, and even sleeping, Sanctorius would calculate how his body weight changed due to each activity.[3] The results were published in his famous historical tome *Ars de Medicina*

Statica. Today, the idea of loading up on fuel, storing it, and burning it away with activity remains the core concept of metabolism.

Despite centuries of studies, however, many of the most important details about metabolism have remained only partially understood. One of the most startling discoveries was made in 2021. A group of bold researchers set out to get definitive answers to two commonly asked questions: How does metabolism change across the human life span? And, what explains the obvious differences in how individuals' bodies store, process, and burn energy (including fat)?

The researchers discovered that all humans are hardwired to have the *exact same pattern of metabolism* over different periods of their lives and that the pattern is not what we once believed. Rather than there being different metabolisms for different people due to "genetics," the differences between people's metabolisms are the result of disruptions—caused by excess body fat—to the standard set pattern.

This groundbreaking research was led by Herman Pontzer, a professor of evolutionary anthropology at Duke University, who worked alongside eighty-one scientists representing forty-seven institutions from nineteen countries.[*] This scientific legion examined 6,421 subjects from twenty-nine countries ranging in age from eight days old to ninety-five years old. It was the largest and most ambitious study of human metabolism ever undertaken.

Pontzer and his collaborators measured the daily metabolism of their research subjects, regardless of their age and location, using the exact same technique. This was the key. They employed a method called doubly labeled water (DLW), in which the subjects drank a special preparation of water (H_2O) made with hydrogen (^2H) and oxygen (^{18}O) atoms that differ from the naturally occurring versions but that are nonradioactive and safe to swallow. The atoms are useful for research because

---

[*] Researchers in this global metabolic study were based in the United States, China, Japan, Austria, Demark, England, Finland, France, Germany, the Netherlands, Norway, Scotland, Switzerland, Ghana, Kenya, Morocco, South Africa, Jamaica, and Mauritius.

they function in the body just like regular water, but they can be measured with a special isotope detector.[4] Like a modern version of the Sanctorius weighing chair, the DLW test allows you to measure the atoms *before* you take a drink and then *after* a period of time to evaluate how those atoms have traveled through the body's metabolic pathways.

Water is essential for metabolism, so the hydrogen and oxygen atoms swallowed by the test subjects are processed by each person's metabolism and excreted in their urine. By collecting the urine at different times and comparing the amounts of these easily identified atoms between measurements, Pontzer and his colleagues could accurately calculate each individual's total daily energy expenditure (metabolism) in an entirely consistent manner. This method takes into account all of the baseline energy each individual expends in just being alive and, beyond that, any energy needed for ordinary daily activities. The results from different countries were entered into a single database managed by the International Atomic Energy Agency based in Vienna, Austria.[5]

Comparing metabolic apples to apples among more than six thousand people is no easy task. To do this, the researchers had to develop a mathematical formula that accounted for differences in age, sex, physical activity, and body composition among all the subjects—small physique versus large, male versus female, very active versus not so active, obese versus lean. Specifically, the formula was able to subtract the differences in body fat among subjects, which allowed them to see what metabolism looks like when fat is removed from the equation. Applying this crucial "fat-free" math equation to the atomic data revealed what true human metabolism looks like when the influence of body fat is removed.

The findings were totally unexpected. Pontzer and collaborators discovered that we humans, *all* of us, have the *same* four phases of metabolism that take place over our life span, from birth through childhood, into adulthood, and during old age. Here's how it breaks down.

PHASE 1: The first phase begins when you are born and lasts until you are one year old. During pregnancy, a fetus's metabolism is similar to its mother's level, which is where it stands at birth. During the first year, however, a neonate's metabolism climbs as they grow into a toddler. Their metabolism revs up and rises to a peak that is 50 percent *higher* than the metabolism of a full-grown adult when adjusted for their smaller size.

PHASE 2: The second phase lasts from age one to age twenty. During this time, metabolism *steadily decreases* from its earlier heightened levels throughout adolescence and finally levels out in adulthood. Believe it or not, there is no metabolic increase during puberty or teenage years when adolescents experience huge growth spurts and their activity levels rocket. Despite the double dinners that teenagers eat, their metabolism is on the downswing as they grow bigger.

PHASE 3: This is the "adult phase" of metabolism, and it is rock *stable* from age twenty to sixty. It does not change during the working years of our lives. Surprisingly, it also does not change during or after pregnancy, nor does it decline after menopause—and there are no differences between men and women.

PHASE 4: After age sixty, human metabolism does begin to decline, but only at a very slow rate: 0.7 percent per year. Remember, this study had data from individuals who were ninety-five years old. Even at that nonagenarian age, however, the person's metabolism was still roaring along at 74 percent of where they were at age twenty during the Phase 3 adult level.

Figure 3.2 shows what the four hardwired phases of human metabolism look like across your life in one diagram.[6] The solid curve in Figure 3.2 shows what your intrinsic metabolism looks like if you do not have "excess adiposity." The dotted vertical lines show the main transition points all humans go through during their lifetime: at ages one, twenty, and sixty. This is your body's natural, hardwired metabolism and what it would be if you were to rid it of extra body fat.

Human Metabolism over a Lifetime

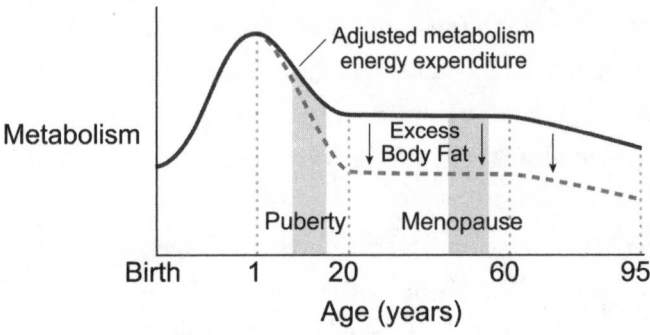

Figure 3.2. Human metabolism over a lifetime.

If you have excess body fat, it can completely alter this normal pattern of metabolism. This is shown in the depressed curve (hatched line). As adipose tissue builds, fat distorts the human metabolism curve by suppressing its normal healthy level. Not coincidentally, a depressed metabolism can contribute to and worsen chronic disease. Fat growth is a primary driver of chronic diseases. Let's take a closer look at how this happens.

Fat Damages Metabolism

The damage to your metabolism and health caused by accumulating excess fat has a name: "metabolic syndrome." This is a serious health condition in which the body's sensitivity to the hormone insulin decreases. Your blood glucose is no longer easily absorbed by your cells, so your blood sugar level rises along with your blood pressure. Your state of being reflects a wobbly, unstable metabolism that is not processing energy properly. Think of it as metabolic drunk driving.

Over time, this imbalance will cause you to develop type 2 diabetes, which is when your cells become less and less responsive to insulin, leading to chronically high blood sugar levels and, eventually, serious damage to your heart, blood vessels, eyes, kidneys, and nerves. If you have metabolic syndrome, this is a giant red flag for your health. It tells you that bad things are going to happen. All of this is tied to excess body fat. Remember how too much fat causes mayhem with your adipose tissue's hormonal and energy functions? This knocks your metabolism off-kilter.[7] Expanding fat slows your metabolism and triggers metabolic syndrome.

Roughly one-quarter of the world's population—more than 2 billion people—suffer from metabolic syndrome.[8] People with this syndrome are at high risk for developing heart disease, type 2 diabetes, and even colon and liver cancer. A long-term study of 2,357 men in their seventies conducted over sixteen years showed that those who experienced increased body weight along with metabolic syndrome had an increased likelihood of an earlier death by 44 percent, while those with full-on diabetes increased their risk of mortality by 86 percent.[9] It's hard to think of a more compelling reason to tame your body fat.

How do you know if you have metabolic syndrome? If you have three or more of these signs:

- fasting blood sugar higher than 100 mg/dL
- blood pressure higher than 130/85
- blood triglyceride levels greater than 150 mg/dL
- low levels of the good HDL cholesterol
- waist size greater than 40 inches for a man and 35 inches for a woman

Like falling dominoes, metabolic syndrome creates waves of impairment that interfere with virtually every function of your metabolism. For example, leaking fuel (triglycerides) from overladen fat cells spills out into your bloodstream and poisons your liver (lipotoxicity), crippling the major organ in your body that is responsible for detoxifying your blood. Excess fat triggers chronic inflammation that interferes with the normal function of all five of your body's health defenses, lowering your shields against disease. Inflammation takes a toll on the delicate lining of your blood vessels, damaging its normally smooth surface.[10] When your vessel lining is damaged, your blood vessels don't relax, so your blood pressure skyrockets.[11] The damaged lining becomes prone to accumulating sticky plaques that narrow the diameter of your blood vessels, which chokes off blood flow to your organs, including your heart. The high blood pressure puts a strain on your heart and places extra demands on your lungs and liver, too. Your metabolism has to divert energy from running the operations of a normal body to compensating for the damage caused by extra body fat.[12]

If you are struggling with any of these symptoms, be reassured that your metabolism isn't permanently broken. You can reverse metabolic syndrome and regain a healthy metabolism by shedding extra body fat and by being physically active.

How You Shed Fat Matters

Shedding fat helps you reset your metabolism and reclaim your health. But it's not just *what* you do but *how* you lose the fat that is important. Surgical remedies like liposuction, bariatric surgery, Lap-Band surgery, and prescription weight-loss drugs do cause large-scale weight loss, but all of them carry significant risks. None of them will bring your metabolism back into balance if you don't also eat the right amounts of healthy foods. Let's take a look at why.

Liposuction removes harmless subcutaneous fat but leaves all the health-threatening visceral fat right where it was—wrapped around your organs. Bariatric surgery makes it harder to overeat by reducing the size of your stomach or by cinching its opening to be smaller, but this interferes with important hormones that are released by your stomach. And drugs that prevent your body from digesting fat not only reduce your ability to receive the benefits of eating healthy fats; they also cause liquid, oily stools to leak out your rear end. Not fun. Other medications used to treat obesity block your appetite or make you feel prematurely full, taking all the joy out of food. Then there are the serious side effects of obesity medications, like suicidal ideation, pancreatitis, and thyroid cancer. These are not worth the risk unless you are struggling with life-threatening obesity.

Besides, you don't need drugs or surgery to reduce harmful fat. You can lose this fat by activating your body's own brown fat.

Brown Fat to the Rescue!

Everyone has brown fat. It is a hidden asset, standing by and waiting for orders to turn on thermogenesis and burn away excess fat to streamline your metabolism. When activated, brown fat draws down on fuel stores found in white fat—it's a natural consequence of brown fat's job as a space heater. Thermogenesis temporarily raises your metabolism at the cellular level as it fires up. Researchers estimate that by activating your brown fat, it can burn the energy equivalent of nine pounds of adipose tissue over the course of a year. Remember there are significant health benefits of losing even five to ten pounds. Switching on your brown fat heals your metabolism and leads to health benefits.

Remarkably, for years, brown fat was not even considered a factor in adult metabolism. Obstetricians and pediatricians have known that newborns have some brown fat between their shoulder blades, but it was thought to be a relic of evolution that was once needed to keep naked newborns warm on the cave floor after they crawled out of the womb. Based on old autopsy studies that looked for brown fat, it was present in childhood, but most experts believed that brown fat disappeared after the age of ten.[13] As recently as 2008, physicians thought that brown fat had reached the end of the line in evolution and was vestigial because humans now live in a world with thermostats, indoor heating, and warm clothing, and no longer need a biological space heater.

But in 2009, Boston endocrinologist Ronald Kahn and his colleagues at Harvard Medical School made a startling and pioneering discovery. They found brown fat—lots of it—in an adult. They weren't even looking for it intentionally. The circumstances were completely unexpected: the brown fat was found in a patient with a tumor.

A sixty-seven-year-old woman had come to a Boston hospital with a mass in her chest. Her doctors used a CT scan to pinpoint the tumor's location, sitting just above her diaphragm at the level of her lower rib cage. Her doctors also performed a PET scan, which is used to find tissues with a high metabolism. Tumors often are highly metabolic, so the colorful images of a PET scan can locate areas where there is unusually high metabolism in the body, typically indicative of cancer.

This patient's tumor lit up like a Christmas tree. But to the researchers' surprise, when the tumor was surgically removed and examined under a microscope, it was not a cancer at all. Rather, it was a rare benign tumor called a hibernoma—and it was made of brown fat! The tumor had lit up brightly on the PET scan because the brown fat was ramping up its metabolism and generating heat through thermogenesis.[14] Now curious, Kahn wondered how much brown fat is actually present in human adults.

With collaborators from four Boston hospitals, Kahn went to the medical records room and reviewed 3,640 PET–CT scans that had been performed on 1,972 patients (no small feat!). These old scans had been ordered for different medical reasons, and some patients even had multiple scans. Kahn and his team scrutinized them for the same brown fat signal they saw in the woman with the hibernoma. Amazingly, the signal was there—but not between the shoulder blades, which is where babies carry their brown adipose tissue. In adults, the brown fat signal was present around the neck and collarbone, pectoral muscles, and shoulder blades, and in the chest and abdomen.

But why had the brown fat shown up on these PET scans and not in others? Kahn knew that brown fat was activated by cold temperatures, so the researchers checked the weather forecast for the days when the PET–CT scans were performed. When they compared the Boston weather report with the positive scans, they found that the brown fat signal was highest in the winter when the outdoor temperature was coldest. There was less signal during the spring and fall, and the signal was lowest during the hot summer months. This correlated to medical reports from Finland in the early 1980s, where outdoor workers such as lumberjacks, painters, and farmers were reported to have more brown fat than people whose livelihood was indoors.[15]

The connection between human brown fat activation and cold temperatures was also demonstrated at the Maastricht University Medical Center in the Netherlands. There, researchers examined twenty-four subjects between the ages of eighteen and thirty-two at both normal room temperature of 22 degrees Celsius and at a chilly 16 degrees Celsius.* Brown fat was not visible in the subjects when they were scanned at the normal room temperature. But in the cooled room, their brown adipose tissue lit up in 96 percent of the subjects (see Figure 3.3).

A research collaboration between Turku University Hospital in Finland and the University of Göteborg in Sweden confirmed that cold exposure increases the brown fat signal by fifteenfold, compared to room temperature.[16] Interestingly, individuals who have a lean build are able to mount more robust brown fat signals than people who are obese.

Recruiting Your Brown Fat

Obviously, chilling your body in a cold environment is not a practical (or pleasant) way to reap the metabolic benefits of your brown fat. But

---

* This is 71 degrees and 61 degrees Fahrenheit, respectively.

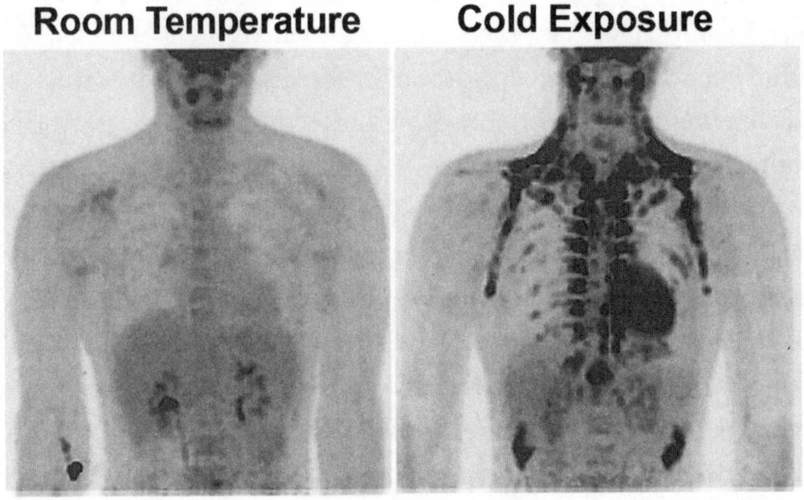

Room Temperature   Cold Exposure

Figure 3.3. Scan showing no brown fat visible when a subject is at a normal indoor room temperature, but under cold conditions, the brown fat reveals itself as dark areas throughout the upper body. (Source: W. D. van Marken Lichtenbelt, J. W. Vanhommerig, et al., "Cold-Activated Brown Adipose Tissue in Healthy Men," *New England Journal of Medicine* 360, no. 15 [2009]: 1500–1508.)

by tracing the pathways that activate brown fat, it's possible to find other more delightful ways to turn on thermogenesis that don't require cold temperatures.

Searching for these kinds of cellular switches is right in my wheelhouse as a scientist. In the part of my work that focuses on new biotech treatments for cancer, chronic wounds, diabetic vision loss, and macular degeneration, my starting point is always to find cellular targets. These are specific molecules or chemical structures on cells that can be "turned off" or "turned on" to get the desired treatment effect. I've used the same approach in my research on food as medicine to find cellular targets that foods can activate to protect health—including how to trigger brown fat and thermogenesis.

Here are the cellular steps that activate brown fat. Chilly temperatures trigger the brain to release a chemical signal called norepinephrine, which mobilizes the body for action. Norepinephrine is both a neurotransmitter and a hormone, which means it can turn on nerves and other tissues, like brown fat. When it is released into your bloodstream, the norepinephrine activates a switch called the β3-adrenergic receptor that is present in the cells of your brown fat. When this switch is turned on, brown fat fires up its fat-burning engine.

There are other ways besides cold temperature to get the brain to release norepinephrine, and you can get your body to trigger the β3-adrenergic receptor without norepinephrine. Foods can do both! I'm going to tell you which foods flip the switch in brown fat to the "on" position and how they do it.

But first, I want to tell you about a pharmaceutical that can do it, too. My research in food as medicine often starts by examining what drug developers have discovered. This can be a powerful jumping-off point to find foods that do something similar or, even better, with greater safety and more enjoyment.

The pharmaceutical is called mirabegron.[17] It is designed to treat an overactive bladder, a condition in which a person feels sudden and frequent urges to urinate because their bladder is spasming.* Mirabegron tames the bladder by triggering the β3-adrenergic receptor—the very same one found on brown fat—that is also located in the wall of the bladder. By activating this receptor, the medication causes the bladder to relax, and this reduces its overactivity.

Researchers at the Joslin Diabetes Center in Boston saw an opportunity to test mirabegron to see if it could turn on brown fat. They conducted a clinical study of twelve lean, healthy men in their early

---

* Mirabegron was approved by regulatory authorities for use to treat overactive bladder in the United States and European Union in 2012.

Placebo   Mirabegron

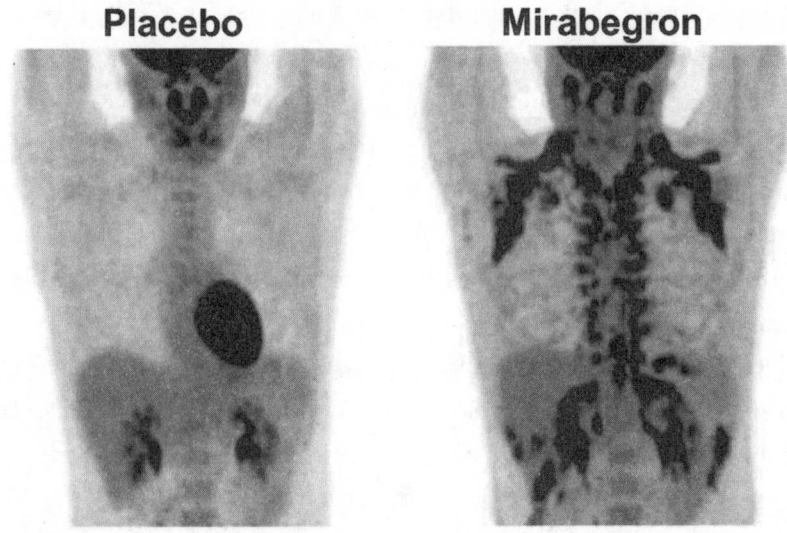

Figure 3.4. The drug mirabegron activates a cellular receptor on brown fat and triggers intense thermogenesis in a clinical study. (Image and permission for use provided courtesy of Aaron Cypess, MD, PhD, US National Institutes of Health.)

twenties. The researchers confirmed that their subjects indeed had brown fat by exposing them to cold temperatures and then performing a PET scan to look for the colorful signals. Then, the researchers measured their baseline resting metabolic rate.

Next, the subjects swallowed 200 milligrams of mirabegron, a high dose that is eight times higher than that normally used for treating an overactive bladder.* Then, researchers scanned them again. They witnessed the mirabegron launch the subjects' brown fat into thermogenesis. Remarkably, the fat-burning activity was elevated by as much as a thousandfold in at least eight areas of their bodies, including the normally hard-to-detect brown fat around the kidneys, spleen, and liver (see Figure 3.4).

When the drug's effects on metabolism were measured, the researchers found that mirabegron had increased it by an average of 13 percent,

---

* The normal dose of the mirabegron is 25 mg orally once a day.

compared to those who took a placebo pill.[18] Their brown fat burned down the fuel that was stored in their white fat. With that rate of metabolism increase, the researchers calculated that mirabegron would result in an eleven-pound weight loss over one year's time and a twenty-two-pound loss over three years.

But mirabegron is not approved for activating metabolism. Furthermore, it can cause side effects such as high blood pressure, swelling of the nose and throat, headache, bloating, and blurred vision even at its usual dose—remember, the dose used in the brown fat study was much higher.

You cannot safely take drugs to activate your brown fat, at least not yet, but I recognized that a far more preferable approach using foods could trigger thermogenesis as well. I began researching foods that can activate the β3-adrenergic receptor to trigger brown fat. I found Mother Nature has provided us with many ways—and many foods—to coax your brown fat to heal your metabolism.

Foods That Activate Brown Fat

Are you someone who enjoys spicy food? Well, here's another reason to relish that hot sauce! The effectiveness of hot chili peppers for weight loss has been studied in human clinical trials. Hot peppers have bioactives that are responsible for their heat and flavor. They are called capsaicin and capsinoids. These chemicals activate pathways in the body that decrease fat production, burn off excess fat, increase your metabolism, and make you feel less hungry.

Researchers from the University of Maryland in Baltimore examined chili peppers in a study of eighty people between the ages of thirty and sixty who were obese. One group of subjects was given an extract from the spicy oil of dried cayenne peppers to ingest twice a day for three months.[19] The extract contained 6 milligrams' worth of capsinoids packed in each capsule.* A second group took a placebo with no chili extract. The subjects were weighed, and their body composition was measured using the dual-energy X-ray absorptiometer (DEXA) scan to identify abdominal visceral fat and total body fat.

The researchers wanted to see if activating the brown fat with chili pepper could burn away harmful fat. All the subjects met with a dietitian to counsel them on how to lower their caloric intake by 300–600 calories per day, based on their typical levels of physical activity. That's not a lot of restriction: a plain bagel topped with cream cheese has roughly 300 calories. The subjects just continued their usual level of physical activity and didn't have to start a workout program.

At the end of three months, the cayenne pepper eaters had a sixfold greater *decrease* in the amount of visceral fat in their belly—the bad stuff—compared to the group who took the placebo (see Figure 3.5).[20] Losing visceral fat has clear-cut health benefits: your body becomes more sensitive to insulin, your metabolism improves, and the amount of inflammation in your body is lowered.

Chili pepper activates your brown fat through your nervous system. Like most physiological processes in your body, brown fat responds to electrical and chemical signals that are sent from one part of the body to another, transmitted from cell to cell like a baton in a relay race. Once the signal is received at its final destination, the cell will respond by taking some action.

The signals that activate brown fat are carried by sympathetic nerves, tiny threads that wind throughout your body. They are especially abundant in brown fat. The ends of each nerve touch the brown adipocytes.[21] Your sympathetic nervous system is best known for its role in flight-or-fight responses—the nerves respond to the hormone

---

* The specific peppers were the CH-19 sweet varietal of *Capsicum annuum* L., known as the cayenne pepper.

Cayenne pepper

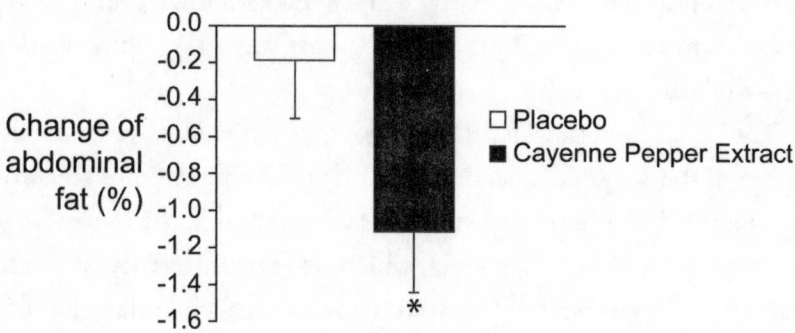

Figure 3.5. An extract from cayenne pepper that is ingested for three months activates brown fat, which then burns away harmful abdominal visceral fat.

norepinephrine you learned about earlier—but these nerves also assist with gut digestion, heart contractions, and thermogenesis.

Here is how chili pepper triggers thermogenesis. Your fight-or-flight nerves are immediately activated the moment the spicy chili peppers hit your tongue. On the surface of your tongue are temperature sensors that live on the ends of special sensory nerve fibers. Their job is to detect hot temperatures (think scalding hot soup) and pain (think the burn of hot chili sauce and wasabi). One of these sensors is known as TRPV1 (pronounced "trip-vee-one"; sometimes called the capsaicin receptor).* As I mentioned earlier, capsaicin is the bioactive found in hot chili peppers. Other bioactives that provoke this receptor are found in black pepper (piperine), ginger (gingerol), and even clove oil (eugenol).

Foods like hot sauce activate this receptor on your tongue and send a powerful signal through the sensory nerves that course from your tongue to your brain. The TRPV1 receptor is also on nerves in the esophagus, stomach, intestines, and colon, so spicy food can send the signal as it

---

* "TRPV" stands for transient receptor potential vanilloid, and it was discovered in 1997. Besides the tongue, this receptor is found in the heart, brain, lungs, and pancreas.

travels all the way through your gut to your tail end.[22] This means that even if you eat quickly, your body will still pick up the signal. You've no doubt heard about spicy food burning on its way in . . . and on its way out—well, this is why.

The signal from the TRPV1 receptor tells the brain to release norepinephrine, the same chemical triggered by cold temperatures to activate brown fat. When the norepinephrine is transmitted to the brown fat cell, it flips the β3-adrenergic receptor, which, as you just learned, is a special switch on the cell surface. This leads to a chemical chain reaction inside the cell, culminating in the activation of a protein called uncoupling protein 1 (UCP1).[23] This very important protein is found in a mini-organ that is inside your cells. The organ is called the mitochondria, and it is your cells' power generator. Just like a mechanical generator, your mitochondria create heat. The UCP1 works like a spark plug and ignites the mitochondria to generate power in brown fat cells. This starts thermogenesis and voilà, your space heater is on, your metabolism increases, fuel from excess fat is burned, and your harmful white fat shrinks. See, this is how using food as medicine can be deciphered—right down to the cellular level.

Beyond Spicy Food

There are other foods that can activate TRPV1 and other points of this thermogenic pathway to activate brown fat. Some foods have bioactives that activate the β3-adrenergic receptor directly on the surface of brown fat cells, bypassing the TRPV1 receptor. Still others directly turn on the UCP1, the ignition switch that ignites your mitochondria.

Foods containing the bioactive resveratrol, for example, can turn on thermogenesis by doubling the amount of UCP1 made by brown fat cells. Resveratrol is famously found in red wine, but it is also present in blueberries, cranberries, grapes, and even peanuts. In the lab, animals fed resveratrol show an increase in their metabolism.[24]

Soybeans also increase UCP1. In the lab, this has been shown to cause a 31 percent loss of body fat.[25] Lab mice fed a soy-rich diet (with bioactive levels proportional to humans eating soy foods) became leaner and weighed 7.6 percent less than mice fed a standard chow. The bioactives responsible for these metabolic benefits are genistein and daidzein, both of which are abundant in soy-based foods typical of Asian cuisine.

Another brown fat–activating food is green tea. The bioactive compound it contains, epigallocatechin-3-gallate (EGCG), also stimulates thermogenesis. But tea is not the only source of EGCG. Apples, cherries, and lemons also contain this bioactive, which increases metabolism and causes weight loss.[26] Just like the capsinoids found in chili peppers, EGCG increases the body's production of norepinephrine, which stimulates the β3-adrenergic receptors on brown fat, activates UCP1, and turns on the mitochondria power generator. You can easily see how foods can activate your metabolism.

Herbs and spices are also a surprising source of thermogenic bioactives. Menthol, which is the bioactive in peppermint, has been shown to increase UCP1 and reduce weight gain by activating brown fat in the lab.[27] Spices like turmeric also activate brown fat by increasing UCP1. Turmeric has another trick up its sleeve: it turns white fat into beige fat, which is a less harmful form of fat that is not quite white but not quite brown. This transformation, known as "beiging," helps rein in the amount of harmful white fat you carry around.[28] Both brown and beige fat cells can burn down excess fat through thermogenesis.

Activating brown fat is just one way that food can be used to improve your metabolism. Next, I'm going to open the floodgates to even more ways that different foods can fight body fat and bring it under control. Get ready for more surprises!

CHAPTER 4

You Can Eat to Beat Fat

Mother Nature is extremely clever and resourceful. Almost all natural biological substances have more than one function. In the case of food, there are tens of thousands of bioactives that are laced into our colorful fruits and vegetables, spices and herbs, nuts and seeds—so many, in fact, that most of them have not been fully researched. That's the fun part, for me, of being a scientist: figuring out what these substances are actually doing inside our bodies when we eat them.

I was inspired by the remarkable letters and emails I received after my previous book, *Eat to Beat Disease*, was published, when readers from around the world wrote me to say that not only were they healthier and feeling more fit; many told me they were also slimming down and losing weight. This observation triggered a startling idea in my mind: What if the bioactives in some of the two hundred foods I wrote about in *Eat to Beat Disease* did more than activate your health defenses—what if they actually could fight body fat and improve metabolism, too?

My medical research had already taken me to explore the deep waters of the field of metabolism, and I knew inflammation, stem cells, microbiome, epigenetics, and circulation were all connected to metabolic health. When I delved into their connections with adipocytes and food, it became clear that many beneficial food bioactives also have fat-fighting and metabolism-enhancing skills to add to their biological résumés. Even more, human studies provide the clinical evidence that eating foods with these bioactives is effective for improving body composition and mending and optimizing metabolism.

I am going to reveal 150 foods with remarkable benefits when it comes to your metabolism, all supported by science and human evidence. You can just trust me and skip to them if you like (they are in Part 3). But I want you to truly understand how to use food to improve your metabolism, so I need to tell you about their bioactives and how they work to combat the harms of excess body fat.

Here's a scorecard of the many ways that food bioactives can aid your metabolism. Each food can have one or more of these benefits:

- reduce the inflammation caused by excess fat
- improve your body's sensitivity to insulin
- activate the pathways that trigger thermogenesis in brown fat
- cause white fat to become brown fat or beige fat (brown fat–like)
- direct stem cells to make more desirable brown fat instead of harmful white fat
- reduce the amount of visceral fat, shrinking waist size
- produce more of the beneficial hormone adiponectin from healthy fat cells
- improve lipid metabolism by restoring the microbiome
- slow fat's ability to grow
- suppress appetite

Let's take a look at some bioactives found in foods that may already be in your kitchen and definitely are at your local grocery store.

Carvacrol

Found in some of my favorite kitchen herbs, like oregano, thyme, and marjoram, this bioactive adds flavor to your food. You don't need to add much of an herb to any food to elevate its palatability. This potency extends to its fat-fighting power. In Chieti, Italy, lab researchers at the National Research Council showed that human stem cells destined to become white adipose cells could be reduced by up to 27 percent using carvacrol.[1]

Quercetin

This is a potent bioactive present in capers, red onions (especially the skin), red apples, tomatoes, shallots, scallion, cabbage, cherries, blueberries, blackberries, and cherries. A powerful fat burner, quercetin fights fat on a number of fronts. In lab studies, adding quercetin to high-fat diets being fed to obese mice reduced their body weight and decreased the amount of harmful visceral fat they carried after eight weeks. Compared to mice eating just the high-fat diet who gained weight and became obese, those eating quercetin weighed 10 percent less, and they had 23 percent less body fat.[2]

Quercetin lowers inflammation in adipose tissue, and it improves your cells' insulin sensitivity, so your metabolism becomes more efficient in using glucose as energy. This bioactive also increases norepinephrine, the hormone that triggers the β3-adrenergic receptor on brown fat cells, setting off thermogenesis. To power this up even further, quercetin also increases the amount of UCP1, the ignition switch that turns on the mitochondria thermal engine that burns fat. One more thing it does: quercetin causes white fat to become beige, thus rendering it less harmful.

Luteolin

A fat-fighting bioactive, luteolin is present in radicchio, green peppers, chicory greens, celery, pumpkin, red leaf lettuce, artichoke, and kohlrabi. It is heat-stable and can survive cooking. In lab studies, luteolin has been shown to prevent weight gain and reduce both visceral fat and subcutaneous fat.[3]

Just like quercetin, luteolin takes a multipronged approach to dismantling the harms of body fat. It sends a signal to brown fat, telling it to make more UCP1, which fires up thermogenesis. Luteolin also causes white adipose tissue to transform itself into brown fat. This bioactive lowers fat inflammation and improves insulin sensitivity, all of which help to improve metabolic health.

Chlorogenic Acid

This is a bioactive found in carrots, artichokes, apples, pears, plums, grapes, kiwifruit, burdock, and coffee beans—and it's a highly potent fat fighter. Lab studies have shown that chlorogenic acid tackles adipose tissue in three ways: it directs fat stem cells to become useful brown fat, it forces white adipose cells to become beige, and it turns on thermogenesis in brown fat to burn away excess fat and increase metabolism.[4]

Ursolic Acid

This bioactive is found in many fruits and herbs, including thyme, rosemary, oregano, marjoram, lavender, elderflower, peppermint, cranberries, bilberries, and hawthorn berries. Ursolic acid increases the amount of brown fat present, improves metabolic efficiency, increases exercise capacity, and decreases body weight, according to lab studies conducted at the University of Iowa.[5] Researchers at the University of Guadalajara in Mexico showed that this bioactive also increases the production of adiponectin, the fat hormone that maintains insulin sensitivity.[6] Ursolic acid also lowers inflammation caused by body fat.[7]

Hesperidin/Neohesperidin

Citrus lovers will be delighted to know that these closely related fat-fighting bioactives are found in oranges, tangerines, grapefruit, lemons, and limes, as well as in peppermint. Hesperidin and neohesperidin can suppress appetite, improve the metabolism of cholesterol in the blood, and turn down the volume control of the genetic switches responsible for creating more fat cells.[8] They also stimulate lipolysis, the process of breaking down existing fat cells. They also increase

UCP1 to improve brown fat thermogenesis and promote the browning of white fat.[9]

Lab studies have shown that neohesperidin can prevent weight gain by improving the gut microbiome, a valuable effect after antibiotics are used to treat an infection and healthy bacteria are knocked out.[10] So, if you are taking antibiotics, be sure to note these bioactives, as well as the next one, that nourish your microbiome.

Beta-D-glucan

This bioactive is a soluble fiber found in mushrooms, oats, barley, wheat, and edible brown seaweed. Beta-D-glucan reduces inflammation caused by fat and improves gut health by nourishing your microbiome.[11] Beta-D-glucan can fight body fat, cause weight loss, and help your metabolism by improving insulin sensitivity. Foods containing beta-D-glucan also slow down the speed at which your stomach empties food. The result is, there is more time for your stomach to signal to your brain the feeling of fullness so it can shut down your appetite.[12]

Lycopene

The colorful red hue of this bioactive alerts you to its presence in tomatoes, watermelon, guava, papaya, persimmons, red bell peppers, and even pink grapefruit. Lycopene counters weight gain by making white fat become brown fat and then activating the brown fat to start thermogenesis.[13] The bioactive also lowers inflammation in body fat, and it blocks new fat cells from developing.[14] There's also a unique fat-fighting trick that lycopene has in its playbook: it shrinks the amount of liquid fat that is stored in adipocytes, so each fat cell gets smaller.[15]

Lignans

These are a family of bioactives found in seeds like sesame, sunflower, pumpkin, flaxseed, and soybeans. A lignan in sesame seeds, called sesaminol, stimulates brown fat thermogenesis in lab studies and is protective against weight gain.[16] Another lignan called secoisolariciresinol is found in pumpkin seeds and flaxseeds. It prevents new fat cells from being formed by inhibiting adipogenesis.[17] Lignans also help fat cells produce adiponectin, the healthy hormone that makes our cells more responsive to insulin and improves the performance of our metabolism.[18] Some vegetables like broccoli and cabbage, and fruits such as apricots, nectarines, and strawberries, also contain lignans.

Ellagic Acid

The tartness of strawberries is the result of different acids present in the fruit, one of which is ellagic acid. This is a bioactive that's also found in cranberries, raspberries, and pomegranates, as well as walnuts, chestnuts, and pecans. Ellagic acid improves your metabolism in a number of ways. It guides fat stem cells to become useful brown fat and causes white fat to undergo browning. It directly affects brown fat cells by increasing the amount of UCP1 to ignite thermogenesis.[19] Ellagic acid also prevents fat cells from getting larger, it improves your body's sensitivity to insulin, and it lowers the inflammation caused by excess fat.[20]

Anthocyanin

This bioactive is a natural pigment whose colors range from blue to purple to black to red. In nature, anthocyanins attract bees to pollinate the flowers, and animals eat the colorful fruits and spread their seeds. Anthocyanins are found in blueberries, blackberries, purple maize, purple potatoes, chokeberries, black raspberries, bilberries, elderberries, and black plums.[21] Lab studies have shown that feeding mice chow that contains anthocyanins can reduce their body weight by 20 percent and lower their total adipose tissue by 18–20 percent.[22] It is also an anti-inflammatory substance and can lower the inflammation caused by excess fat. In the lab, anthocyanin stimulates fat cells to release adiponectin, which improves metabolism.[23] It also causes the beiging of white fat cells and initiates thermogenesis by stimulating the β3-adrenergic receptor on brown fat cells.[24]

Hydroxytyrosol

Olives are the source of this potent bioactive. Hydroxytyrosol is made by the fruit as it matures. It's mostly present in the watery liquid pressed from olives during the making of extra virgin olive oil, but it is also found in the oil. Lab studies show that hydroxytyrosol prevents the growth of visceral fat in the belly. This effect is tied to its beneficial effect on the gut microbiome, which is to increase the diversity of bacteria present, a sure sign of gut health.[25] Hydroxytyrosol prevents stem cells from producing more white fat, and it also has anti-inflammatory effects.[26]

Sulforaphanes

This is another family of bioactives that are found in cruciferous vegetables such as broccoli, broccoli sprouts, cabbage, bok choy, mustard greens, kale, collard greens, and Brussels sprouts. They cause the browning of white fat, incite thermogenesis in brown fat, and reduce the inflammation caused by excess body fat.[27]

Sulforaphanes are unique because they can reverse leptin resistance.[28] Recall that leptin is the hormone released by fat cells that acts on the brain to suppress your appetite. As excess fat accumulates, the brain becomes resistant to leptin, which results in you feeling hungry all the time. Sulforaphanes reverse this resistance, so your brain can do the right thing for your metabolism and turn down your feeling of hunger—an important move that helps you combat body fat.

Omega-3s

Omega-3 polyunsaturated fatty acids are well-known, healthy bioactives that are found in seafood, especially oily fish like salmon, sardines, and anchovies. They originate from marine algae and plankton but are found in the many fish and shellfish that eat them as part of the food chain. Omega-3s activate brown fat by stimulating the TRPV1 receptor in the gut, just like chili peppers and green tea, and this sends a signal to the brain that it's time to release norepinephrine, the trigger for thermogenesis. Omega-3s also increase UCP1 in brown fat and turn harmful white fat into useful brown fat.

Foods That Activate Your Health Defense Systems to Fight Fat

Recall that your fat cells are tethered to your five health defense systems. The cells rely on an adequate blood supply (angiogenesis), are formed from stem cells (regeneration), and are influenced by your gut bacteria (microbiome). Their DNA can be impacted by your environment and behavior (epigenetic changes of your DNA), and fat cells coexist with immune and inflammatory cells within fatty tissue (immune defenses). Well, it turns out that the foods that activate your health defenses also use these connections to help rightsize your body fat. In fact, many of the foods that counter excess body fat are the same ones I wrote about in *Eat to Beat Disease*. This is extraordinarily good news because it means you can literally eat to beat your diet and beat disease at the same time.

Foods That Starve Fat

Your angiogenesis defense system provides the lifelines to bring oxygen and nutrients to your healthy body fat. It keeps your fat in a healthy state so it can do its job as body padding, as a fuel depot, as a heat generator (thermogenesis), and as a hormone-producing organ. These same blood vessels transport important fat hormones like leptin, adiponectin, and resistin to your brain, muscles, and other organs.

When there is excess adipose tissue, however, the fat cells are crippled and can't function normally. Hormones are not made in normal amounts, inflammation rages within fat, and the blood vessels in fat transport high levels of inflammatory cytokines made by the fat to the rest of the body. Not good.

Just like antiangiogenic foods can starve a cancer by cutting off its blood supply, they can also rein in growing fat by limiting its circulation. Many of the fat-fighting food bioactives I discussed earlier have this antiangiogenic power: quercetin, chlorogenic acid, hydroxytyrosol, sulforaphane, genistein, daidzein, anthocyanin, beta-D-glucan—they all can help control and throttle back the harmful blood vessels that feed excess fat (just like a tumor!), and this can improve your metabolism.

Another move that helps your metabolism, fasting, also starves cancer cells and can shrink excess fat by pruning away their blood supply. Bioactives are multitaskers; they can turn on thermogenesis to burn away fat while at the same time controlling its blood supply. An example is capsaicin, the thermogenic protein found in chili peppers, which is also a powerful antiangiogenic substance.[29] Eating to fortify your angiogenesis defenses also strengthens your body's ability to control excess fat.

Regenerative Defenses Fight Fat

Your regenerative defenses can be tasked with combating excess fat. A fat stem cell, the preadipocyte, can morph into any type of cell. This is called plasticity, and it's a very useful property to know about because you can eat certain foods that redirect the fate of preadipocytes away from creating harmful fat. The chlorogenic acid found in apples, pears, artichokes, kiwifruit, and capers—and ellagic acid that's found in pomegranates, cranberries, chestnuts, and walnuts—can do this. They tell stem cells to make useful brown fat instead of white fat.

Other foods can stop stem cells from turning into fat cells of any type, like hydroxytyrosol from olives and extra virgin olive oil, and capsaicin found in chili peppers and hot sauce. What's remarkable is that all of these fat-fighting foods also simultaneously direct stem cells to repair and regenerate healthy organs. Making more good fat and halting the production of bad fat, while repairing and regenerating your organs, are the benefits of eating regenerative foods.

Turn Your Microbiome Against Fat

Your microbiome is responsible for gut health, but it can also create metabolic health—both are influenced by what you eat.[30] It's known, for example, that the greater the diversity of bacterial species in your gut, the better your health. Lean people tend to have more bacterial diversity than people who are overweight or obese. Eating prebiotic foods containing dietary fiber, such as broccoli, bok choy, kiwifruit, mushrooms, and even pears, encourages more diverse types of bacteria to grow, matching the "lean profile."[31]

Eating probiotic foods such as yogurt, kimchi, sauerkraut, and even pickles can directly put more strains of healthy bacteria into your gut. Although diversity is valuable, there is one bacterium that you really want to grow because it is a guardian of your health: *Akkermansia mucinophila*.[32] This oval-shaped organism makes up only 3–5 percent of the gut bacteria in healthy people, but despite this, *Akkermansia* helps maintain your metabolism, control your body weight, power up your immune defenses, and even support your mental well-being. Take note: this bacterium is found in the gut of lean people, but it's mostly absent in the gut of people who are obese.

A study of *Akkermansia* involving 10,534 people ranging in age from twenty to ninety-nine by researchers from Beijing Hospital, Kunming Medical University, and the Chinese Academy of Sciences[33] found that the presence of *Akkermansia* in the gut was protective against obesity but that levels of this bacterium decline with age.[34] They also showed that having a mere 10 percent higher level of *Akkermansia* would reduce the risk of obesity by 26 percent. This may help explain why some people battle more against weight gain as they get older: less *Akkermansia*, more body fat. Foods that help grow more *Akkermansia* in the gut include pomegranate, cranberry, Concord grape, turmeric, green and black tea, and chili pepper.

Another gut bacterium that is beneficial for your metabolism is *Lactobacillus reuteri*. This organism has anti-inflammatory, antitumor, wound-healing, and immune defense–supporting effects in your body. In the lab, *Lactobacillus reuteri* also causes white fat to become brown fat, and it increases the UCP1 protein that ignites brown fat to start thermogenesis.[35]

A clinical study of *Lactobacillus reuteri* supplementation was conducted among seventy-one young people ranging in age from six months to twenty-two years. All the subjects had Prader-Willi syndrome, a rare genetic condition that causes life-threatening childhood obesity, cognitive impairment, and behavioral problems.[36] The researchers gave their subjects either a *Lactobacillus reuteri* probiotic every day for twelve weeks or a placebo capsule. Body fat measurements were taken at six and twelve weeks after beginning the study. The results showed those taking the *Lactobacillus reuteri* probiotic had decreased their body mass index by 7 percent, while there was no significant change in subjects taking the placebo.* Some probiotic foods that contain *Lactobacillus reuteri* include cheeses (Parmigiano Reggiano, Grana Padano, Toma, Gruyère, Roncal, Idiazabal), sourdough bread, Korean kimchi, sauerkraut, and some forms of yogurt.[37]

DNA Defenses Counter Fat

Your DNA defenses protect your genetic code against damaging forces, especially oxidative stressors, the chemicals that act like rogue samurai slashing at your DNA. Excess fat increases oxidative stress, and it also

---

* People with the rare Prader-Willi syndrome also experience developmental delays and neuropsychiatric symptoms. The clinical study also showed that subjects receiving *Lactobacillus reuteri* experienced improved social communications and social interactions, compared to placebo. This fits with beneficial gut-brain interactions known to be associated with *Lactobacillus reuteri*.

stokes chronic inflammation. Both can lead to harmful DNA damage.[38] Foods with antioxidant and anti-inflammatory properties counter these effects and are protective. Some of the best examples are kiwifruit, tomato, watermelon, broccoli and broccoli sprouts, citrus, papaya, red bell pepper, and seafood rich in omega-3 fatty acids—all can help keep your DNA shielded from the effects of having too much fat.

Certain foods can also turn on or turn off your DNA in ways that protect you against the harms of fat. This is called epigenetic change, and foods like dark leafy green vegetables, beans and legumes, and beets are known to do this. They bring about a process called DNA methylation. This epigenetic change is associated with slimming down abdominal fat, weight loss, and improving metabolism.[39]

Another epigenetic tactic that is useful for combating fat involves turning on the genes that cause undesirable white fat cells to become more desirable brown and beige fat cells.[40] There are at least twenty-seven genes that can be activated in brown and beige fat but not in white fat.[41] By flipping on the switch for these genes, white fat becomes brown. Foods like chili peppers (capsaicin), apples (quercetin), onions (luteolin), peppermint (menthol), coffee (chlorogenic acid), oregano (ursolic acid), tomatoes (lycopene), strawberries (ellagic acid), blueberries (anthocyanins), and bok choy (sulforaphanes) can activate these useful fat-fighting genes to improve your metabolism. You can perform gene therapy in your own kitchen!

Immune Defenses Rally Against Fat

Your immune defense system tackles bacteria, viruses, and cancer cells—and it also puts the brakes on excess body fat. This defense also lowers the inflammation that is caused by all of these insults. While most of your immune system is based in your gut (living right next to your microbiome), part of your immunity is actually situated right within your adipose tissue.[42] An entire army of immune cells, in fact, live in a giant piece of fatty tissue called the omentum, which is in your belly.

This fat slab has a protective function as it moves and molds itself around areas where your intestines may have been damaged to wall off the rest of your body from a dangerous infection. Once it has spotted and roped off an infectious spot, your omental fat focuses a blast of inflammation like a flamethrower into the infected area to destroy any harmful organisms. When the danger is over, your omentum turns off the inflammation using specialized immune cells called M2 macrophages and regulatory T cells (Tregs).* The job of these cells is to bring the immune defenses in fat back to normal healthy levels.

Excess body fat wrecks the delicate balance between immunity and inflammation and causes inflammation to dominate and rip dangerously through your body.[43] Even worse, your defensive immune cells—the ones that protect you against infection—malfunction when they are caught in this wildfire, and they release proteins called cytokines, which spark even more inflammation. This vicious cycle of more and more inflammation is a dangerous biological trap that sets you up for inflammatory diseases ranging from diabetes to atherosclerosis to cancer.

Eating foods containing anti-inflammatory bioactives, such as quercetin, luteolin, lycopene, ellagic acid, anthocyanin, hydroxytyrosol, ursolic acid, and sulforaphane, can help control and extinguish these fat-fueled fires within adipose tissue. Some foods are able to do double duty and calm inflammation while activating immune cells that protect you against infection and cancer at the same time. Blueberries, green tea, and foods containing vitamin C, such as citrus, red cabbage, and kiwifruit, are just some examples of these immune multitaskers that can intercept the dangers of too much body fat and help restore your metabolism.[44]

---

* You may recognize macrophages as immune cells that are normally part of the proinflammatory response. This is true in most of the body, most of the time. In fat, however, they play a different role. They are on standby as anti-inflammatory cells. Technically, they are called "M2 macrophages."

Avengers Assemble!

In the famous comic books and in the cinematic Marvel Universe, superheroes like the Avengers unite as a team and use their combined efforts and various superpowers to defeat galactic enemies that threaten the planet.* By eating the right foods, you can assemble your own super-hero team of bioactives inside your body. Remember the scorecard I gave you at the beginning of this chapter? These natural chemicals act on the body in multiple ways to improve your metabolism, burn away harmful excess fat, and help you maintain a healthier body weight. Some foods can prevent more white fat from growing, others can trans-form white fat into useful brown or beige fat, and still other foods can send a signal to the brain commanding it to release hormones that trig-ger brown fat cells to start thermogenesis and burn away fat. And there are even some foods that can work from within brown fat cells and prompt them to make more of the protein that ignites thermogenesis.

These same foods also boost your body's five health defenses and recruit their powers to help you fight the villainy of fat overage. Each health defense system combats fat in its own way—by starving your fat cells through antiangiogenesis or by preventing more fat from forming from your stem cells, which can be redirected to making more useful brown fat, or by shoring up your gut microbiome to counter the damage fat inflicts on your metabolism, to lowering the inflammation released by fat.

Getting all these elements to join forces might sound complicated, but it is actually very simple when you do it using food. I'm going to show you how. In Part 2, I'll start by telling you about the foods that

---

* The Marvel Comics team Avengers was originally composed of six superheroes: Iron Man, Hulk, Thor, Captain America, Ant-Man, and the Wasp. Other superhero teams from com-ics included the Fantastic Four, X-Men, and the Defenders. The concept of multiple powers from bioactives in natural products combining for a desired effect has been coined the "entourage effect."

have human evidence for improving your metabolism and fighting body fat. Then, in Part 3, I'll give you a highly customizable protocol that you can follow and refine to fit your life and suit your own preferences and tastes.

The foods that improve your metabolism and the foods that boost your health defenses are often one and the same. Better yet, they are all used as ingredients in delicious traditional recipes and most are easy to find and cook. Eating these foods is a joyful and healthful way to live your life while you improve your metabolism, trim away harmful body fat, and gain better health.

PART 2

FOODS FOR METABOLISM

The secret powers of nature are generally discovered unsolicited.

—*Hans Christian Andersen*

CHAPTER 5

Eating the MediterAsian Way

B ecause of my research, many people assume that I must be following a special diet myself. They ask, "Dr. Li, what do *you* eat?" I suppose years of conditioning by gurus and their books have led folks to assume that I follow strict eating habits. The truth is that I love to enjoy my meals, especially when it comes to healthy eating.

Everything I shared in the last few chapters may tempt some people to fight fat by becoming a "biohacker"—someone who uses do-it-yourself biology to improve well-being, perhaps by taking a capsule or creating a meal replacement that manipulates your metabolism and fat so that you don't need to think about the benefits of real food. But I strongly recommend taking the food-based approach. Some of the greatest food cultures in the world—Mediterranean and Asian—have for centuries used delicious combinations of natural ingredients in their cuisines that contain the very bioactives that improve metabolism, burn down harmful fat, and activate your health defenses. Eating these types of cuisines is far more satisfying than taking a capsule or guzzling down a shake.

My number-one priority is that my meals must taste great. And because of my childhood, travels, and life experiences, as well as my research on food and health, I naturally gravitate toward the traditional cuisines from the Mediterranean and Asia. Their cuisines are delicious! And both the Mediterranean region and Asia have areas known as Blue Zones, where people age better, live longer, and are overall healthier.* Their cuisines are abundant in whole foods—fruits, vegetables, herbs, nuts and legumes, and whole grains—and in coastal regions, they're plentiful in seafood. One study of people ninety or older in one of these Blue Zones, the island of Ikaria in Greece, showed that 87 percent had normal levels of cholesterol, 82 percent were at a healthy weight, and 80 percent were free of diabetes.[1] Even at this super senior age, 30 percent had no chronic diseases at all and excellent metabolism!

I don't follow any diet—instead, I follow a food *approach*. I call it the MediterAsian Way because it brings together the healthiest foods and the most tantalizing flavors from these two culinary worlds. MediterAsian eating incorporates the fat-fighting and health-promoting compounds we discussed in the previous chapter, but it doesn't require you to memorize the names of chemical compounds or follow complicated rules about food combinations. My approach is an intuitive way of putting all of that scientific research to work for you, without needing to analyze all the beneficial actions that happen at the molecular level.

The MediterAsian Way allows you to delight in a variety of delicious foods while you boost your health defenses, optimize your metabolism, and fight harmful body fat. It is a philosophy that will help you enjoy the pleasures of food—not struggle with them—throughout your entire life.

The Path to MediterAsian

I've always been an enthusiastic and curious traveler, exploring different cuisines, cultures, and approaches to well-being, many of which I've incorporated into my own life. The world's varieties of foods are vast, and some of the most delicious ones I've encountered also correlate with some of the healthiest people I have met. From the monks on Mount

---

* The Blue Zones in the Mediterranean are Ikaria, Greece, and Ogliastra, Sardinia, in Italy. Asia's Blue Zone is Okinawa, Japan.

Athos in Greece to villagers in Lazio, Italy, to tea farmers in Jiangsu, China, a healthy style of eating involving nutrient-dense, whole foods and relatively unprocessed foods are common denominators.

Another traditional value I have observed in Mediterranean and Asian cultures is eating in moderation. The practice of moderation is based on the ideas that deliberate restraint is a virtue and that quality always triumphs over quantity. These ideas align perfectly with current research showing that high-quality foods contain more healthful bioactives.

Whenever I travel, I especially enjoy exploring new foods—ones that I do not recognize. It's how I learned about horned melon, hon-shimeji mushrooms, and slipper lobster. (Go ahead, look them up. They are delicious!) My friends from all around the world, some of them chefs, often invite me to try a new dish or ingredient, and my taste buds have been rewarded on many occasions. For me, the discovery of a new favorite flavor is an exciting and memorable life experience.

The MediterAsian Way draws on everything I have seen, eaten, enjoyed, learned, and researched. It integrates the lessons of healthy eating from different parts of the world with ingredients and cooking styles that allow one to enjoy good health and good meals at the same time. My MediterAsian approach is inspired by revered food traditions and is supported by cutting-edge biomedical research. It is also guided by my mission to tear down destructive misconceptions about food as something to be feared. Healthy eating is available to everyone, everywhere, no matter what you do for a living and no matter where you may be in your health journey—and it can and should be delicious.

From the Silk Road to Your Kitchen

Both Mediterranean and Asian cuisines are the result of millennia of exploration and experimentation with foods. Long before anyone coined the term "fusion" in relation to cuisine, people were combining the best ingredients they could find from far-flung regions. The reason you have cinnamon and oranges in your kitchen is because of the Silk Road, a two-thousand-year-old trading route that once connected China with the Mediterranean Sea. If you'd taken a road trip along what was actually a series of paths centuries ago, you would have eaten at rest stops along the way and experienced MediterAsian food. The transport, sale, and exchange of foods along the Silk Road marked the beginning of our modern culinary melting pot from East to West, and vice versa.

Many foods you'll find in this book are in your kitchen but had their origins along the Silk Road. The summer peaches and apricots you enjoy originated in China. Their trees were cultivated along the Silk Road before they eventually made their way to the fruit bowls of the Mediterranean and Europe and later to the Americas. The apple was once a wild fruit growing in the forests of Tian Shan, a mountain range on the border between Kazakhstan and northwest China. Apples were picked, sold, and eaten along the Silk Road, as were walnuts, almonds, grapes, melons, and cucumbers.[2] Chickpeas, barley, and wheat were exchanged by traders who carried them to destinations east and west, along with fermented and pickled foods.

According to archaeobotanists who conduct research expeditions along what remains of the Silk Road today, traders experienced different styles of cuisine using the exact same ingredients, dried and fresh, as they made their journey from one end of the route to the other.* They intermingled and swapped recipes. Spices such as turmeric, ginger, pepper, saffron, and cinnamon are now common to the cooking of China, India, Central Asia, and the Mediterranean countries of Italy, Greece, Spain, and France. Fresh vegetables, fruits, herbs, spices, and dried and fermented foods were a cultural currency that has connected these cuisines over two thousand years of ingredient exchange.

---

* This research is conducted by archaeobotanists who search for dried remains of pits, seeds, stems, and flesh of produce and other foods in the ruins of old settlements along the Silk Road and identify their origins.

MediterAsian Is More Than Meets the Eye

Because of this cross-pollination, there is no clear dividing line between an "Asian diet" and a "Mediterranean diet" when it comes to healthy eating. These labels were coined by scientists who needed to come up with a simple name while comparing the health advantages of one dietary pattern to another. The labels were then propagated by journalists reporting on the research. Once spread by the media, they were adopted by nutritionists, wellness influencers, and even academics citing the original research. The truth is, the terms "Mediterranean diet" and "Asian diet" are part of a nutrition slang that gives eating patterns that once existed from one end of the Silk Road to the other almost a false identity. The MediterAsian Way gets rid of these artificial divisions and embraces the full range of dietary traditions that emerged along this great trade route; this breadth and inclusiveness is the very antithesis of the narrowness of the typical "diet book" approach.

Take a look at the map of the Silk Road in Figure 5.1, and you'll see it's not possible to easily split the highly diverse styles of food of all the regions that were traversed into just two simple categories.

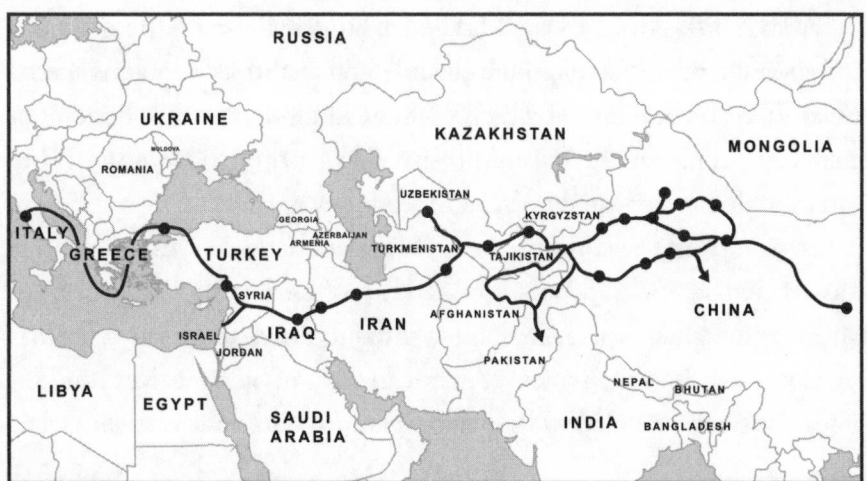

Figure 5.1. Main routes of the Silk Road connecting Asia to the Mediterranean. (Map by Diana Saville.)

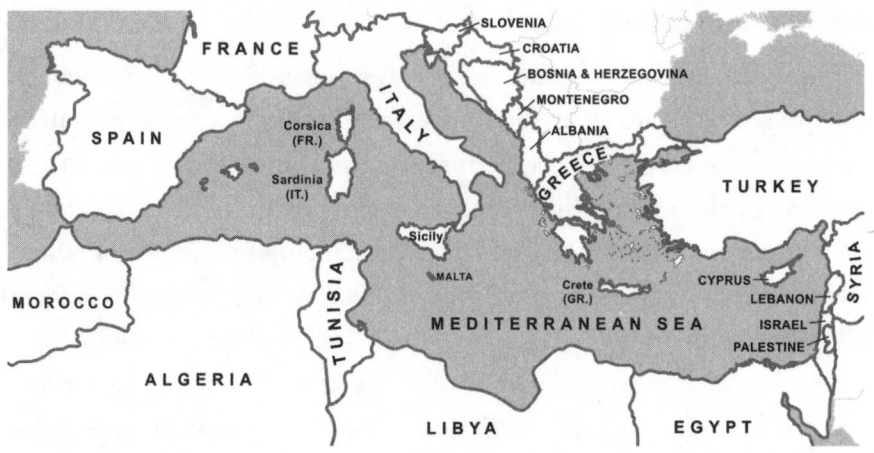

Figure 5.2. Map of countries in the Mediterranean. (Map by Diana Saville.)

Now let's take an even closer look to see what countries are actually in the Mediterranean today. You will probably quickly call out Italy, Greece, and Spain as being Mediterranean, but you might not be aware of all the other countries that complete the ring of land surrounding the Mediterranean Sea. Check out the map in Figure 5.2 and you will see there are actually twenty-one surrounding countries!*

From North Africa to the Middle East to the Balkans, these regions and their countries have unique cuisines and traditional cooking methods of their own, many of which comingled along the Silk Road. You might not consider the cuisines of Israel, Egypt, or Slovenia as being part of a Mediterranean diet—but indeed they are.

So where did the concept of the "Mediterranean diet" come from? It was created in the 1950s by a research professor at the University of Minnesota named Ancel Keys. He wanted to prove there was a healthier way to eat than the typical "American diet" of his time. Keys and his wife, Margaret, traveled to Italy and Spain in 1952 to investigate what

---

* The twenty-one Mediterranean countries are Albania, Algeria, Bosnia and Herzegovina, Croatia, Cypress, Egypt, France, Greece, Israel, Italy, Lebanon, Libya, Malta, Montenegro, Morocco, Palestine, Slovenia, Spain, Syria, Tunisia, and Turkey.

they perceived to be a superior diet compared to what Americans were eating, which was loaded with red meat, sodas, and ultraprocessed foods, with sparse amounts of fresh vegetables and fruits. Spurred by what he and his wife observed and ate in those two countries, Keys began the first long-term global epidemiological research study of diet and health, known as the Seven Countries Study.* This research included only three of the twenty-one Mediterranean countries: Italy, Greece, and the former Yugoslavia.**

Still, the Seven Countries Study was a breakthrough in the scientific investigation of food and health. It showed that eating less fat is associated with lower blood cholesterol, which in turn is associated with a reduced risk of heart attack and stroke. Even though the Seven Countries Study omitted most of the countries surrounding the Mediterranean Sea (and oddly included the decidedly non-Mediterranean nations of Finland, Japan, and the Netherlands), Ancel Keys coined the term "Mediterranean diet" in a popular book that he and his wife cowrote about their research.[3] The traditional diet they described as beneficial contained mostly plant-based foods, and the diet is abundant in fruits and vegetables, legumes, nuts and seeds, healthy oils, and whole grains. It was the diet of villagers in the countryside, low in saturated fat and red meat and with only moderate amounts of fish and poultry.[4]

The twenty-one Mediterranean countries each have highly distinctive regional cuisines that can't be summarized with a shorthand name. Even the term "Italian food" is a crude generalization, with meaning only for people who do not live in Italy (Italians do not refer to their own meals as "Italian"). Italy has twenty regions, and within each is a trove of culinary traditions based on locally grown, raised, and caught

---

* To learn more about the Seven Countries Study, see www.sevencountriesstudy.com.
** The seven countries studied by Ancel Keys were Finland, Greece, Italy, Japan, the Netherlands, the US, and Yugoslavia. The former Yugoslavia is now six countries: Bosnia and Herzegovina, Croatia, Macedonia, Montenegro, Serbia, and Slovenia. So in today's world, the Seven Countries Study included eight Mediterranean countries.

ingredients.* This is also true in Spain and France, where regional reci-pes feature unique flavors and styles. And nowhere is this specialization more evident than in Greece, where each of its 227 inhabited islands has its own unique food traditions. All this is to say that to fully enjoy Mediterranean cuisine, you'd have a lot to explore.

The term "Asian diet" is even less precise. Asia is a continent that is much larger and more diverse than the Mediterranean region. It's made up of forty-seven countries, including some you might not normally identify as part of Asia, such as Turkey, Georgia, Jordan, and Kazakh-stan, but the people from those countries consider themselves "Asian."** Each country has its own culinary identity that is unique. It's hard to confuse the food of Japan with that of Thailand, India, or Turkey.

Similar to Mediterranean countries, within each country in Asia there is enormous diversity in cuisine. When I did my treks across China, I saw that as the landscape changed, so, too, did the products in the market and the dishes cooked in homes, restaurants, and night mar-kets. The diversity is amazing. I learned there are eight basic Chinese cuisines: Cantonese, Jiangsu, Hunan, Shandong, Anhui, Zhejiang, Fujian, and Sichuan. Each uses many of the same ingredients, but they are combined and prepared in distinct ways to create local specialties. While traveling through Sichuan Province, I savored foods that were intensely fragrant, with fiery chilis, garlic, and Sichuan peppercorns. While in Jiangsu Province, I ate foods that were mild, slightly sweet, brimming with flavors brought out by braising, simmering, and stewing.

---

* The twenty regions of Italy are Abruzzo, Basilicata, Calabria, Campania, Emilia-Romagna, Friuli Venezia Giulia, Lazio, Le Marche, Liguria, Lombardy, Molise, Piedmont, Puglia, Sar-dinia, Sicily, Trentino-Alto Adige, Tuscany, Umbria, Valle d'Aosta, Veneto. Each area has its own traditional dishes.
** The countries of Asia are Afghanistan, Armenia, Azerbaijan, Bahrain, Bangladesh, Bhu-tan, Brunei, Cambodia, China, Cyprus, Georgia, India, Indonesia, Iran, Iraq, Israel, Japan, Jordan, Kazakhstan, Kuwait, Kyrgyzstan, Laos, Lebanon, Malaysia, Maldives, Mongolia, Myanmar, Nepal, North Korea, Oman, Pakistan, the Philippines, Qatar, Saudi Arabia, Sin-gapore, South Korea, Sri Lanka, State of Palestine, Syria, Tajikistan, Thailand, Timor-Leste, Turkmenistan, United Arab Emirates, Uzbekistan, Vietnam, and Yemen.

The cuisine of Guangdong (once known as Canton) is stir-fried, roasted, and steamed, full of natural flavors enhanced by garlic and ginger.

The food traditions throughout Asia are notable in that they embody basic principles that are important for metabolic health and fighting body fat. First is the variety of foods that is part of the culture. Eating diverse foods, especially fiber-rich vegetables, benefits your microbiome, which streamlines your metabolism. Second, many of the cooking methods used—stir-frying, simmering, stewing, and steaming—are healthier and less damaging to your metabolism than deep-frying and grilling. Third are the condiments, which often include fermented foods that are probiotic in nature, and a wide variety of sauces with spices like chili that activate your brown fat. And finally, the format of meals usually involves many small plates of food shared among a group, which increases the diversity of ingredients any diner can eat at each meal, and allows each individual to control their portion sizes. The communal nature of eating together also fosters a more relaxed pace for each meal, which helps to prevent overeating.

Mediterranean cuisine likewise is built on dietary principles that encourage healthy eating. This includes eating in harmony with the seasons by using ingredients available from the fresh market. Simplicity of preparation is key for extracting the full flavor and health benefits of food. Insisting that the food is savored and eaten with restraint is another aspect. A balanced meal is produce-centric and light on meat and includes legumes, herbs, and extra virgin olive oil, along with fish and other seafood.

All these principles come into play with MediterAsian-style eating. But you don't need to be a food historian, food critic, or chef to eat this way. All you have to do is draw on the thousands of traditional and modern recipes found across the countries of the Mediterranean and Asia—and pick the ones you enjoy, whether you prepare your own meals or you dine out. Just pay attention to seasonal ingredients and look up the traditional, time-honored methods of preparation that villagers have been using to cook for thousands of years. Embracing this approach does require some mindfulness—you have to choose quality ingredients and make the time to prepare a recipe to create a delicious and healthy meal—but the rewards can be tremendous for your taste buds and your metabolism.

The Evidence for MediterAsian Benefits

Beyond the fact that it includes great-tasting food, there is abundant evidence that the MediterAsian Way of eating is beneficial to your metabolism. Researchers from Sapienza University and the Paracelso Institute in Rome found that, given the same number of calories, people who eat healthy Chinese food lose significantly more weight.[5] The team studied the body composition of 694 middle-aged white adults who were obese but did not have active cardiovascular disease, high cholesterol, or diabetes. All the subjects reduced their food intake to 1,200 calories per day to trigger weight loss, but half were given a basic traditional Chinese diet for lunch and dinner, while the other half were given a modern "Western diet."*

The Chinese diet included soybeans, black beans, sesame, shallots, mushrooms, ginger, a variety of green vegetables, seaweed, and fish. The Western diet contained chicken, veal, pork, beef, eggs, and cheese, and was heavier in meat and dairy, with some fish and vegetables. Everyone was also encouraged to exercise for fifteen minutes each day.

After six weeks of lower calorie intake, everyone lost weight. Those who ate the traditional Chinese diet lost 0.8 pounds, while those eating the Western diet lost only half a pound, or 62 percent as much. When

---

* Similarly, it's inaccurate to refer to all less healthy patterns of eating as "Western." There are many traditional North American and Western European food traditions and recipes that are in fact quite healthy. Nonetheless, nutrition researchers have chosen to use the term "Western diet" as shorthand for foods containing less than healthy ingredients prepared using less than healthy methods.

each group's "sense of hunger" was compared before and after each meal, hunger pangs experienced by those on the Chinese diet decreased by 88 percent, while the Western diet resulted in only a 50 percent decrease in hunger. This suggests the Chinese meal was more satiating.

The traditional Chinese dietary pattern of eating also has long-term benefits when it comes to weight loss.[6] The same researchers enrolled 284 adults aged twenty-five to seventy who were overweight or obese and repeated the earlier study using a basic Chinese diet or a Western diet for six weeks. Again, they found more weight was lost with the Chinese diet. But a year later, twice as many people who ate the Chinese diet *maintained* their decrease in body weight. In contrast, 35 percent more people on the Western diet gained back some of their initial weight. This effect had an even longer tail. At five years, more than 25 percent of the subjects who ate the Chinese diet were able to keep their weight off, which was four times more than those on the Western diet.

The benefits and risks of how you eat start early in life. Researchers from China Medical University examined diet and health outcomes from the China Health and Nutrition Survey, which collected data from thirty thousand individuals across fifteen Chinese provinces.[7] They analyzed eating patterns in 489 children ranging in age from six to fourteen and looked at their risk of becoming obese five years later. They compared the effects associated with eating a modern Chinese diet, which includes fast food, red meat, and ultraprocessed foods, versus a traditional Chinese diet. Their analysis showed that those who ate a traditional diet when young had a 71 percent lower risk of developing obesity later in life. In contrast, those eating the modern diet had as high as a threefold *increase* in the risk of becoming obese.

Parallel benefits have been documented with Japanese cuisine. The food of Japan goes far beyond the sushi, maki rolls, and ramen with which you may be familiar. Japanese cuisine is wonderfully diverse, famous for its delicacy and precision, the harmony of its ingredients, and its seasonality. It features an abundance of vegetables and fish and is sparse on meat and dairy products. On the island of Okinawa, where many inhabitants still live a traditional lifestyle and eat traditional foods, the citizens' health is exceptional, as is their longevity.

As in China, the old ways of Japan contrast with the modern ways. Contemporary Japanese diets incorporate many Western elements—namely, less vegetables and fish and more bread, dairy, meat, and oil.[8] Researchers from Tohoku University in Japan showed that the traditional Japanese diet was superior for improving body composition in young adults.[9] They conducted a study of this effect by recruiting thirty-two healthy university students between the ages of twenty and thirty. All the subjects were of normal weight and were assigned to eat either a traditional or a modern Japanese diet three times a day for twenty-eight days.* A menu was prepared by a registered dietician following specifications for a traditional versus a modern Japanese diet. The makeup of the traditional diet featured 14 percent more variety than the modern one. It contained 30 percent more plant-based foods and 43 percent more condiments, including fermented sauces.

The results at one month showed that those eating the traditional Japanese diet lost 2.4 pounds, while those on the modern diet actually *gained* 0.2 pounds. When body composition was analyzed, these losses and gains were all in fat. The traditional diet eaters lost 7 percent body fat, while the modern eaters gained 1 percent more body fat.

These benefits also translated to the subjects' metabolism. Blood tests taken at the beginning and end of the study showed that the traditional eaters had lowered their harmful LDL (low-density) cholesterol and simultaneously increased their beneficial HDL (high-density) cholesterol levels. The pattern was exactly the opposite among those who ate the modern Japanese diet—they had more harmful LDL and lower beneficial HDL.

---

* Specifically, they modeled the diet on the attributes of a diet typical of Japan in 1975, which adhered to traditional cultural values.

To find out if the same benefits are seen in older people who are overweight, the same study was performed on sixty people ranging in age from twenty to seventy.[10] After four weeks, the traditional eaters had lost 2 pounds, while the modern diet eaters gained 1.1 pounds. When it came to body fat, traditional eaters lost 1.7 pounds of fat, which was four times more than the modern eaters lost. The same benefits in blood lipid levels that had been seen in younger nonoverweight people—lower harmful LDL and higher protective HDL—were also seen in the older overweight group.

The older traditional Japanese food eaters had a reduction by two-thirds of inflammation markers in their blood, which had been elevated because of their excess body fat. Those same inflammatory markers *doubled* over the study period in people eating the modern Japanese diet. The traditional eaters had a modest reduction in their waist size, but modern eaters expanded their waist circumference by 0.4 inch. Waist circumference is a convenient measurement of abdominal adiposity, reflecting the amount of harmful visceral fat that has developed in your belly.

Crossing to the other side of the Silk Road, the same kind of evidence shows that eating the traditional diets of Mediterranean countries is beneficial when it comes to body fat. Many of the ingredients in traditional cuisine—tomatoes, onions, garlic, chili peppers, seafood rich in omega-3 fats—turn on brown fat and thermogenesis to improve metabolism and burn down harmful white fat. Not surprisingly, eating patterns that fight fat reduce the risk of developing chronic diseases, including cancer.

An extensive epidemiological study called the European Prospective Investigation into Cancer (EPIC) was designed to find associations between diet and specific cancers.[11] The data collected also included information about body composition, weight, height, waist size, diet, physical activity, and other lifestyle factors of the participants, who live in ten European countries: Denmark, France, Germany,

Greece, Italy, the Netherlands, Norway, Spain, Sweden, and the United Kingdom.

Researchers have examined the EPIC database to analyze the dietary patterns and body composition of 497,308 men and women ranging in age from twenty-five to seventy. To evaluate the food they ate, the researchers used a rating system called the modified Mediterranean Diet Score to assess how closely each subject's eating habits matched a "healthy Mediterranean diet." For every food the subjects ate that corresponded to a healthy Mediterranean ingredient, points were assigned. Then they correlated this score with body measurements. The outcome of the analysis showed that those whose eating patterns had a high Mediterranean Diet Score had a significantly smaller waist circumference, correlating to lower body fat and better metabolic health.

This benefit is further supported by the results of a study that involved 3,042 men and women in Greece. Known as the ATTICA study, it revealed that those whose food consumption adhered most closely to the Mediterranean diet had a 51 percent lower chance of being obese and a 59 percent lower chance of having abdominal obesity, when compared to people whose eating patterns veered away from healthy Mediterranean-based foods.[12]

The Mediterranean diet's effect on weight loss was studied by researchers from the University of Naples in Italy and Harokopio University in Greece. They analyzed sixteen well-designed clinical trials in which the subjects were randomized and there was a comparator diet.[13] The trials lasted anywhere from one month to two years and took place over a span of sixteen years in different locations, including the United States, Greece, Italy, France, Spain, Israel, Germany, and the Netherlands.

A total of 3,436 subjects were included in the researchers' analysis, which showed that eating the Mediterranean diet was associated with a greater weight loss by 3.86 pounds more than any diet to which it was compared, across the sixteen studies. These comparator diets included a low-fat diet; a high-carb diet; the American Diabetes Association diet, or "prudent diet"; and the "usual" diet. The weight loss was greater when the number of daily calories was restricted and when the subjects were more physically active. When they looked at the fat content of Mediterranean food, which is mostly healthy omega-3 polyunsaturated fatty acids and extra virgin olive oil, the researchers found that in no case were these healthy fats commonly present in the Mediterranean diet associated with weight gain in any of the sixteen studies.

Just as was found in studies of traditional Chinese food, the Med-Weight Study in Greece—which involved 565 adults—showed that those who stuck most closely with a traditional Mediterranean diet were twice as likely to be a "maintainer" of their weight loss over one year.[14] The study also found that eating fruit high in dietary fiber can make a difference. For every serving of whole fruit that people consumed per week, there was a 3 percent increase in the odds of maintaining their weight reduction.

Get Started on the MediterAsian Way

How do you start eating the MediterAsian Way to tap into all of its benefits? It's easy! The first step is getting the right type of high-quality ingredients. Your local grocery store will likely stock a decent selection. Even better, hit up a farmers market or, if you are lucky enough to have one nearby, a local village market. Start with the produce section and get to know the fresh foods that are available right now so you can connect your meals with the season. Identify the fat-fighting foods that you already enjoy eating and take note of the ones you see but have yet to explore. Buy a bottle of pure extra virgin olive oil and keep it on your counter for cooking and to use as a condiment. If you can't find the ingredients near where you live, don't worry; almost everything can be ordered online and delivered right to your doorstep.

The MediterAsian Way is not about rigid rules, so I want to emphasize that this is not a formula for creating a medically tailored meal. The approach is flexible and personal. You get to choose what you enjoy. For inspiration, select recipes and ingredients from any of the twenty-one Mediterranean and the forty-seven Asian countries—a total of sixty-eight culinary cultures to choose from, spanning east to west. You could spend several lifetimes exploring the cuisine in these countries. You probably already have favorite recipes that fit into the MediterAsian genre, but if you need ideas, a simple way to match a seasonal ingredient with a recipe is to do an online search. Just type "Recipe" "[Your main ingredient]" and "[Mediterranean or Asian cuisine you are interested in exploring]." When I do this, I look for videos in the search results. When you search this way, you'll be rewarded with a large selection of appetizing dishes from which to choose and videos from enthusiastic home cooks or professional chefs who are excited to show you exactly how to prepare them along with practical cooking tips. You can meal plan this way, and before long, you'll find yourself with your own favorite list of MediterAsian dishes. Later, in Chapter 12, I'll give you several recipes from my own kitchen that will get you started.

This approach is endlessly varied and can be adapted to any palate, but there are some useful basic guidelines to keep in mind. I call these the "Principles of MediterAsian Eating." They will help you use foods that benefit your metabolism and activate your health defenses to your best advantage, all while allowing you to enjoy the pleasure of eating.

Ten Principles for Eating MediterAsian

1. Eat with Intention

Choose your food wisely. Approach each meal as a chance to enjoy something you truly value that is good for your health. You have only so many meals left in your lifetime, so make each one meaningful. Cut down or cut out the foods that harm your health. Eat with the intent to improve your health. Can't find what you need or really want to eat? See the next principle.

2. Skip a Meal (or Two)

If you are busy or you can't find anything healthy you really want to eat, go ahead and miss a meal. Don't worry; you'll still have enough energy in your body from your last meal. Skipping a meal has been shown to activate your health defenses, and because doing so limits the calories you eat and lowers your insulin levels, it will also help you improve your metabolism and burn body fat. This is actually so beneficial for your health, I recommend you consider making it a habit to skip a meal or two each week. Just be careful not to overeat, though, when you sit down at your next meal.

3. Go for Fresh

Fresh foods are the backbone of MediterAsian eating. They contain the bioactive compounds that activate your health and help you fight harmful fat. Avoid the temptation of convenient but ultraprocessed foods that can be associated with weight gain and health loss.[15]

4. Personalize Your Food Choices

It's all about you: your preferences, your tastes, your circumstances, and your health concerns. Choose what you like and what you need based on what is available to you. Have it your way. Don't settle for less. Follow your instincts on what is good for you—and what is not.

5. Respect Tradition

When it comes to MediterAsian eating, respect traditional recipes and methods of preparation. This means buying the right ingredients, preparing them from scratch, and making sure to develop full flavors in your meals. Take advantage of the wisdom of centuries. When it comes to healthy food, newer inventions are rarely better.

6. Eat in Moderation

When there is a bounty of food, such as at a celebration, special event, or buffet, practice restraint and moderation. Eat for enjoyment, but do not overload your body. Portion control is key. Overeating stresses your metabolism, and this has the long-term consequence of impairing your health defenses.[16] Listen to your body. The Japanese saying *Hara hachi bun me*, "Stop eating when you are 80 percent full," is good advice.

7. Drink the Trinity

No MediterAsian meal is complete without a beverage. Three have uncontested health and metabolic benefits that help you fight body fat—water, tea, and coffee. They are the number one, two, and three most-consumed beverages in the world. Drink them before, during, or after a meal, or any time of the day.

8. Eat Together

Eating the MediterAsian Way is convivial. In both Mediterranean and Asian countries, people tend to eat with family or friends. If you have a choice, don't solo a meal. It's better for your health to eat with others—social bonds lower your stress, and you tend to eat more slowly with company. Sharing food helps you better appreciate what's on the plate. If you live alone, invite a friend over. If there is a communal table, join it.

9. Open Your Mind and Explore

Be adventurous when it comes to MediterAsian food. Expand your horizons by trying new foods you do not recognize. Variety helps you become healthier. Open your mind and dare to try something new. Take the opportunity to discover your new favorite healthy dish.

10. Live to Eat

Eating to live is for survival. The MediterAsian Way goes beyond this basic instinct and allows you to be a bon vivant and *live to eat*. Give yourself permission to enjoy the pleasure of food. Feed the hedonic center in your brain. Take great delight in tantalizing your taste buds with great food. Share your enjoyment of food with others.

A Day in My MediterAsian Life

If you follow these basic MediterAsian principles, you will enjoy food the way I do. Rather than narrowing your dietary horizons, the MediterAsian Way expands them.

In the next chapters, I will identify the foods, with evidence for their benefits, that are staples of MediterAsian eating. But first, here's a glimpse of a typical day in my life, showing the choices I make and the ways I think about food. This is how I eat, combining pleasure with health—it's an approach and not a diet.

Breakfast

I keep my breakfast light and quick. I start my mornings with a small cup of strong coffee, usually an espresso. There are many ways to make a great cup—using a French press or an old-fashioned Italian moka pot are my favorites—but the method matters less than using really good beans. I don't add dairy because dairy fat forms soap bubble–like units around the healthy bioactives like chlorogenic acid in coffee and makes them less absorbable in the gut. One Brazilian clinical study showed that adding dairy cuts down chlorogenic acid absorption by 42 percent.[17] Nut milks and soy milk are okay to use because they don't have this effect. To protect my microbiome, I never use artificial flavors or sweeteners in my coffee.

Fresh fruit is a must for my MediterAsian breakfast. This is how I get my fruit bioactives and a good dose of dietary fiber at the beginning of each day. I choose ripe, seasonal fruits from a fruit bowl I keep stocked in the kitchen, like oranges, apples, or pears in the fall and winter; kiwifruit or strawberries in the spring; and figs or peaches in the summer. Blueberries, raspberries, or blackberries are favorites, too. Eating what is in season offers me the brightest flavors and most bioactives. If fresh fruit is not on hand, I will substitute with cut-up frozen fruit or sometimes dried fruit, which are inexpensive and still retain healthy bioactives. I prefer to eat my fruits plain, but they can be added to yogurt with some honey, which is good for the microbiome.[18]

Occasionally, I'll cook a single egg, organic and cage-free if I can find them, usually a quick scramble with a little olive oil. Studies have shown eating an egg a day can raise levels of good HDL cholesterol, lower inflammatory markers, and reduce harmful visceral fat in people with type 2 diabetes.[19] The carotenoid bioactives in the egg yolk are beneficial to your vision and can lower the risk of age-related macular degeneration.[20] I try to buy the highest-quality eggs I can find, and I'm conscious that the hens that lay them should be humanely raised.

I'm also inspired by the light breakfasts I've eaten in Japan and China. Although it may take a little more effort to create, I love a morning bowl of soba noodles in a light vegetable broth. Soba is made with buckwheat, a whole grain that has a low glycemic index and contains the bioactives quercetin and rutin.[21] These have anti-inflammatory, antiangiogenic, antioxidant, and metabolism-activating properties.[22] Another light Chinese breakfast is a bowl of hot congee, a rice porridge cooked with ginger and bone broth and topped with chopped scallions and other savory tidbits.* They both go well with a fried or scrambled egg cooked with extra virgin olive oil and fresh fruit. These options pair

---

* Pickled vegetables are often served with breakfast in Asia. I avoid them because studies have suggested they are associated with a twofold increase in the risk of esophageal cancer, possibly due to fungal contaminants. (Source: F. Islami, J.-S. Ren, et al., "Pickled Vegetables and the Risk of Oesophageal Cancer: A Meta-Analysis," *British Journal of Cancer* 101, no. 9 [2009]: 1641–1647.)

better with a cup of green or oolong tea than coffee. Soy milk is also a good accompaniment.

If my schedule is extremely busy, I may just down a cup of coffee and skip breakfast, knowing this is essentially a way to keep my insulin low, restrict my caloric intake, and boost my metabolism.

Lunch

I do enjoy eating lunch but try to keep the food simple and unfussy. If I have leftovers from dinner, I will heat them up to save time. It also gives me another chance to enjoy a tasty dish from the night before. Sometimes it even tastes better the next day! If I skipped breakfast, I remind myself to practice restraint, so I don't overeat at lunch.

If I'm preparing lunch, I choose one or two healthy ingredients to build the meal around. I make sure one of them is a plant-based ingredient, whether it's a legume or a leafy vegetable. I don't usually spend much time cooking lunch, but I enjoy a salad, and olive oil with lemon or balsamic or apple cider vinegar makes a tasty dressing. Add some protein to this, and it's a quick and healthy lunch. A soup or stew is a convenient and warming meal that I can make beforehand and just heat up. These can provide several meals. This is *my* definition of fast food.

Lunch is also the perfect time to add seafood to my diet. I will sometimes open a tin of fish packed in olive oil and eat it with some condiments like a pickle, or capers, or kimchi along with a small slice of sourdough or whole-grain bread or brown rice. I avoid creamy foods and pastas for lunch, as they are too rich and heavy. I know they also would spike my insulin levels, which is not good for metabolic health.

If I go toward an Asian-style lunch, it might be a composed lunch. The Japanese bento box is perfect for this: it is a to-go container with small amounts of balanced food choices placed into their own neat compartments. It's a great way to enjoy a modest and healthy variety of food. For a free-form approach, a container of steamed brown rice with a sautéed vegetable and a small amount of fish or chicken is another option.

For lunch, I eat small portions. If I am at a restaurant, I look for the healthiest items and choose the one that is exactly what I want to eat that day, making sure it has healthy ingredients. If it is a large portion, I shamelessly do not finish it all. Sometimes I will only order an appetizer as my lunch. When I am out with friends or colleagues, we may order different dishes and share.

If I'm on the go or can't find something flavorful and healthy, I will sometimes skip lunch (but I never skip both breakfast and lunch on the same day). This is a conscious choice. This is part of the basic practice of intermittent fasting, and I know that it's beneficial to my health defenses and metabolism. We'll explore intermittent fasting in detail in Chapter 11.

Dinner

I typically make dinner the focal point of my day. This is where I like to put everything all together in one meal: fresh ingredients, flavor, texture, and aroma. I'll decide which type of cuisine from the MediterAsian choices I feel most like eating and prepare (or order) that meal. It is an opportunity to select just the right combination of items so that the overall result is more than the sum of its individual parts but also not overly complicated. Here's how I do it:

I design my dinner starting with the plant-based food that will be the star of the meal. It could be a fresh green vegetable like bok choy, radicchio, or asparagus. Or it could be a legume like lentils or navy beans, or a mushroom, or a taproot like carrots or beets. In the summer, it could be fresh tomatoes. Next, I come up with a recipe that will make it tasty and have other metabolism- and health defense–activating ingredients, such as garlic, onions, ginger, shallots, extra virgin olive oil, or herbs or other seasonings. I might then build a meal around a vegetable stir-fry, a beet salad, roasted carrots, sautéed mushrooms, a lentil or bean stew, sliced fresh tomatoes, or maybe a flavorful *sugo* (tomato sauce). I go with what's available in the market and what inspires me when I see the produce display at the grocery store.

If I am dining at a restaurant, I will scan the menu using the same basic approach. What is the tasty vegetable that I would like to eat that evening? It may be listed as an ingredient in an appetizer, it may be a component of an entrée, or it could be a side dish. This is my starting point, and in my mind, I regard it as the star of the meal.

Next, I think of the foods that could pair well with the vegetable dish. It could be fish, shellfish, or other seafood on the menu. It could be poultry, like chicken or duck. It could also be rice or pasta. I want it to be flavorful and to complement the vegetable I choose.

If I'm dining with others, I might ask my dining partners if they would be game to order multiple dishes off the menu that can be shared. This allows everyone to taste and sample different flavors and preparations and enjoy variety while we serve ourselves smaller portions.

If it's an Asian-style meal, there is a cultural sensibility for ordering dishes for the table. There should be varied ingredients using different cooking techniques, like steamed, sautéed, baked, and roasted. As tasty as they might be, I steer away from deep-fried foods and red meats. Ordering one dish per person is typically the right amount and diversity of food for everyone to share. Sample the dishes, and don't feel like you have to eat everything that's on the table. If I am cooking and hosting dinner at home, I try to do the same thing and make one type of dish per person to be served family style.

I practice restraint and moderation at dinner. Whether I'm eating at home, dining at a restaurant, or attending a dinner as a guest in someone's home, I remind myself *not to overeat*. If there are multiple offerings on the table, I will quickly eye the items containing the healthiest ingredients and take a (modest) serving of those foods first. I eat slowly, so my brain will have time to turn down my appetite as food enters my body. I pay attention to how my body is feeling as I eat so that I can stop eating *before* I am full. Even if the food is amazing, I do not go back for a second helping of food, no matter how delicious it tasted.

I try to make dinner a delight for my senses. Researchers have shown that eating for pleasure is not only more fun, it is also associated with a higher quality of diet, healthier food choices, more restrained portions, and, importantly, an improved sense of well-being.[23]

After Dinner

I wind down my evening with a cup of tea. Green tea is my go-to and very calming. The caffeine does not bother me, but if it did, I would choose a decaffeinated version, with the caffeine removed using the "water process," which preserves the bioactives. I will sometimes instead sip pu'er tea as a probiotic drink. I often use loose-leaf tea to brew my cup, but tea bags are convenient to dunk. Dunking helps more of the tea's catechins seep into the beverage.

The ideal temperature for brewing tea is 180 degrees Fahrenheit (82 degrees Celsius). But you should allow the tea to cool a bit, so it's not scalding when you drink it. Sipping scalding-hot water injures the cells of your esophagus. A study by the Tehran University of Medical Sciences involving more than fifty thousand individuals showed that drinking scalding-hot tea is associated with a 90 percent increased risk for esophageal cancer.[24] The hot liquid damages the cell lining of the esophagus, and repetitive injury like this can cause malignant cells to develop. It's the temperature, not the tea. Researchers from the Guangzhou University of Chinese Medicine examined twenty clinical studies and concluded that green tea, when consumed at nonscalding temperatures, has an overall 35 percent *protective* effect against esophageal cancer.[25]

I sometimes have a tiny cup of espresso after dinner. It's a habit I picked up when I lived in Italy—and, strangely enough, I've never had insomnia from the hit of caffeine. In Italy, it is believed that drinking an espresso after dinner aids your digestion.

*   *   *

The MediterAsian Way allows you to enjoy a broad range of foods with different cultural origins, a modern version of the experience Silk Road traders had more than two thousand years ago.*

Like any journey, this one can seem daunting when you are first getting started. With so many ingredients, which ones do you choose, and how do you select the best versions? With so many different cuisines, where do you even begin with recipes and meal plans?

Don't worry. I have a strategy to help you get started. Come with me to the first stop on your journey: the supermarket.

---

* According to archaeobotanist Robert N. Spengler III of the Max Planck Institute for the Science of Human History, there was evidence of East-West food exchange going back even earlier, four thousand years, before the Silk Road; specifically, Chinese and Kazakhstan food intermingled as long ago as 2200 BCE, in a settlement in the Dzungar Mountains. (Source: Robert Spengler, *Fruit from the Sands: The Silk Road Origins of the Foods We Eat* [Oakland: University of California Press, 2019].)

CHAPTER 6

The Fresh Market

Healthy eating begins with smart shopping—and pleasurable eating also begins with smart shopping. I particularly enjoy picking out produce at a farmers market or a village market. I like to arrive early, before the crowd builds, and watch the vendors set up for the day. I hear the *beep, beep, beep* of trucks backing up to empty wooden stalls and see the farmers unloading their freshest goods of the season. They carefully set down the crates full of fruits and vegetables they've grown and proudly organize them to look beautiful on display.

Once the stands are set up, the throngs of shoppers start strolling in. It's a privilege to buy produce from vendors who have a direct connection to the goods they sell. If you have access to a local market like this, I strongly encourage you to make use of it. But even the most basic grocery store is a marvel when you think about it: items from around the world, brought to you by truck, train, plane, and ship, laid out for you to pick and choose.

Whether you shop at a farmers market or a supermarket, produce is probably the first food you will see. Sellers know what makes a dramatic first impression, after all. And while you revel in the colors, shapes, and diversity of the fruits and vegetables, I'm going to show you the biochemical beauty hidden within and help you spot the most beneficial items for your health. In this chapter, I will focus on foods with clinical studies that have shown their benefits on body composition and metabolism.

Overwhelming scientific evidence shows that eating fruits, vegetables, legumes, root vegetables, and mushrooms as whole foods provides crucial resources that help the body defend itself against disease. Mother Nature loaded plants with the bioactives that give them their color and flavor. These bioactives serve to protect the plant. Some attract pollinators to help the plants reproduce so their species has a future. Others are natural pest repellents that keep insects from eating their leaves and stems. There is a misconception that these repellents are "antinutrients." Quite the opposite: many of the bioactives that keep bugs away are also the ones that activate your health defenses and metabolism.

When humans came along and began consuming plant-based foods, these same plant bioactives took on another job: to interact with your cells in ways that protect your health—including fighting body fat and improving your metabolism.

By choosing the right produce to eat using the MediterAsian approach, you can counteract excess body fat in multiple ways. Some foods in the produce section contain bioactives that reduce harmful visceral fat, while others cause browning of white fat. Yet others trigger thermogenesis that improves metabolism. Certain produce can counter the harmful consequences of obesity by lowering inflammation or by increasing insulin sensitivity (which reduces the odds of diabetes) and lowering leptin resistance (which makes you less likely to overeat). Foods in the produce section also can reduce the disease risks associated with excess body fat, such as metabolic syndrome, cardiovascular disease, and cancer. Some foods do all of these things in one fell swoop.

As your guide through the produce market, I've chosen specific foods to highlight. I'll single out foods that have been studied for their ability to cause weight loss, reduce waist circumference, and improve metabolism—where the fat-fighting bioactives they contain are known, and where the data clearly demonstrate they have health benefits. Some items, like herbs, contain useful bioactives, but it is not practical to eat them in large quantities. I've also selected foods that are used in Mediterranean or Asian cuisine that fit the MediterAsian theme.

The foods I'm about to describe are not *like* medicine; they *are* medicine—natural "farm-aceuticals"—so I am going to talk about them that way. I will describe the scientific and clinical evidence supporting their benefits, along with the associated "food dose" from the research study. I first introduced the concept of food doses in *Eat to Beat Disease*. This is the amount and frequency of a food needed to achieve a desired outcome, based on clinical research. Just as prescription medicines have a dose, so, too, do foods that improve your metabolism.

You are going to appreciate some familiar foods in an entirely new way based on their ability to fight body fat, as shown in human studies. But there is an important caveat: I am not giving you this information intending that you eat every food I describe, every day, and I don't want you to become obsessed with any single food as "the solution." At the end of this chapter, I'll provide a summary of the food doses from each study, but you should not limit yourself to those amounts—they are for reference purposes only.

Eating to beat your diet recognizes that your body is designed to favor diversity and that everyone has different tastes and preferences. Pick the foods you like, mix and match them, and try new ingredients or use the old standbys in new ways. Food as medicine is wonderful because of its vast flexibility. The more variety, the better it is for your metabolism. A study of 7,370 men and women in the US National Health and Nutrition Examination Survey program found that people who ate more diverse foods had a whopping 50 percent lower chance of becoming obese.[1]

More good news is that the quantities of fruits, vegetables, herbs, and spices you need to eat to get meaningful health benefits are not ridiculous. The food doses are easily achievable. Keep in mind that the first principle in fighting fat is to eat in moderation. Don't put it all in your shopping cart (or your belly) at one time. Focus on quality over quantity or frequency. For the produce section, do your best to select foods that are in season. Better to have ripe strawberries in summer and juicy pears in the fall than think you need to have strawberries or a pear every day of the year.

In this chapter, we are going to first explore the fruit section, often the first products you see in the grocery store, before checking on the vegetables such as brassica, Asian greens, and beans. Then we will look at carrots, mushrooms, onions, garlic, and chili peppers. Sound familiar? What I'm about to tell you about these common produce items will give you new insights into everday foods that can help your metabolism.

Fruits

I need to address a common misconception up front: that one should avoid eating fruits because of their natural sugar content. On the contrary, eating modest amounts of fruit actually decreases weight gain and combats obesity.[2] Fruit fiber feeds the gut microbiome, helping this health defense to improve your blood glucose utilization and overall metabolism—and also lower triglycerides and total cholesterol. As you are about to learn, the bioactives present in fruit have their individual actions on adipose tissues, impeding the development of harmful fat or activating thermogenesis to burn it down. Fruit also promotes satiety, so you do not feel ravenous throughout the day.

Apple

An apple a day might keep the doctor away, but three apples a day can help reduce body fat. I love apples for their sweet and tart flavor. They are versatile, great for salads or as a snack, baked in a dessert, and even cooked in a main dish (try adding some chopped apple to a curry dish). To me, apples evoke the crisp air and fiery colors of autumn.

You may be surprised to learn apples did not originate in North America or Europe but in the forests of the Tian Shan mountains in Central Asia, alongside the Silk Road. Packed on caravans and planted along the trail, the apple made its way to the Mediterranean and the rest of the world.

One of the bioactives in apples is chlorogenic acid, which I discussed in Chapter 4. Chlorogenic acid increases your metabolism and causes white fat to transform into useful brown fat for thermogenesis and fat burning. Apples also contain a hefty amount (4–5 grams) of dietary fiber that feeds the gut microbiome. As one of your health defenses, a well-tended gut microbiome produces short-chain fatty acids that can lower inflammation caused by excess body fat. The metabolic benefits don't end there. The short-chain fatty acids made by healthy gut bacteria also improve the body's insulin response and lipid metabolism.[3]

The metabolic benefits of apples have been studied by researchers from the State University of Rio de Janeiro.[4] They recruited forty-nine Brazilian women aged thirty to fifty who were overweight and gave half the subjects a snack consisting of three apples a day. The other half were given calorie-matched oat cookies instead. All the subjects were weighed at the beginning and end of the study. At the end of twelve weeks, the apple eaters had lost 2.7 pounds, compared to the cookie eaters, who consumed the same number of calories. The apple's ability to help weight loss was confirmed in three large clinical studies involving a total of 133,468 people in the United States.[*] From a meta-analysis of the results of these studies, apple eating lowered body weight by 1.24 pounds per daily serving.[5]

Even dried apples are efficacious for weight loss. Researchers from Florida State University gave 160 postmenopausal women two dried

---

[*] The three studies were the Health Professionals Follow-Up Study, Nurses' Health Study, and Nurses' Health Study II.

apples to eat every day for one year. The resulting weight loss over that time was 3.3 pounds.[6] The apple's benefits were also detectable by blood tests. Apple eaters had lower total cholesterol levels in their blood, and the decreases were seen as early as three months after the women began eating the dried fruit.

Those weight-loss numbers might seem incremental but remember that small metabolic changes can have big health impacts. Recall that losing a mere two pounds can lower the risk of heart failure by 3 percent and the risk of stroke by 5 percent. Every improvement counts, and the benefits add up.

Eating an apple along with its peel is beneficial, because the peel contains ursolic acid, a bioactive that lowers fat-associated inflammation. Ursolic acid increases your body's production of adiponectin, the hormone that aids metabolism by making cells more sensitive to insulin, which makes your metabolism more efficient. Ursolic acid also activates your health defenses—it protects your circulation, stimulates regeneration, improves gut health, and can starve tumors by cutting off their blood supply (antiangiogenesis) while it kills cancer stem cells.[7] Fruit skin can be quite powerful.

The topic of fruit peel inevitably raises the question of whether you should choose organically grown fruits. The short answer is yes. It is very difficult to scrub away pesticide residue on the surface of any fruit. In one study by scientists at the University of Massachusetts in Amherst, researchers exposed whole apples to commercially used pesticides for just twenty-four hours.[8] They found that the standard postharvest washing of fruit—using bleach for two minutes—was ineffective for removing the pesticide. In fact, it took up to fifteen minutes of soaking the apples in a sodium bicarbonate (baking soda) solution to completely remove pesticides from just the surface of apples. Even this was insufficient. When the researchers examined the fruit skin itself, they discovered 20 percent of the pesticide had soaked so deeply into the apple peel that it could not be washed away at all.

The benefit of choosing organically grown produce is not just "less bad" chemical residue. Organic fruits also contain *more* beneficial polyphenols—the very bioactives that boost your health defenses and metabolism—than conventionally grown ones.[9] One study showed the difference was 10 percent more.

Apples activate your angiogenesis and immune defenses.[10] Both are useful for cancer prevention. The evidence was seen in the Nurses' Health Study and the Health Professionals Follow-Up Study, two large real-world studies of diet and health. In these studies, researchers examined 125,061 people's fruit and vegetable consumption and analyzed their risk of various cancers. The results showed that those who increased their apple intake by one serving per day had a 37 percent decrease in the risk of developing lung cancer.[11]

Which apples are the most potent? More than seventy-five hundred varieties of apples exist in the world, but there are three varietals that have been shown to have the highest levels of polyphenols: Granny Smith, Red Delicious, and Reinette.[12] These are the ones I look for when I go apple shopping (or picking).*

Pear

The Tian Shan mountains were also the ancestral home to pears. I enjoy ripe pears, slicing them into a salad, incorporating them into entrées, and enjoying them as part of a healthy dessert. They are an excellent source of dietary fiber (a medium-sized fruit has 6 grams) for gut health and supporting immunity. Like their genetic relative the apple, pears are a significant source of chlorogenic acid.

Pears can shrink your waistline. Researchers at Florida State University studied the effects of eating pears in forty men and women aged forty-five to sixty-five. They all had metabolic syndrome, which is a

---

* Reinette is a medieval varietal from Europe, and it is commonly found in European markets.

prediabetic condition characterized by the "4 H's": high blood pressure, high blood sugar, high blood cholesterol, and high amounts of body fat.[13] In the study, half the subjects were given two pears (Bartlett or Anjou cultivars) to eat each day.* The other half received a calorie-matched placebo drink to consume. Everyone maintained their normal diet and physical activity.

After twelve weeks, the pear eaters had a two-inch reduction in their waist circumference and an eight-point beneficial drop in their systolic blood pressure (the top number in your blood pressure reading). Pear eaters lost 1.32 pounds. By contrast, the placebo group *gained* a little more than half a pound. A blood test showed that eating pears lowered blood levels of leptin by 5 percent. Recall that leptin is produced by adipocytes (fat cells), so the more fat the body has, the more leptin is produced. A reduction in fat cell mass leads to less leptin, which helps to control your appetite.

Of the three thousand types of pears in existence, the ones you are most likely to find in your market are Anjou, Bartlett, Bosc, Comice, and Seckel. Fall and winter are their seasons, so look for the best fruit in these months. Pro tip: to find a ripe pear, hold the fruit by its base with one hand, and with the other, pinch the flesh at the bottom of the stem. If the flesh gives slightly, the pear is ready to eat.

Grapefruit

This popular breakfast fruit was named after the clusters it forms on its tree, which resemble a bunch of enormous grapes. It is a relatively new fruit, created only in the seventeenth century in the Caribbean West Indies as a hybrid of the pomelo, a citrus fruit from Southeast Asia, and the Jamaican sweet orange. Grapefruits are known for their bittersweet juice, which has a tartness between that of an orange and a lemon.

---

* The Bartlett pear was named by Massachusetts native Enoch Bartlett (after himself), not realizing that it was previously known in Europe as the Williams pear. A famous fruit brandy called Poire Williams is made from Williams pears.

Grapefruit flesh contains many bioactives, including the fat-fighting flavonoids hesperidin and naringenin, as well as vitamin C, which is a powerful DNA-protecting antioxidant and anti-inflammatory substance.[14] Pink grapefruit also contains the bioactive lycopene, which gives the fruit its reddish color and has potent antiadipose benefits. It is also a good source of dietary fiber that supports the microbiome.[15] Together, grapefruit bioactives have antiadipose and health defense–activating benefits.[16]

Eating grapefruit (without sprinkling sugar on top!) can promote weight loss. Researchers from the Scripps Clinic in California tested the grapefruit effect by recruiting seventy-seven individuals who were obese, whom they divided into four groups. The groups received one of the following: half of a fresh grapefruit to eat three times each day, eight ounces of grapefruit juice to drink, a dietary supplement made with freeze-dried Florida-grown grapefruit including the peel, or a placebo pill with no grapefruit content whatsoever.[17]

All the participants were asked to walk for thirty minutes three to four times each week to stimulate weight loss during the study. After three months, body measurements showed that grapefruit-half eaters lost 3.5 pounds. Those who consumed the other grapefruit products (juice and supplement) also lost some weight, but whole-fruit eaters lost the most. Bottom line: the whole grapefruit delivers more benefits than juice or a supplement.

Blueberries

Small, plump, and delightfully sweet, blueberries have several aliases. In parts of North America, they are known as wild huckleberries or whortleberries. In Europe, they are called bilberries. These berries are in season during the summer, although as with many fruits, international growers and transportation make them available in the grocery store year-round. I often eat a handful of plain blueberries for breakfast. They are lovely to add to yogurt, salads, muffins, or pie.

The blue color of blueberries comes from bioactives called anthocyanin and proanthocyanidin. These compounds improve your metabolism by helping your body respond to insulin. They are also anti-inflammatory. In addition, blueberries have the bioactive quercetin, which transforms white fat into useful brown fat. Blueberries also boost your immune defenses.[18]

Can eating blueberries help fight body fat? This question was answered by researchers from Bursa Uludağ University in Turkey.[19] They enrolled fifty-four adults who were overweight or obese into a twelve-week weight management program. During the first six weeks, they had everyone reduce their daily calorie intake to lose one-half to one pound per week. After six weeks of caloric restriction and exercise, half of the group were given one-quarter cup of frozen organic blueberries to add to their diet every day. They ate the blueberries for the next six weeks. The other half of the group were given a calorie-matched placebo to eat.

At week twelve, everyone was weighed. The blueberry eaters lost a substantial eight pounds, on average. This was 21 percent more than the subjects who ate the placebo. The researchers found that eating blueberries also resulted in a 5 percent greater reduction in body fat, as well as better insulin sensitivity and overall metabolism, compared to the placebo group.

Blueberries can also influence where fat is distributed in your body. When the diets of 2,734 female twins, eighteen to eighty-three, were examined by researchers at the University of East Anglia and King's College London, a clear link was observed between how much polyphenol was in their diet and body fat distribution. Researchers found that people who ate more foods containing anthocyanin and proanthocyanidin had less central fat, the harmful visceral fat packed inside the belly.[20]

Shopping tip: look for plump, dark-colored blueberries with a silvery surface. Avoid berries that are green, which are unripe, or mushy ones that are damaged. Lemon adds a delicious complementary flavor to

---

Other Berries with Anthocyanins

Dark blue, almost black colors are the telltale sign of anthocyanins in a berry. Blackberries, black raspberries, black currents, and açai berries all have this bioactive. So do some red-colored berries, such as strawberries and red raspberries, lingonberries, and cherries. The chokeberry, also known as aronia, is chock-full of anthocyanins. These berries can be found fresh in the market but are very tart, so they are not often eaten plain. Aronia berries also come frozen or powdered. Try them in a smoothie or baked into muffins or bread.

---

blueberries. Try zesting a lemon on a bowl of berries for a simple, mouthwatering treat.

Strawberries

Strawberries are one of my favorite fruits. When I was a kid, their bright-red color, pleasing shape and aroma, and sweet-more-than-tart juicy taste reminded me of candy. Not all strawberries are equal, however, when it comes to their taste or health benefits. Woodland strawberries, called *fraises des bois* ("from the woods") can be found in European summer markets. Small and ragged looking, these are highly aromatic and sweet; in an open-air market you can smell them long before you see them on display. On the other end of the spectrum, many commercially cultivated strawberries have been bred for appearance—large, uniformly shaped, and brightly colored—but often, disappointingly lacking in flavor. Between these extremes are berries that look and taste delicious, including hydroponically grown berries. A simple test to find great strawberries is simply to smell them. They *must* be fragrant.

Most of the bioactives in strawberries are found in the tiny seeds (called achenes) that dot the strawberry skin.[21] Each seed contains ellagic acid and vitamin C, which activate your health defenses and combat body fat.[22] Ellagic acid triggers the browning of white fat and causes brown fat to make more uncoupling protein 1 (UPC1) for igniting thermogenesis and increasing metabolism.[23] Similar to vitamin C, ellagic acid is anti-inflammatory and counters the inflammation incited by excess fat.[24] In the lab, freeze-dried strawberry powder slowed the growth of adipose cells and lowered inflammatory markers associated with fat.[25]

When it comes to potency, organic strawberries have substantially more ellagic acid than conventionally grown berries. This was shown in a landmark study from Texas A&M University in which researchers compared the ellagic acid levels of organic strawberries with that found in conventional berries. Ellagic acid is produced by the strawberry plant as a natural wound-healing response when its leaves or stem are injured by insects nibbling on them. It is a natural insecticide that helps the strawberry plant repel pests.[26]

The Texas A&M researchers replicated leaf-chewing injury by creating holes in the leaves. They found this produced four times as much ellagic acid than is produced when there was no leaf injury (no pests).[27] Because conventional strawberry plants are sprayed with pesticides to repel pests, their berries contain less ellagic acid. I had been skeptical about the true superior health value of organic foods, but this discovery changed my thinking completely. The claim was typically grounded on organic food containing fewer chemical pesticides. The strawberry study led me to realize that, as a general rule, organic fruits contain both higher levels of bioactives and no pesticides—more good stuff *and* less bad stuff—which makes them a clear winner when it comes to health.

Eating strawberries is associated with weight loss. A study led by the Harvard School of Public Health and the Tufts University Friedman School of Nutrition in Boston examined the intake of plant-based foods, including strawberries, in a group of 133,468 healthy men and women.[28] Researchers found that eating the equivalent of one cup of strawberries per day was associated with a 1.5 pound weight loss over four years.

Strawberries also protect against the threats that can occur from having too much fat: metabolic syndrome, inflammation, and insulin resistance. Eating strawberries can improve the body's sensitivity to insulin, thus improving metabolism.[29] Researchers at the University of Nevada and Oklahoma State University enrolled thirty-three men and women who were obese and gave them a controlled diet plus either a powdered strawberry mix (equivalent to two and a half cups of strawberries) each day or a placebo powder that was strawberry-flavored. The powder was mixed into water and consumed outside of a meal, so any strawberry effect would not be diluted by other foods. Blood samples were taken at the beginning and the end of the four-week study.

The real-strawberry eaters had a beneficial 40 percent decrease in their blood insulin levels. But there was no change in their blood glucose levels, which means eating the natural sugar in strawberries did not elevate their blood sugar. The decline in insulin was due to strawberries' lowering their insulin resistance—when their body responded more normally to insulin, less insulin was needed, so its level went down. The placebo eaters had no changes in their insulin levels.

The researchers noted a particularly interesting finding from the blood tests: strawberry eaters had lower amounts of a protein called plasminogen activator inhibitor-1 (PAI-1). This protein is made by fat cells and aids their growth. The PAI-1 protein also causes inflammation within fat.[30] The strawberry eaters had a 23 percent drop in PAI-1 levels, which reflects the berry's fat-busting power. Another berry benefit was seen through improved blood lipid levels. Strawberry eaters lowered their total blood cholesterol by about 5 percent, likely due to the fruit fiber that fed their healthy gut bacteria.[31]

Lab studies also show that the ellagic acid in strawberries can help activate your angiogenesis defenses to starve cancer and prevent liver cirrhosis.[32] In the gut, ellagic acid is metabolized by healthy gut bacteria to generate a chemical called urolithin A, which protects the gut against inflammation.[33] Ellagic acid also reduces blood markers of inflammation sparked by osteoarthritis in obese adults.[34]

I love eating ripe strawberries on their own, but they are also delicious sliced into a salad. Adding some good-quality balsamic vinegar to strawberries will intensify their flavor. Another great pairing combines strawberries with the herb basil to create a sophisticated taste. Of course, you can use strawberries to make a smoothie, alone or combined with other fruits like banana, kiwifruit, or mango, or even in a green smoothie made with spinach or kale.

Watermelon

If there is one fruit that embodies the summer, it is the watermelon. With ancestral roots harking back five thousand years ago to Northern Africa, the watermelon was once used as a natural canteen for hydration—its juicy flesh is 92 percent water surrounded by a thick, protective rind. Watermelon flesh was originally yellow and bitter, not red and sweet like it is today. Farmers cultivated it to perfection by breeding genes for color and sweetness as the melon migrated from Africa across the Mediterranean and to India and China.

Watermelon's red flesh (called the pepo) contains lycopene, the same bioactive responsible for the hue of tomatoes. Lycopene is an antiadipose powerhouse. It causes white fat to become brown fat and triggers thermogenesis to increase metabolism. Lycopene is also antiangiogenic and can starve fat as well as tumors. It also protects DNA from damage by ultraviolet radiation.

In addition, watermelon is loaded with vitamin C and vitamin A, both of which are anti-inflammatory and beneficial for your circulation.[35] Both the pepo and the rind contain the amino acids L-citrulline and arginine that help the body produce nitric oxide. Nitric oxide (NO) is a chemical signal that dilates your blood vessels and lowers your blood pressure. In addition, NO activates your body's regeneration defenses to call in stem cells that repair and heal your organs.[36] As a metabolic fringe benefit, NO turns on thermogenesis in brown fat cells.[37]

Eating watermelon can aid weight loss. Researchers from San Diego State University recruited thirty-three men and women who were overweight and obese and gave everyone two cups of fresh-diced watermelon to add to their usual diet every day for four weeks.[38] Then, after a two-week gap, the same subjects were given a calorie-matched processed food snack (92-kcal low-fat cookie) for another four weeks to compare the effects.

At four weeks, the watermelon eaters lost 1.1 pounds, and their waist-to-hip ratios (think belly circumference to hip measurement) shrank. Eating the watermelon kept the subjects feeling full for two hours, which also helped to decrease their daily calorie intake. In contrast, those who ate cookies dampened their appetite for only twenty minutes before they felt hungry and were ready to eat again. Not surprisingly, cookie eaters gained 1.3 pounds, and their waistlines expanded. When their blood was analyzed, the watermelon eaters also had lowered triglycerides and harmful LDL cholesterol levels, while their protective HDL cholesterol levels increased.

Serving watermelon slices is a wonderful way to end a summer meal, but don't be afraid to use watermelon in a salad, a smoothie, or a gazpacho. If you're feeling adventurous, you can even pickle the rind, prepare it as a chutney, or cook it into a curry.

Avocado

The name "avocado" comes from the Aztec *ahuacatl*, meaning "testicle." Avocados are pitted fruits that grow on trees dangling in pairs. Their skin is thick with a pebbly texture and can range in color from green to purplish-brown. I love the light green color of avocado flesh and its soft, creamy texture and mild flavor. The avocado is not a classic Mediter-Asian food—it originated from Mexico and Central America—but these fruits are delicious fat fighters that are now available in the global market, including Italy, China, and Japan.

Avocados contain an array of fat-fighting bioactives including chlorogenic acid and proanthocyanidin, just like apples and blueberries, as well as carotenoids like lutein and zeaxanthin, all of which can counter the growth of adipose tissue by stimulating thermogenesis and burning down harmful fat.[39]

Eating avocados can slim your belly. Researchers at the University of Illinois in Urbana recruited 105 adults aged twenty-five to forty-five who were overweight or obese.[40] Half of the subjects were given one avocado to eat every day for twelve weeks. The other half received a calorie-matched food. Their body composition was measured using a DEXA scan to determine the amount of fat in different parts of their bodies. The results showed that women (but not men) who ate avocados reduced their abdominal visceral fat by 5 percent.

The fats in avocados are healthy monounsaturated fatty acids, which can reduce blood levels of bad LDL cholesterol and lower your risk of heart disease.[41] They are also rich in dietary fiber (a whole avocado contains 10 grams of fiber, half of the recommended daily intake for women and 25 percent of that recommended for men). This means avocados are prebiotic foods that nourish your microbiome to foster gut health. Avocados are satiating; their fiber makes you feel fuller and less hungry later.

A unique bioactive in avocados, called avocatin B, has been shown in the lab to fight diet-induced obesity.[42] Researchers found that AvoB improved insulin sensitivity in mice fed a high-fat diet, and it also slowed the speed of their weight gain. Initial human studies of AvoB as a potential drug showed that it was safe and well tolerated with evidence for weight loss.

Tomato

The tomato is a core ingredient of MediterAsian eating and a personal favorite of mine. Summer is tomato season, and many varieties are found in the market. While they are considered culinary vegetables, botanically, they are fruits. There are urban legends suggesting that tomatoes are toxic, but I want to dispel that myth right here.

Originating in South America, tomatoes have been used in cooking for at least two thousand years. In the Aztec language Nahuatl, they were called *tomatl*, meaning "swollen fruit." Spanish conquistador Hernán Cortés encountered the tomato in his journeys and introduced it to Europe in the early 1500s, where it became established in Spanish and Italian society. The early tomatoes that reached the Mediterranean were yellow-orange, however, not red. This color, together with their round shape, led to the name *pomme d'oro* (pomodoro); literally, "golden apple."

So where did the myth of toxic tomatoes come from?

In the sixteenth century, tomatoes were initially available only to wealthy European families. The myth of toxic tomatoes started when the fruits were displayed by these families on pewter trays made of tin and lead. The acid from the tomatoes leached the lead from the trays, which was then absorbed into their fruity flesh. Those who ate the tomatoes then suffered lead poisoning. Unaware at the time that lead was the cause, the people mistakenly identified tomatoes as the culprit. As a result, the upper class shunned tomatoes, and they were instead given to peasants, who did not own leaded trays. The peasants did not suffer any toxicity. Hence, the use of tomatoes in traditional cooking often originated in rural recipes.

The myth of tomato toxicity is amplified by its botanical classification. Tomatoes are part of the Solanacae, or nightshade, family, which includes more than two thousand different plant species. Some of these species are indeed poisonous, like the deadly *Atropa belladonna* nightshade and the mandrake root, but both plants also have been used in medicine. One of their so-called toxins is called atropine, a chemical that cardiologists use to treat a slow heart rate. It's also used by ophthalmologists to dilate the pupil, and by military medics to treat nerve gas poisoning. Another use is the drug scopolamine, which is used to treat seasickness.*

Tomatoes do not contain toxins. Abundant clinical data and eons of human experience have *proven* that tomatoes are safe to eat. So are other Solanacae foods, like eggplants, potatoes, bell peppers, and chili peppers. So long, urban legend.

Although tomatoes originated in the Americas and then traveled to the Mediterranean, they also made their way to Southeast Asia via Spanish colonialism through the Philippines and eventually to China. You might not associate tomatoes with Asian cuisine, but in China tomatoes are scrambled with eggs, stir-fried with beef, and added to soup, especially in home cooking.

Tomatoes contain numerous bioactives, including lycopene, chlorogenic acid, and quercetin. Among these, lycopene has been most studied. Lycopene activates thermogenesis in brown fat and staves off the creation of new fat cells. It is also anti-inflammatory and can starve cancer and fat by reducing their blood supply.[43] Cooking tomatoes makes it easier for your body to absorb lycopene into your bloodstream.**

Eating tomatoes has even been shown to reduce body fat in people who are of healthy weight. This was studied by researchers from the University of Porto in Portugal who gave thirty-five young women, university students between eighteen and twenty-five, one ripe raw tomato to eat before lunch each day for thirty days.[44] Their body composition was measured, and blood samples were drawn at the beginning, middle, and end of the study.

The measurements showed that eating a pre-lunch tomato decreased body weight by 2.4 pounds after one month, with changes seen as early as two weeks. When fat mass was measured, the tomato eaters had a

---

* Both atropine and scopolamine are on the World Health Organization's Model Lists of Essential Medicines.
** The chemical form of lycopene, called trans-lycopene, is found in tomatoes picked off the vine. This form is harder for the body to absorb. Cooking tomatoes converts the trans-lycopene into a form called cis-lycopene, which is readily absorbed by the body. Tomato sauce is cooked, and eating it generates higher blood levels of this bioactive.

decrease of 1.5 percent. All of the weight loss came from body fat, with no loss of muscle or bone mass. Eating tomatoes also decreased blood cholesterol by 7.7 percent, and there was a 7 percent decline in blood triglycerides. Fasting blood glucose, an indicator of metabolism, improved after eating tomatoes. Taken together, these beneficial effects are remarkable because they occurred in women who were not over-weight or obese—and resulted from eating only one tomato before lunch, without any other change in diet or activity.

I am interested in food doses, and the positive results in one form of food translates into other forms of the product. The amount of lycopene in the tomatoes the women ate was analyzed. Each pre-lunch tomato contained 10.7 milligrams of lycopene per 100 grams of tomato. Trans-lating this into other tomato products, the same amount of lycopene can be found in tomato paste (one heaping tablespoon), tomato sauce or soup (three-quarters of a cup), or tomato powder (one and a half table-spoons)—these are very reasonable amounts that anyone can consume.

Why are tomatoes so effective? One reason could be that lycopene dissolves in fat. It is sopped up like a sponge in body fat. Researchers at Tufts University in Boston wondered where in the body the lycopene accumulates the most. They recruited twenty-five adults in their late twenties and early thirties, all within normal weight range, and recorded the foods they ate, including tomatoes and other dietary sources of lyco-pene, such as watermelon, papaya, pink grapefruit, red bell peppers, and persimmon. They found that the group consumed the lycopene equiva-lent of about five fluid ounces of tomato juice per week.

The researchers then biopsied fat in the abdomen, thighs, and but-tocks of each subject.[45] The biopsy showed that abdominal fat contained the most lycopene, about 41 percent more than the buttocks, and 74 percent more than thigh fat.* So, when you eat a tomato, the lycopene

---

* The form of lycopene measured by the Tufts researchers is cis-lycopene, which is the chem-ical form that is most easily absorbed by the body.

in it concentrates around your belly, which is a very convenient place to start its fat-fighting activity.

Lycopene has many benefits when it comes to health defenses. The buildup of lycopene in body fat may help its cancer-starving (antiangiogenic) properties. When consumed in the diet, specifically in tomato sauce, lycopene has been associated with a 20–50 percent lower risk of prostate cancer.[46] A study of 2,102 men with prostate cancer in the American South showed that those who ate the most lycopene-rich food had stored most of it in their fat as a kind of depot for this cancer-fighting bioactive.[47] Those with more lycopene in their fat had a 44 percent lower risk for aggressive prostate cancer.[48]

Beyond lycopene, there are other health-promoting bioactives found in tomatoes. Beta-cryptoxanthin is another tomato carotenoid (also found at high levels in satsuma mandarin oranges) that prevents fat from growing larger. This bioactive improves metabolism in lab studies of obese mice.[49] Rutin is another bioactive found in tomatoes. Lab studies at the Beijing University of Chinese Medicine showed that rutin increases the UCP1 trigger for thermogenesis in brown fat. It also improves the gut microbiome's production of anti-inflammatory short-chain fatty acids that aid in improving metabolism.[50] Besides tomato, rutin is also found in buckwheat, peaches, asparagus, and citrus peel.

All three of these tomato bioactives—lycopene, beta-cryptoxanthin, and rutin—activate regenerative defense systems to support health and healing.[51] A practical tip: researchers have discovered that adding onion and olive oil—as is done when making marinara sauce in Italian-style cooking as well as the flavorful base sauce called sofrito—protects the tomato bioactives from being degraded by heat while cooking.[52]

When buying tomatoes, look for firm, brightly colored tomatoes with intact skin. If you are not eating them right away, or if you need to further ripen them, place them stem-side down for a few days. Never refrigerate a tomato. The cold temperature changes the activity of their DNA that is responsible for flavor, which is why chilled whole tomatoes are never as tasty as when they ripen on your kitchen counter.[53] Always store tomatoes at room temperature.

Vegetables

Broccoli

The broccoli plant belongs to the *Brassica* genus of vegetables that also includes Brussels sprouts and leafy greens like kale, mustard, and bok choy. Broccoli originated from a type of wild cabbage in the Mediterranean. As a crop, it was first cultivated in Calabria, at the southern tip of Italy. Its name comes from the Latin *brachium*, which means "arm," referring to the multiple branches that fork at its top to create the tree-like florets.

A taste for broccoli originated two thousand years ago with the Etruscan and Roman civilizations in what is today Italy. The vegetable migrated to France in the sixteenth century, then went on to England (where it was called Italian asparagus) in the eighteenth century. In the early 1900s, it began to appear on dinner plates in the United States.

The characteristic flavor of broccoli can be described as "sulfurous" due to its potent bioactives known as sulforaphanes, which combat fat and activate health defenses. I've conducted, with colleagues at the Angiogenesis Foundation, studies on broccoli for its cancer-starving properties. We showed that while the broccoli florets do have abundant cancer-starving sulforaphane activity when it comes to angiogenesis defenses, the stem contains even more of the bioactive ingredients than the florets. Broccoli sulforaphanes also activate your other health defenses. They protect stem cells, stimulate beneficial epigenetic changes in your DNA that protect health, improve gut health and metabolism, and amplify beneficial immune responses.[54]

Add to all these benefits the effect that sulforaphanes have on adiposity. Recall that sulforaphanes can battle body fat by increasing the amount of brown fat and by turning on thermogenesis to improve metabolism. By helping the brain become more sensitive to leptin, sulforaphanes also help you feel less hungry. Mom had no idea how right she was when she told us kids to eat our broccoli!

Researchers at Harvard and Tufts Universities identified the contribution of broccoli to weight loss. They used the data in the Nurses' Health Study and the Health Professionals Follow-Up Study, analyzing the fruit and vegetable intake of 117,918 men and women. When correlated to weight loss, this study found that eating the equivalent of just one-half cup of broccoli per day was associated with losing about one pound over four years.

Young, three- to four-day-old sprouts of broccoli have up to one hundred times more sulforaphane power than the adult plant. This high potency has been seen in clinical trials that studied the ability of sprouts to stimulate immune cells that protect the body against viruses.

When it comes to fighting fat, broccoli sprouts protect the body against the inflammation caused by excess fat. This was studied by scientists at the Catholic University of Murcia and the CEBAS-CSIC research center in Spain.[55] They recruited forty overweight adults aged thirty-five to fifty-five and gave them one-third cup of fresh broccoli sprouts to eat daily for ten weeks. Throughout the study, blood tests were performed to measure inflammatory markers associated with excess body fat, specifically interleukin-6 (IL-6) and C-reactive protein (CRP). Their urine was collected to see the amount of sulforaphanes present from eating sprouts.

At the end of ten weeks, the broccoli-sprout eaters decreased their body fat mass by 6 percent. What was remarkable was this reduction in fat persisted for *another* twenty days after they stopped eating the sprouts. Then, slowly, their body fat built back up to its pre-sprout baseline levels.

In the urine taken from the subjects during the ten weeks of broccoli-sprout eating, the researchers found high levels of sulforaphane. In their blood, the inflammatory markers declined, with IL-6 falling by 38 percent. Just like with their body fat, there was a continuing anti-inflammatory benefit after they stopped eating sprouts. In fact, the IL-6 levels kept declining until day ninety. The other inflammatory marker, CRP, declined by 40 percent and slowly returned to baseline by day ninety.

Sulforaphanes can prevent weight gain. This has been studied in the lab using lean mice fed a high-fat diet.[56] When sulforaphanes were injected into the mice, their appetite decreased. This led to 30 percent less weight gain, compared to mice who did not receive sulforaphane. The sulforaphane increased their brain's sensitivity to leptin, which dampened their appetite, and, as a result, the mice ate less. When a higher dose of sulforaphane was given, the mice gained even less weight, a phenomenon known as a dose-response. When the researchers analyzed the effects more closely, they discovered that the sulforaphane itself *increased* metabolism even as the mice ate less food.

When buying broccoli, look for firm green stems. Broccoli sprouts are usually packaged in containers. Look for sprouts that have small light-green leaves and yellow-white roots. They should smell like adult broccoli, with no strange odors that might indicate spoilage.

Soy

First described in China more than four thousand years ago, soybeans are one of the most important protein sources in our global food supply. Soy is eaten as a bean, made into tofu (bean curd), fermented, mashed into a paste, and can even be transformed into wine. Soybeans form in green, hairy pods that hang like bats from a stalk, which is how you'll often find them in the produce section of Asian markets. They can also be found preshelled (removed from their pods) and frozen.

Eaten whole, soybeans have a mild, slightly sweet, nutty flavor. Tofu is found fresh, packaged, frozen, or dried. Soy pastes, like miso and

---

Other Brassica

You can find many edible brassica vegetables in the market, all containing sulforaphanes. The ones with the highest levels are cabbage, Chinese kale, and Brussels sprouts. Broccolini, a thinner version of broccoli with smaller florets, is a cross between broccoli and Chinese kale (*gai lan*), and it possesses sulforaphanes (most people do not know that the name "broccolini" is not botanical but rather is a trademark of the Mann Packing Company).[57] Rapini (broccoli rabe) is another delicious brassica with bioactives.[58] It has thin stalks and leaves and flowering buds. With a slightly bitter taste that mellows with blanching and cooking, rapini is a classic green found in Mediterranean cuisine. Romanesco broccoli is mild tasting, with a chartreuse flower bud that has a striking, almost hypnotic geometric pattern. As noted previously, Brussels sprouts and collard greens also belong to this family of vegetables, as does arugula. Some Asian brassica are bok choy (a good source of dietary fiber), gai choy, choy sum, napa cabbage, mustard greens, watercress, and wasabi—all with sulforaphanes.

---

doenjang, and soy sauces are popular ways to add flavor to food or as a condiment. Regardless of its form, soy has always played a central role in Buddhist and other vegetarian cuisines. Fun fact: soybeans are also used to make crayons, and the colors they produce are brighter than traditional wax crayons!

The fat-fighting bioactives in soybeans are genistein and daidzein. These activate brown fat thermogenesis and increase metabolism. They also lower appetite and can suppress fat deposition.[59] Genistein and daidzein also activate all five of the body's health defense systems. Indeed, eating soy is associated with lowering the risk of many diseases, including breast cancer (by 30 percent), cardiovascular disease (by 20 percent),[60] and diabetes (by 23 percent)[61]—all conditions associated with excess body fat. Lab studies have shown that eating soy over a lifetime reduces the risk of obesity in mice.[62]

Can soy cause weight loss? This question was investigated by researchers from the Shiraz University of Medical Sciences in Iran.[63] They recruited 107 women between twenty and forty with "normalweight obesity," meaning they had excess visceral fat packed around their organs, despite having a normal body mass index (BMI). Half of the women were given a soy snack that was equivalent to one-quarter cup of boiled edamame (50 grams) to eat every day for six months. The other half received a comparator snack, which was made of caloriematched fruit (3.5 servings). Both groups were instructed to eat their snacks three hours before lunch, but no other changes were made to their routines. The women ate their usual diet and maintained their usual level of physical activity. Body measurements were taken, and their appetite was assessed throughout the study.

At the end of six months, the researchers found that the soy eaters lost 6.4 pounds and four times more body fat, versus the fruit snack group. Soy eaters also shrank their waist circumference by 1.7 inches, which was five times more than the fruit eaters. This all came from losing fat. There was no change in lean muscle mass in either group. The soy eaters had less of an appetite, and they reported feeling greater satiety, or sensation of fullness, after their snack, which led them to eat less with their meal. A meta-analysis of other soy clinical trials showed similar benefits on shrinking waist circumference in people who are obese, older, and female.[64]

Carrots

The carrot is an ancient root vegetable that originated in Southwest Asia. The earliest carrots were not orange as we know them today but purple on the outside with a yellow interior. The outer hue was due to fat-fighting anthocyanins, the same bioactive found in blueberries. You can still find eye-catching purple carrots in some farmers markets and grocery stores today.[65] Orange carrots came about as the product of cultivation by Dutch farmers in the seventeenth century. By lore, they were grown as a tribute to William of Orange, a Dutchman who led an independence campaign to free the Netherlands from Spanish rule.[*]

Carrots are a good source of dietary fiber for gut health. A half cup of grated carrot has 2 grams of fiber. They also have the fat-fighting and health defense–activating bioactive chlorogenic acid.[66] Carrots contain bioactives that are eponymously called carotenoids, specifically beta-carotene and beta-cryptoxanthin.[67] The latter is a bioactive that increases UCP1 in fat cells, thereby increasing thermogenesis to burn fat.[68] In the lab, beta-cryptoxanthin also reduced body weight and visceral fat by 20 percent when fed to obese mice.[69] Conversely, not eating enough foods containing carotenoids, like carrots, is a risk factor for obesity. To this point, an analysis of dietary intake and obesity by Jilin University in China showed that people with low blood levels of carotenoids had a 73 percent increased risk of obesity.[70]

Eating more carrots may also lower your risk of developing metabolic syndrome. Researchers at the University Medical Center Utrecht in the Netherlands studied this in 374 middle-aged and elderly men, aged forty to eighty, by asking them to report their intake of carrots and other foods containing carotenoids (bell peppers, broccoli, mangoes, cantaloupe) using a standard food frequency questionnaire.[71] The researchers also asked the subjects if they had signs of metabolic syndrome: high blood pressure, high blood sugar, high blood cholesterol, and large waistline. They then brought the subjects into a medical center where they directly measured these same key features of metabolic syndrome: waist circumference, body fat distribution, insulin levels, blood cholesterol levels, and blood pressure. Metabolic syndrome was

---

[*] This was the Dutch War of Independence, also known as the Eighty Years' War. It lasted from 1568 to 1648.

found in 22 percent of the men. When everyone's diet was compared with whether they had metabolic syndrome, the analysis showed that eating more foods with carotenoids—equating to three medium orange carrots per day—lowered the risk of metabolic syndrome by 58 percent. At that dose, the average waist circumference of subjects was 1.6 inches smaller and the overall amount of visceral and subcutaneous fat was half that of people who ate few to no carrots.

Why do some people like carrots more than others? There might be a genetic explanation. Researchers from the University of Niigata, the University of Toyama, and the University of Tsukuba in Japan studied carrot-eating behavior and genetics. They recruited 12,225 adults and asked them to report their intake of carrots, pumpkin, and green vegetables (broccoli, spinach, green pepper, green beans, cabbage).[72] Everyone's height and weight data were collected. Not surprisingly, the researchers found that those who ate more plant-based foods were more likely to have a lower body mass. Next, saliva samples were collected so the researchers could extract each individual's DNA and evaluate 285,387 genes in their samples. Then, a genome-wide association study analysis was performed.[73] This is a research technique in which high-speed computing analyzes correlations between specific genes and health patterns or behaviors—in this case, carrot eating.

The results revealed a surprise: a link was found between one human gene (rs4445711) and high carrot consumption (three or more per day) and a lower chance of obesity in both men and women under the age of sixty. The mechanisms of this gene and carrot preference are unknown. Interestingly, this rs4445711 gene is also associated with better physical functioning in people over age eighty-five.[74] Talk about winning the genetic lottery: more carrots, less fat, and greater agility as you reach your twilight years. But you don't have to have this gene to love carrots!

There are many ways to eat carrots—raw or cooked, alone or as part of a recipe with other ingredients—but the key is to make sure you buy good product. Carrots should be firm and look even on the outside.

Select ones with a bright-green leafy carrot top still attached. These will be the freshest because the tops quickly spoil after picking. The bottom is called the taproot. It should be intact and uniform in color. My research group at the Angiogenesis Foundation conducted studies on the cancer-starving antiangiogenic properties of carrots. We found that the orange taproot is potent, but the green carrot tops have twice that potency. Use the whole plant and find a recipe that uses carrot tops, like in a salad or for making a pesto.

The "baby-cut" carrots you see in bags at the store? They are not young taproots but rather large and disfigured full-grown carrots that have been deemed unsuitable for display, so they are shaved down to bite-sized bits. Look closely at them: this is why they have no skin and no stalk. You can easily recognize true baby carrots that are harvested before maturity—you'll be able to see their stalk on one end.

Mushrooms

I love the meaty, earthy flavor of mushrooms. They are one of my favorite foods. You can roast, sear, sauté, and even grill fresh mushrooms. They can be served alone or incorporated into a more complex dish. You'll find tasty mushroom recipes in every great food culture.

More than two thousand kinds of edible mushrooms grow in the forest, but you'd be well advised to leave wild foraging to professionals. Poisonous ones can resemble those that are safe to eat.[75] You can feel confident about the mushrooms stocked in the grocery store or on display at farmers markets.

Mushrooms contain a soluble fiber called beta-D-glucan. This bioactive fights fat and activates your health defenses.[76] Beta-D-glucan stimulates angiogenesis defenses to grow new blood vessels needed for wound healing; at the same time, it can prevent harmful blood vessels from feeding cancers—or expanding fat.[77] The fiber also supports your immune defenses by feeding your gut microbiome. Just as with angiogenesis, beta-D-glucan performs double duty for the immune defenses.

It can boost protective immunity while it simultaneously reduces inflammation.[78]

Eating mushrooms can help you lose weight. Researchers from Johns Hopkins University conducted a clinical study to show this effect. They recruited seventy-three adults who were obese and gave half of the group about fifteen white button mushrooms to replace any red meat they would otherwise eat, twice a week for one year.[79] The mushrooms could be eaten raw or prepared in any way the subject chose. They could also be mixed into other foods. The other half of the group were given lean ground beef to eat three times per week (equivalent to one quarter-pound beef patty each meal).

At the end of one year, the researchers performed clinical measurements on all the subjects and compared them to their starting point. The mushroom eaters lost 7 pounds and shrank their waist circumference by 2.6 inches. In contrast, the beef eaters lost only 2.2 pounds and actually grew their waistlines by 3.3 inches. Mushroom eaters saw their systolic blood pressure (top number) lowered by 7.9 points. The inflammatory markers in their blood also decreased.

Mushrooms can reduce your appetite, too, so you feel like eating less. Researchers from the University of Bonn in Germany studied mushrooms and appetite.[80] They enrolled twenty-two middle-aged adults who were obese. All suffered from glucose intolerance, which means they had higher-than-normal levels of blood sugar. This was the result of an unstable metabolism as a result of having too much body fat.

The researchers gave all subjects a two-course meal that included a smoothie and potato soup, to which mushroom powder was added. The powder contained 8.1 grams of beta-D-glucan. In mushroom terms, this same amount of beta-D-glucan can be found in fresh, diced oyster mushrooms (one and a half cups), white button mushrooms (six cups), porcini (three cups), chanterelles (five cups), shiitake (one cup), cremini (one cup), diced portobello (three and a half cups), and fresh enoki mushrooms (three and a half cups).* The researchers assessed the sub-jects' satiety after the meal and drew their blood to measure hunger hormones.

After eating the meal, they were not allowed to eat any more mush-rooms for the next month. Then, all the subjects were called back to eat a second test meal, this time containing no mushrooms. Again, the researchers drew blood to evaluate hunger hormones and assessed their satiety in comparison with the mushroom meal period.

The mushrooms in the meal made everyone feel less hungry for ninety minutes after eating, which helps to prevent overeating. One hormone, glucagon-like peptide-1 (GLP-1), was 15 percent higher after the mushroom-spiked meal. This hormone is made by your gut, and it acts on the brain's satiety centers to turn down appetite. Notably, there are obesity drugs that are designed to mimic the effects of GLP-1. Two of them, semaglutide and liraglutide, are injections that, like mushrooms, help to reduce hunger and lower calorie intake, leading to weight loss. But eating mushrooms is a much tastier option.

Onion

Onions belong to the *Allium* genus, a group that also includes shallots, scallions, garlic, chives, and ramps, along with the decorative allium flowering plants seen in gardens. Allium are cornerstones for cooking in MediterAsian cuisine. They are packed with bioactives that help fight fat and improve your metabolism.

Onions are the quintessential allium. They are the bulbs of the onion plant wrapped with paper-thin skin that can be white, yellow, or a purplish-red. Beneath the skin, the outer peel and flesh of an onion are packed with bioactives. When you chop an onion, some of those bioac-tives leak from damaged cells and mix together to produce a sulfurous chemical that wafts through the air and causes your eyes to sting and

---

* The mushroom powder contained 8.1 grams of beta-D-glucan, and equivalent amounts in other common culinary mushrooms were calculated from this amount.

tear up.[81] Practical tip: chilling the onion for thirty minutes before cutting will slow the chemical reactions and lessen the tearing.[*]

Allicin is a potent sulfurous bioactive found in onions. It activates brown fat to start thermogenesis and increase metabolism. Lab studies show that allicin prevents weight gain and improves metabolism by lowering insulin resistance.[82] Allicin also activates angiogenic defenses and can grow blood vessels to help heal wounds, while it also stops the growth of the kind of harmful blood vessels that feed cancers.[83] And it activates NO, which helps to lower blood pressure and stimulate regeneration.[84]

Onions are a good source of quercetin, the bioactive that stimulates your health defenses. Quercetin activates stem cells for regeneration, promotes gut health, is a potent DNA protector, and supports healthy immunity.[85] Quercetin also turns on brown fat thermogenesis and prevents fat from expanding.[86]

Clinical studies have shown that eating onions can reduce body fat. Researchers from Hokkaido Information University and the National Agriculture and Food Research Organization in Japan recruited seventy healthy adults who were overweight and assigned them to eat onion in powder form that was added to their food.[87] Two types of onion powder were created, one with quercetin and one in which the quercetin had been removed by the researchers. Each day, for a total of twelve weeks, the subjects incorporated the onion powder into their usual meals. They could eat anything and use any cooking method they desired. The amount of onion consumed each day was equivalent to half a bulb of the Quergold varietal of onion or a third of the Sarasara-gold varietal. These onions have high levels of quercetin, about three times the amount found in typical red onions.

At the beginning and end of the study, blood samples were collected from all the subjects. Their blood pressure was measured, and their

---

[*] The chemical in onions that makes you cry is syn-Propanethial-S-oxide, and it is known as a lachrymatory factor, meaning it causes you to tear up.

abdominal fat was assessed using a CT scan. The results after twelve weeks were eye-opening. In subjects who were at higher risk for cardiovascular disease because their good (HDL) cholesterol was low (less than 74 mg/dL), eating onion led to an 8.2 times decrease in the amount of visceral fat in their belly.

The blood tests analyzed in the study found that onions helped restore liver health. A liver marker called alanine transaminase (ALT) can be elevated in the blood of people who are obese.[88] ALT is an enzyme found in liver cells that helps convert protein into energy. When the liver is injured, the ALT leaks out of the cells. In the onion eaters, their ALT decreased by 98 percent during the course of the study, reflecting a healing of the liver.

A study by researchers at Changwon National University in Korea tested just the onion's outer peel, the first few layers beneath the paper-like skin. These layers have the highest levels of quercetin.[89] Researchers enrolled seventy-two subjects who were obese and had metabolic syndrome.[90] Half of the group received an extract made from onion peel containing 50 milligrams of quercetin (equivalent to the amount in four whole red or yellow onions). They ate this twice a day. The other half received a placebo capsule. Body measurements were taken at the beginning and end of the twelve-week study. A DEXA scan was used to document everyone's body fat. The results showed that onion-extract eaters lost 1.8 pounds, and their waist circumferences declined by about three-quarters of an inch. Their hip circumference also shrank by half an inch, and they lost 0.7 percent of their arm fat.

When buying onions, choose ones that are heavy, firm, and dry, with no soft spots. Avoid any bulbs with green sprouts, which can make the onion taste bitter. Once you get home, store onions in a dry, cool location. At room temperature, an onion will last up to a month. Chopped or sliced onions should be stored in the refrigerator in a resealable bag. They will last seven to ten days. To get the benefit of as much quercetin as possible, keep in mind that the outer peel is packed with

Other Beneficial Alliums

Shallots, sometimes known as the cook's onion, are smaller than conventional onions and have an elongated egg shape with a thin, dry skin. The edible portion grows in clusters like garlic cloves. Similar to an onion, the shallot has a strong pungent scent when chopped but a sweeter, milder flavor when cooked. Shallots have six times the quercetin and four times as much DNA-protecting antioxidant potency as onion, making it an advantageous choice when it comes to fighting body fat.[91] Shallots can be sautéed to build layers of flavor in a dish, or they can be roasted, used raw in a mignonette sauce, or even pickled.

Scallions are another important culinary allium. Also known as green onions, scallions have thin green stalks with a small white bulb at one end. They are workhorses in Asian cooking and are found in stir-fries, braises, and marinades, and are used as a garnish to add a peppery, onion-like flavoring. Like all members of the allium family, scallions contain quercetin, which can combat body fat. Lab studies show that scallion extracts also have anti-inflammatory and cancer-starving (antiangiogenic) properties.[92]

One of my all-time favorite finds in the spring market is the ramp. In case you are not familiar with ramps, they are wild leeks. They have a small white bulb and thin white stalk with narrow, flat green leaves. Due to their allicin content, they have a pungent garlicky flavor. They contain a hefty amount of quercetin, about three times as much as a scallion and half as much as a red onion. Ramp season is very short, lasting only about one month, so buy them when you see them in the market. Tip: pick through them carefully, look for ones that are intact and not mushy (they are harvested wild), and wash them well to remove the dirt. I cook ramps very simply: I heat a small amount of extra virgin olive oil in a cast-iron pan or plancha, wait for the oil to be hot, add the ramps and cook for literally one minute, and eat immediately.

the bioactive. Use as much of the peel as possible for cooking. Onion peel is also useful for making stock and for seasoning soups. The peel can be cooked with rice to impart a nice flavor to it.

Garlic

Known for more than four thousand years, garlic is another food with origins in Central Asia. Reflecting its spread via caravans, garlic is mentioned in the ancient manuscripts of Greece, Egypt, and India as both a cooking ingredient and a treatment for illness. The medicinal properties of garlic are legendary. It was used to treat colic, menstrual cramps, liver disease, parasitic infections, influenza, snakebite, and skin diseases.[93] Folklore in Eastern Europe regarded garlic as an apotropaic, a food that could ward off evil spirits, demons, and vampires.

Garlic is one of the most common ingredients in Mediterranean and Asian cooking. It is a crucial element in many recipes. Popular dishes that you enjoy would taste utterly bland if garlic were removed. The pungent bulb is peeled, sliced, chopped, or minced and sautéed to flavor cooking oil before adding other ingredients. Garlic is also added directly into soups and stews, and it can be baked as cloves alongside or stuffed in foods.

Like onions, garlic contains allicin, which imbues it with fat-fighting and health defense attributes. Researchers in Iran studied the effect of garlic on ninety middle-aged men and women who were obese and had metabolic syndrome.[94] They gave half the group garlic powder equivalent to half a tablespoon of fresh crushed garlic (one and a half to two cloves) to consume each day. The other half received a placebo with no garlic.

After three months, the garlic eaters had a significant half-inch reduction in their waist circumference, compared to those taking the placebo, who had no change in waist size. Remember that a shrinking waistline reflects a reduction in the amount of harmful visceral fat inside your belly.

Garlic is found year-round as bulbs with a cluster of cloves bound together beneath parchment-like skin. During the summer, you may find garlic scapes in the market. These are the green tops of garlic plants that form artistic curls resembling a cowboy's lasso. Although they do not contain as much allicin as the cloves, scapes are delicious—eating them is a way to sustainably use the entire garlic plant.

Chili Peppers

Many people enjoy spicy food made with chili peppers. It is the chili that gives it the heat. We'll learn about dried chilis in the next chapter, but fresh chilis are a delight to find—and cook. A chili pepper is technically a berry, with hundreds of different varieties that originated more than six thousand years ago in Latin America.[95] Chilis were first brought from their homeland to Southeast Asia, China, and Europe by Spanish and Portuguese explorers. Because they were prized for their spicy taste, chili plants became domesticated and now are found in virtually all food cultures.

The fiery heat of chili pepper is due to its bioactives, capsaicin and capsinoids. Contrary to popular belief, the burning sensation does not come from the seeds. Instead, the spicy bioactives are mostly concentrated in the pithy white membrane called the "placenta" that holds the seeds. Recall from Chapter 4 that capsaicin and capsinoids wear multiple hats when it comes to your metabolism: they activate brown fat and trigger thermogenesis, burn down white fat, improve your blood sugars, and curb your appetite.[96]

The spiciness of chili helps turn on your metabolism. Capsaicin and capsinoids make you feel "the burn" because they attach to TRPV1, the pain receptor that is found on nerve endings throughout your digestive tract but that is especially numerous in your mouth and on your tongue. Eating chili peppers triggers these nerve endings, which technically causes a "pain" sensation (the wincing reaction you have when you eat something really hot is caused by this) and sweating. Pain is a hardwired response to danger and tells the body and brain to go on red alert.

The signal from capsaicin and capsinoids is sent from your tongue to your brain, which responds by releasing proteins called endorphins.[97] These endorphins are natural opioids that give you a sense of euphoria to counteract pain. The love for spicy foods that many have is in part due to this pleasurable brain response. Those who can't stand spicy food react instead to the pain. Personally, I love spicy food, so long as it's not torturously hot.*

Does eating fiery-hot foods affect body composition? A nine-year epidemiological study examined this among 12,970 people living in nine provinces across China. The researchers documented the amount of chili each person ate annually and rated them in four categories: none (0 grams per day), little (1 to 20 grams), medium (20.1 to 50 grams), or large (more than 50 grams). The researchers then followed the individuals' weight over nine years. They wanted to determine if there was any correlation between the amount of chili pepper they ate and the risk of becoming overweight or obese.

Compared to those who did not eat any chili, those who ate a "little" chili every day were 19 percent less likely to become overweight or obese over nine years. Those who ate "medium" amounts were 23 percent less likely, and those who ate "large" amounts were 27 percent less likely to have a weight problem. The pattern suggests a dose-response, which means the higher the quantities of spicy food you eat, the more benefit you get.

The specific dose of capsinoids for weight loss was studied by researchers from the University of Maryland in Baltimore.[98] They recruited eighty adults between thirty and fifty who were overweight or

---

* The scale used to measure the spiciness of chilis, called the Scoville scale, ranges from zero (the sweet red bell pepper) to more than 16 billion. The world's hottest pepper, according to *Guinness World Records*, is the Carolina Reaper, which is 2.2 million Scoville units and so hot that it put one eater in the hospital with a condition called the "thunderclap headache."

obese. Half of the subjects were given an extract containing capsinoids from a type of chili pepper called CH-19 Sweet to eat every day for twelve weeks. The other half received a placebo capsule. The subjects swallowed three capsules (3 milligrams of capsinoids) in the morning and three at night, for a total of 6 milligrams of capsinoids each day. This is equivalent to one-quarter teaspoon of dried chili flakes or two fresh Anaheim, Hatch, or serrano chilis per day. The subjects' weight and body composition were measured using the DEXA scan.

After twelve weeks, subjects who ate the capsinoids had a decrease in their abdominal fat that was sixfold greater than the placebo group. This decrease in belly fat correlated with a twofold greater decrease in body weight. Their lean body mass remained stable, so the weight loss came from fat, not muscle. There was also an increase in resting metabolism with the capsinoid group, whereas the placebo group experienced the opposite and had a decline in their resting metabolic rate.

When buying fresh peppers in the produce section, look for ones with smooth skin that feel heavy in your hand. Avoid wrinkled skin or soft, brown spots—signs that they are going bad. You can store your chili peppers in the refrigerator. Safety tip: when preparing chili peppers, wear a pair of rubber gloves to prevent burning your skin with capsaicin or capsinoid oil. Never touch your eyes after handling a chili pepper until after you thoroughly wash your hands.

* * *

Now you've met some of the best metabolism-revving, fat-fighting fruits and vegetables in the produce section. Table 6.1 summarizes the foods and their doses from clinical studies. Next, we will move on to a part of the market that you might be surprised I'm steering you toward: the middle aisles. Yes, the middle aisles are where you will find chips, cookies, sodas, and artificially flavored snacks. But science tells us there are also important fat-fighting foods in that section that you should bring home. Let's go find them.

TABLE 6.I. FOODS AND DAILY DOSES

This table is a summary of the data you've read and is for reference only. It is not a recommendation for you to eat all these foods every day.

Food	Daily Doses
Apples (fresh)	3 whole
Apples (dried)	¾ cup
Blueberries (fresh or frozen)	¼ cup
Grapefruit	1 ½ fruits total (eat ½ 3 x per day)
Pears	2 whole
Strawberries	1 to 2 ½ cups
Watermelon	2 cups diced (4 medium slices)
Avocado	1 whole
Broccoli	½ cup
Broccoli sprouts	⅓ cup
Carrots	3 medium carrots
Chili peppers	2 fresh Anaheim, Hatch, or serrano peppers
Garlic	½ tablespoon crushed garlic or 2 fresh cloves
Mushrooms	15 white button mushrooms, 2 x per week 1 ½ cups freshly sliced oyster mushrooms 6 cups white button mushrooms 3 cups porcini 5 cups chanterelle 1 cup shiitake 1 cup cremini 3 ½ cups portobello (diced) 3 ½ cups fresh enoki
Onions	2 medium red onions
Soy	¼ cup edamame, equal to ½ cup tofu or miso, or 4 tall glasses of soy milk
Tomato	1 raw medium-sized tomato or its equivalent: tomato paste (1 heaping tablespoon), tomato sauce or soup (¾ cup), or tomato powder (1 ½ tablespoons)

CHAPTER 7

Treasure Hunt

The middle aisles of the supermarket get a bum rap. This is completely understandable, with their endless shelves of nonperishables packed in boxes, bags, bottles, and cans. Many of the products here contain added sugars, unhealthy fats, stabilizers, artificial preservatives, artificial coloring, fillers, and other chemicals that can not only weaken your metabolism and cause you to gain weight; they can also degrade your health defenses.

And yet, the commonly heard healthy shopper's advice to avoid the middle aisle is oversimplified—and wrong. The secret is to know how to distinguish the "great for you" from the "not so good" for you and choose accordingly.

Preserved whole foods are an important part of both Mediterranean and Asian culinary traditions. For tens of thousands of years, people have preserved whole foods to extend their edible life. Foods were dried, salted, fermented, and packed away in containers. Preservation enabled people to eat during the winter months between harvests and allowed travelers to carry nourishing foods with them during long journeys.

Two thousand years ago, the merchant stalls that lined the Silk Road routes connecting China to Southern Europe through Central Asia sold boxes and ceramic vessels filled with these foods. While the process of food dehydration dates all the way back to the Middle East in 12,000 BCE, preserving and sealing foods in jars didn't begin until the early 1800s, and canning didn't catch on until one hundred years later. Today, some of the most highly rated delicacies among the cultures of Spain, France, and Italy are packaged in jars and tins. Visit any town in those countries, and you will find these items artfully displayed in specialty stores where dried spices; oils; and preserved legumes, condiments, and canned seafoods are sold.

Now it's time to begin our treasure hunt in the middle aisles of your grocery store (you'll also find them on your next visit to a village market). I'll highlight those foods that are best to include on your shopping list.

Legumes

Keep an eye on the cans and sacks in the middle aisle: dried and canned legumes are delicious and metabolism-enhancing offerings in both Mediterranean and Asian cuisine—well worth adding to your diet.[1] Legumes have been grown since ancient times (archaeologists found them to be part of the diet of Roman gladiators), and their fruits or seeds are excellent sources of protein, fiber, and healthy omega-3 fats.* White beans, lentils, fava beans, peas, chickpeas, soybeans, and peanuts are examples of legumes. When sold in dried form, they are called "pulses."[2]

Modern science has discovered that legumes contain useful bioactives such as polyphenols, phytoestrogens, and plant-based peptides that can activate your health defenses and your metabolism.[3] Let's look more closely at the health benefits and the fat-fighting power of some specific legumes.

White Beans

The common white bean has many names. One of them is "navy bean" because, since the 1800s, the US Navy has been serving them to sailors

---

* Gladiators were not vegetarians or vegans, despite popular lore. The totality of evidence shows that the ancient Roman diet was omnivorous. Gladiators were slaves and were fed the least expensive food, which included beans.

on battleships.[4] This is the white bean that is used to make Boston baked beans, and it is the star ingredient in the famous Senate Bean Soup, which has been served in the US Senate cafeteria since the early twentieth century.[5]

White beans can be found dried or packed in cans in the middle aisles. Canned beans, packed in a little water with salt, can keep for two to three years and still retain their nutritional value. The shelf life of dried beans when properly stored in a cool environment is, well, indefinite. Dried beans dating back ten thousand years have been found by archaeologists in the Galilee in northern Israel.[6] They might not be as tasty as they were originally, but they were intact.

Beans are rock stars when it comes to macro- and micronutrients. They are a great source of plant-based protein and soluble fiber that nurtures a healthy gut microbiome. The result is a nutritious food that reduces cardiovascular risk factors by lowering blood cholesterol and improving blood-lipid profiles. They also contain iron, zinc, magnesium, and folate—valuable micronutrients, especially for people eating a vegetarian diet.

Beans can shrink your waist size.[7] Researchers from the University of Toronto studied this effect by recruiting fourteen overweight and obese adults, aged thirty-five to fifty-five, and giving them five cups of canned ready-to-eat navy beans each week, added to their regular diet for one month.[8] Each person kept a food diary that was checked by a dietician, and they had to present the empty bean cans to confirm that they actually ate the beans. Body measurements were taken at week one and week four of the study. The results were striking. After one month, the women who ate the beans had a one-inch reduction in their waist size. The men in the study also benefited, with waistlines that shrank an average of three-quarters of an inch.

Multiple studies have shown that your waist circumference is a good indicator of the amount of visceral fat in your body.[9] In an analysis of twenty-nine studies involving fifty-eight thousand people, researchers from Wageningen University in the Netherlands found that waist girth is a predictor of mortality, even for people who are considered underweight.[10]

Lentils, Chickpeas, and More

Lentils are a classic, versatile legume from Mediterranean cuisine. Look for them on different shelves in the middle aisles, since they can be dried or canned. Any home cook can use lentils to make a hearty soup or salad, and they can be cooked with rice. Lentils are packed with microbiome-feeding dietary fiber. One-half cup of dry lentils contains 18 grams of fiber, which is more than half of the recommended daily intake for both men and women. The fiber feeds healthy gut bacteria, which then produce the short-chain fatty acids that help to streamline metabolism, control weight, and lower inflammation.[11] A lab study showed that when lentils were fed to rats, their body weight dropped by 14 percent, compared to rats eating standard chow.[12] The lentil-fed animals had a superior microbiome with more beneficial bacteria and fewer harmful bacteria—a pattern we all should develop.

I also recommend chickpeas (used for Middle Eastern falafel, hummus, and Provençal *socca*), yellow split peas (for Indian dal), gigante beans (used in gigantes plaki, the Greek version of baked beans), and mung beans (in Chinese soups). They all share the protein, polyphenol, and fiber benefits of white beans and lentils.

Eating legumes reduces the risk of metabolic syndrome caused by excess body fat. This was shown by a study from the University of Toronto, which recruited forty middle-aged men and women who were obese.[13] The researchers compared two interventions—caloric restriction versus beans—for weight loss. Half of the subjects were given five cups per week of a legume mix (lentils, chickpeas, yellow peas, navy beans) to add to their regular diet for a total of eight weeks. The other half were coached by a dietician to reduce their caloric intake by 500 calories per day, but they did not eat any legumes and kept to their usual diet. Body measurements and blood tests were taken at the beginning and end of the study.

After eight weeks, both groups had smaller waistlines. The calorie-restricted group lost 1 inch of waist circumference, while the legume eaters lost 0.66 inch. But remember, the legume eaters *did not restrict their calories* like the other group. Instead, they *added* legumes to their usual diet—and still lost visceral fat, showing the power of these middle-aisle products.

Legume eaters lowered their elevated blood pressure and improved their fasting blood glucose levels, attributes of metabolic syndrome. Fasting blood glucose was six times better in the legume-eating group than in the calorie-restricting group. The legume eaters increased their microbiome-feeding dietary fiber by 5 percent each day with the beans. In contrast, the calorie-restricted group actually *decreased* their fiber intake by 12 percent. This is a prime example of how *adding* a fat-fighting food can offer more health benefits than going on an elimination diet.

The ability of legumes to cause weight loss has been observed time and time again. In 2016, a group of Canadian researchers conducted a meta-analysis of twenty-one clinical trials involving 940 people who were obese and not eating legumes. The scientists found that adding just one serving per day of legumes for six weeks resulted in an average weight loss of three-quarters of a pound, even if the diet was not calorically restricted.[14]

The PREDIMED (PREvención con DIeta MEDiterránea) study from Spain showed that legumes are also protective against cancer. This study tracked a group of 7,216 participants in their late sixties who were overweight. Those eating the most legumes had a 49 percent lower risk of death from cancer. The researchers attributed this benefit to the dietary fiber and other bioactives such as lignans found in beans.[15]

Eating beans for health is easy. There are countless recipes you can explore using beans in soups, salads, chilis, stews, and curries. They are great additions to almost any other dish you can think of. Beans are also a great high-fiber substitution for rice or pasta.

Grains

Barley

Barley is usually found as dry kernels, stocked near the dried beans and rice. It is sold hulled (shell-less), and when cooked it has a chewy texture and a nutty taste. You can cook barley in a soup or stew. It can be used in a whole-grain salad or served as an accompaniment to vegetables, chicken, or fish. Barley can be also substituted for Arborio rice to make a healthy "risotto" that is called orzotto in Italy.

Barley is an ancient grain that grew wild ten thousand years ago in the Fertile Crescent, the part of the Middle East that borders the Mediterranean Sea, and also Tibet. Its hardiness makes it one of the most important whole grains in agriculture, along with corn, rice, and wheat. Barley is a great source of vitamins, minerals, and the bioactives lutein and zeaxanthin, which protect stem cells. It also contains beta-D-glucan, the soluble fat-fighting fiber that is also found in mushrooms.[16]

Barley was studied for its antiobesity effects in Shizuoka, Japan.[17] The researchers recruited forty-four men, aged thirty to fifty, who were considered obese by Japanese standards. Half of the group received a daily meal containing rice plus pearl barley for twelve weeks. The meal contained 7 grams of beta-D-glucan each day, the amount in about one cup of cooked barley. The other half received a meal with rice and no barley. Body measurements and blood samples were taken before and after the study. An abdominal CT scan was performed every four weeks to assess changes in body fat.

After twelve weeks, blood tests showed that the barley eaters had lowered their total cholesterol by 5 percent, and their bad LDL cholesterol declined by 4 percent, compared to their baseline measures. The rice-only eaters had no changes in their levels of blood cholesterol. Barley eaters shrank their waist size by half an inch, while rice eaters' waist size increased. The CT scans of their belly fat revealed the most significant effects of all. The visceral fat of barley eaters decreased by 11 percent, which was five times greater than what the only rice eaters lost.

Store your barley in an airtight container and keep it in a cool, dry location. Barley kept this way will last for a year. Before you cook barley, it's a good idea to rinse the grain with cold water to remove any dirt and debris. Toasting the barley in a pan will give it more flavor. So will cooking the barley in a vegetable stock or a bone broth rather than water. Be aware that the barley kernels will double in size when cooked! In a well-stocked supermarket, you may also find roasted barley, which is used to make a traditional light and nutty tea in China (where it is called *damaicha*), Korea (*boricha*), and Japan (*mugicha*).

Purple Maize

Nestled among the dried grains and legumes in the middle aisle, you might spot a bag of unusual-colored dried kernels: purple maize. This is a type of corn from the Andean Mountains in Peru, Bolivia, Colombia, and Ecuador that has an intense dark-purple and black-blue color. The pigment comes from anthocyanin, a bioactive that combats body fat and improves metabolism.[18] In the lab, mice fed an extract made from purple maize do not gain weight as fast, even if they are fed a high-fat diet. In fact, by adding purple maize, they reduced their weight gain by 28 percent, and their blood glucose was 27 percent lower. Their blood triglyceride levels were also 22 percent lower on the purple maize diet. The antiobesity effect of anthocyanin has also been seen in studies of purple sweet potatoes.[19]

The kernels of purple maize are larger, chewier, and less sweet than those of yellow corn. To make them edible, the dried kernels must first be soaked or boiled. This is the corn from which blue tortilla chips are made. A delicious traditional Peruvian beverage, *chicha morada*, is made from purple maize seasoned with spices like cinnamon and cloves, which have their own antiobesity effects.[20] A dessert called *mazamorra morada* is a pudding made with purple maize and fruit. If your supermarket carries any traditional Latin foods in the middle aisles, you might find these kernels as a specialty item, or you can order purple maize kernels online.

Buckwheat

You will find buckwheat near rice and dried grains, although sometimes it is on supermarket shelves near dried oats and breakfast cereals. Despite its name, buckwheat is not related to wheat. It's not even a grain. It's known as a pseudocereal, and it is gluten-free. Buckwheat is a plant whose seeds—called groats—contain a bioactive called rutin, which has antiadipose effects. Rutin activates brown fat and increases thermogenesis.[21] It also stimulates the gut microbiome to produce beneficial anti-inflammatory short-chain fatty acids that streamline the metabolism.[22] Adding buckwheat to chow has been shown to prevent obesity-induced inflammation and to lower blood cholesterol in lab rats.[23]

Buckwheat groats have a mild nutty taste that toasting enhances. They can be simmered in water or broth and served similarly to a rice pilaf or added to a salad or soup. In Japan, roasted buckwheat is used to make a tea called *soba-cha* and also thin soba noodles. Roasted buckwheat groats are used to prepare a fluffy, gluten-free rice-like Eastern European dish called *kasha*.

Dried Fruit

Dried Apple

Dried apples are found in the healthy snacks section of the middle aisles. They are sold prepackaged, so read the ingredient list carefully to make sure there is no added sugar, artificial preservatives (such as sulfites), or coloring. The advantage of dried apple and most types of dried fruit is that you can quickly consume a whole fruit, peel and all. The peel contains ursolic acid, and the flesh has chlorogenic acid. Both are fat-fighting bioactives. Eating the peel also gives you the benefit of even more dietary fiber than just the flesh.

A study conducted at Florida State University involving 160 post-menopausal women (one to ten years after menopause) showed that eating three-quarters of a cup per day of dried apple led to 3.3 pounds lost over a one-year study.[24] The total cholesterol levels in their blood tests also improved. The researchers also measured the inflammatory marker C-reactive protein (CRP). By the end of the study, their blood levels of CRP had declined by 32 percent. All these benefits are desirable, but you want to be careful not to overindulge in dried fruits, as they do contain all the natural sugars of a whole fruit shrunken into a tiny size. Eat them in moderation.

Dried Prunes

Even a supermarket with a meager dried fruit section is sure to have prunes. A prune is simply a plum with its pit removed then dried into a sweet, soft, purple-black nugget. They are made from the variety of plums known as freestone, meaning the pit is easily separated from the flesh. Freestones are distinct from clingstone plums, in which the flesh adheres to the pit. The clingstones are better for eating when they are fresh and ripe. The fiber and fermented sugars of prunes have a laxative effect, which is why they are so famously known as a home remedy for constipation. They really do work! The efficacy of prunes has been confirmed in a clinical study showing improved stool mass and frequency.[25]

Prunes contain chlorogenic acid, anthocyanins, and abundant dietary fiber.[26] One cup of pitted prunes has 12 grams of fiber for your gut microbiome. An analysis conducted by Harvard and Tufts University researchers examined fruit and vegetable intake in 117,918 healthy men and women and found an association between those people who ate six prunes per day and weight loss of 1.3 pounds over four years.[27] A lab study showed that a concentrated extract from prunes can stop new fat cells from developing, and it caused white fat cells to turn into useful brown fat cells.[28]

You can eat prunes as a snack or cook or bake them into sweet or savory dishes. They pair well with spices like ginger, cinnamon, nutmeg, clove, and allspice. An ultradried prune that is found in Asian markets is *li hing mui* (or *huamei*), which means "traveling plum." This salty, sweet-and-sour plum originated in China as a snack. Its unique mouth-puckering flavor can keep you awake if you are taking a long road trip. As a student, I sometimes sucked on these while I stayed up late studying.

Fungi

Dried Mushrooms

If you like fresh mushrooms, you'll love their dried versions, too. Dried mushrooms can be found in the middle aisles of the grocery store, often situated near the spice racks. In a large Asian market, you will find entire shelves dedicated to these fantastic fungi. From Chapter 6, you already know that clinical studies have shown that eating mushrooms can reduce waist size and lower body weight, inflammatory markers, and blood pressure.[29]

Some of the more common dried mushrooms you will find are porcini, morel, chanterelle, and shiitake. Asian markets carry a variety of dried shiitake mushrooms that are instantly recognizable because of the white tic-tac-toe-like crosshatched pattern on their caps. The drying process concentrates the unique flavors of each type of mushroom and amplifies their umami flavor. Oyster mushrooms have a mild, earthy note, while shiitake mushrooms have a deeper, richer flavor. Dried shiitake caps are used in Chinese and Japanese cuisine, often for braised dishes. Dried porcinis are potent and rich, and their robustness in flavor makes them the king of dried mushrooms. All of these types can be used for sauces, stews, and soups as well as for stir-fries, risotto, pasta, and other noodle dishes.

To reconstitute dried mushrooms, simply place them in a bowl, pour boiling water over them, and let them soak for at least twenty to thirty minutes. Thick-capped mushrooms may take up to one hour. Once softened, the mushroom can be chopped and cooked. The water in which they were soaked will become a dark, flavorful broth you can use to intensify the flavor of the dish you're cooking.

Bottles and Jars

Extra Virgin Olive Oil

An entire section of the middle aisle is often dedicated to olive oil. Sometimes you'll find it near other cooking oils or by the vinegars or condiments. There is a lot of history behind this product. Olives originated from Western Asia five thousand years ago and became established in the Middle East and Mediterranean regions as a staple food. The oil from pressed olives was used for religious ceremonies, as oil for lanterns, to make soap, and for cooking. What might surprise you most is that olive oil also fights fat.

Extra virgin olive oil (EVOO) is the most desirable form of olive oil. It is pressed from different olive varietals. The "extra virgin" refers to oil that is not refined, and, as a result, it will contain small particles from ripe olives. These bits are the source of potent polyphenols like hydroxytyrosol. This bioactive activates your health defenses, and it also fights fat by preventing preadipocyte stem cells from making more fat. Hydroxytyrosol also reduces inflammation caused by excess fat.

The effect of EVOO on weight loss was studied by researchers from Universidade Federal de Viçosa in Brazil.[30] They recruited forty-one women aged nineteen to forty-one who were overweight or obese and who did *not* habitually use olive oil for their cooking. The researchers gave half of them EVOO and the other half soybean oil to add to their breakfast every day for nine weeks.* The amount of oil they consumed was just under two tablespoons per day. The women were then placed on an 1,800-calories-per-day restricted diet.

All of the women lost weight due to the calorie restriction, but the EVOO drinkers lost 6 pounds, 62 percent more weight loss than the soybean oil drinkers. The EVOO participants specifically lost 5.3 pounds of total body fat, 82 percent more than soybean drinkers. The group receiving EVOO also had a decrease in their diastolic blood pressure (the second number in a blood pressure reading) by 5 points. This level of blood pressure reduction has been estimated to reduce the risk of stroke by 34 percent and coronary artery disease by 21 percent.[31]

There are more than a thousand varieties of olives grown around the world, but only a fraction are used for olive oil production. The olives themselves range in skin color from green to reddish-brown to black. When olives are first pressed, the oil that results is intensely green, which comes from the chlorophyll present in the fruit. The chlorophyll helps fuel the metabolism of the olives themselves.

When I buy EVOO, I scan the label on the bottle to identify which olive varietals were used. Many oils are made from multiple varieties of olives, which can taste very nice, but I prefer monovarietal oil, which is pressed from a single type of olive. There are three olive varietals known to have the highest levels of polyphenols: Picual olives (from Spain), Koroneiki olives (Greece), and Moraiolo olives (Italy). The higher the polyphenol levels, the more spicy, peppery, and fruity the taste.

Another reason I prefer monovarietal EVOO is that it is less likely to be counterfeit or diluted with cheaper oils.** You want the real deal. Check the harvest date of the olives pressed for the oil. It should be

---

* The EVOO was Andorinha, from Algés, Portugal.
** There is an entire industry of counterfeit or adulterated low-quality olive oil being sold as "high-quality" extra virgin olive oil on the market.

printed on the label. EVOO is perishable and should be kept in a cool, dark place. A bottle will last about two years from the time of harvesting and should be consumed within two months after opening. I recommend buying the very best EVOO you can afford and using it every day for cooking as well as a condiment.

One last myth-busting tidbit: there is a widely held belief that EVOO should not be used for high-temperature cooking because of its supposedly low smoke point, the temperature at which the oil begins to burn and change its chemical properties. In reality, the smoke point of EVOO is almost the same as canola oil (both around 200 degrees Celsius), which is routinely used for frying. High-quality EVOO is very heat-stable even at deep-frying temperatures (160 degrees Celsius), although I don't recommend that method for healthy cooking. So don't worry: EVOO can safely be used for sautéing and even stir-frying in a wok. The polyphenols in EVOO actually protect the oil from forming dangerous petroleum by-products. In addition, when you cook with EVOO, some of its beneficial fat-fighting olive polyphenols are transferred from the oil into the food itself.[32] Cooking with EVOO can make healthy food even healthier.

Apple Cider Vinegar

Many people do not realize how many types of vinegar exist in the middle aisle. Along with apple cider vinegar, white vinegar, red wine vinegar, white wine vinegar, sherry vinegar, balsamic vinegar, and rice wine vinegar, you might also find black vinegar and malt vinegar. Distilled white vinegar can be used for cleaning (and sometimes is stocked alongside cleaning products) because the acetic acid (which is the chemical name for vinegar) is good for breaking down dirt and scum. Vinegar has a similar effect in your gut. Because of its acidity, vinegar has an antibiotic property.[33]

The history of vinegar dates back five thousand years to the Babylonians, when it was a fermentation product used for both culinary and medicinal purposes. Its creation was also recorded in China three thousand years ago. The name "vinegar" is derived from the French *vin aigre*, which means "sour wine." When red or rice wine goes sour, the bacteria growing in the liquid create the vinegar. Vinegar is primarily water plus 4 to 8 percent acetic acid, a natural acid produced by bacterial fermentation that is used for pickling. Fruit vinegars are commonly made from apples, raspberries, quince, persimmons, kiwifruit, and raisins. Although the flesh of all of these fruits have fat-fighting bioactives, only trace amounts remain in their vinegars.

Zhenjiang black vinegar from Jiangsu Province in China is made with rice, wheat, or sorghum, and it is aged until it becomes an inky-black color. The result is a smoky, malt-flavored vinegar. Italy's prized version is balsamic vinegar from Modena. This is a concentrated vinegar, made with the sweet must of Trebbiano grapes and aged for up to twenty-five years. In England, malt vinegar (the mild vinegar used in British pubs as the traditional condiment for fish and chips) is made by germinating and drying barley, then fermenting the maltose into a vinegar.

Medically, the acetic acid in vinegar improves insulin sensitivity and lowers blood sugar.[34] In the lab, acetic acid prevents the accumulation of fat droplets in adipose tissue by turning down several genes related to lipogenesis (fat creation), and it decreases body weight in obese diabetic rats.[35] It's the acetic acid of the vinegar that promotes metabolic health.

In one clinical study on vinegar and weight loss, researchers from the Mizkan Group in Aichi, Japan, recruited 155 people aged twenty-five to sixty who were considered obese by Japanese standards but were otherwise healthy.[36] The Japanese have stricter criteria for obesity, which is defined as a body mass index (BMI) of 25 or above, while in the United States, obesity is defined as a BMI of 30 or above. The subjects were given beverages in which either one tablespoon ("low dose") or two tablespoons ("high dose") of apple cider vinegar had been mixed into a water-based beverage each day for twelve weeks. A third test group received a placebo beverage that contained no vinegar. The subjects drank half their daily beverages after breakfast and the other half after dinner. Everyone ate their usual diet.

Vinegar drinkers began to lose weight after four weeks and continued until week twelve. People drinking the high-dose vinegar lost more weight (4.2 pounds) and fat mass than people drinking the low-dose beverage (2.7 pounds). All vinegar drinkers lost more weight than the placebo drinkers. High-dose vinegar drinkers lost three-quarters of an inch from their waist circumference, while low-dose drinkers lost half an inch. In the placebo group, both body weight and waist circumference *increased* over the duration of the study.

Both visceral and subcutaneous fat decreased in the vinegar drinkers, compared to the placebo group. High-dose vinegar drinkers also had lower triglycerides (by 17 percent), lower total cholesterol (by 6 percent), and lower systolic blood pressure, by just under 5 points. These changes occurred with modest consumption of vinegar—which is surprising but very practical.

Another weight-loss study involving apple cider vinegar was conducted by the Shahid Beheshti University of Medical Sciences in Iran. Researchers recruited thirty-nine men and women, aged twenty-seven to forty, who were overweight but not obese. The subjects received two tablespoons of apple cider vinegar each day, along with a calorically restricted diet for twelve weeks. The vinegar was divided into one tablespoon at lunch with a salad and one tablespoon with dinner. A control group ate the same calorie-restricted diet without any vinegar. Everyone in the study lost weight because of the caloric restriction, but the vinegar drinkers lost 8.8 pounds, 42 percent more than those who did not consume any vinegar. The vinegar drinkers also lost 2.3 inches from around their hips, 74 percent more than the control group. By measuring the waist and hip circumference as a reflection of the amount of visceral fat in each subject, the researchers concluded that apple cider vinegar reduced visceral fat by 44 percent in males and by 33 percent in females. By contrast, the control group who had no vinegar increased their visceral fat by 44 percent in males and by 33 percent in females, despite the calorie restriction.

Keeping a supply of vinegar on hand is convenient since it is self-preserving and lasts indefinitely. Vinegar does not need to be refrigerated. That said, it's best to store vinegar in a dark place, and avoid light and heat exposure. Always make sure the bottle is tightly sealed after each use. If too much air enters the bottle, the vinegar may form a "mother," an otherworldly-looking gelatinous disc of airborne acetic acid bacteria (*Mycoderma aceti*) that ferments the vinegar. To remove the mother, pour the vinegar through a strainer or cheesecloth and rebottle it in a clean glass container. Tip: if you are like me and don't like the taste of a pure shot of vinegar, you can add it to a beverage, such as tomato or pineapple juice or even kombucha—the sharp vinegary taste will blend into the background.

Fermented Bean Paste

Stroll through the middle aisles of any Asian grocery store, and you will see many types of fermented bean paste—or you can order bean paste online. These savory pastes deliver a rich umami taste and are used as a concentrated base ingredient or as a seasoning to dramatically enhance the flavor of a vegetable, seafood, or poultry dish. The Chinese version is called *doubanjiang*, made with fermented fava beans and chili pepper. Harking from Sichuan Province, it is spicy-hot. In Korea, it is called *doenjang* and is made with fermented soybeans, but it is not hot. When red chili pepper and glutinous rice flour are added, it is called *gochujang*, which tastes like a slightly sweet blend of miso with spicy sriracha sauce.

Fermented soybeans contain higher levels of the bioactives genistein and daidzein than fresh soybeans. These bioactives combat fat cells and activate your health defenses. The chili in the paste contains capsaicin and capsinoids, making spicy bean paste a powerhouse for fat fighting. Because they are fermented products, doubanjiang, doenjang, and gochujang are also probiotic foods, meaning that they contain beneficial bacteria that contribute to gut health and help lower gut inflammation.[37] Lab studies have shown gochujang increases *Akkermansia muciniphila*, the bacteria associated with lean bodies, a healthy metabolism, and cancer-fighting immunity.[38]

Can gochujang fight harmful body fat? Researchers from Jeonbuk National University in Korea studied fifty-three healthy men and women, aged nineteen to sixty-five, who were at the top end of normal weight but not overweight.[39] Half of the subjects were given the equivalent of two and a half tablespoons of gochujang, the amount typically consumed daily by someone living in Korea. The gochujang was packed into a capsule like a supplement, which was taken each day for twelve weeks. The other half of the group received a placebo capsule containing vegetable powder that was matched in calories. Both groups were instructed to maintain their usual diet and lifestyle. Body measurements and blood tests were taken. A CT scan was performed at the beginning and end of the study to measure body fat.

After twelve weeks, the gochujang eaters lost an average 6 percent of their visceral fat. By contrast, the placebo eaters lost virtually no fat. Blood lipid markers also improved with gochujang, with an 18 percent decline in serum triglyceride levels. In contrast, the placebo group had a 13 percent increase in their triglyceride levels.

Many versions of commercial fermented bean paste are available to please any palate, each with slightly different spice combinations and levels of heat. The way to find the best version for you is simply to try a few until you find one that suits your taste. You only need a small amount of gochujang for any dish, so once the jar is opened, seal and store it in the refrigerator—it will last for months.

Kimchi

Kimchi is a two-thousand-year-old pickled food from Korea, made with different ingredients with fat-fighting power: napa cabbage, daikon radish, onion, carrots, garlic, and even more garlic! Modern kimchi contains hot chili pepper, although peppers were not introduced to Asia until the 1600s by Portuguese explorers who brought them from South and Central America. Asian markets carry many brands of factory-made kimchi, and it has also become a common item in regular grocery stores.* Which version is best depends on your preferences because different kimchis have varying amounts of salt, garlic, chili, and acidity.

The health benefits of kimchi come from multiple properties. The fiber in the napa cabbage, shredded radish, and fermented anchovy makes kimchi a pre- and probiotic food. The hot red pepper contains fat-burning capsaicin and capsinoids to activate your TRPV1 receptors that signal the brain to trigger thermogenesis. Garlic has fat-fighting allicin. Kimchi has even been studied as an antiobesity intervention. Lab mice eating kimchi have lower body weight, less inflammation in their fat, and lower blood cholesterol.[40]

The probiotic property of kimchi is important. It contains *Lactobacillus* bacteria and many other probiotic species, especially in the fermented versions. When the number of bacteria in the kimchi preparations was analyzed, researchers found four-thousand-fold more bacteria in the fermented version (4.3 billion per milliliter), compared to fresh kimchi (1.4 million per milliliter).

Another bacterium found in kimchi, *Lactobacillus sakei*, has been discovered to have antiobesity properties. Researchers at Seoul National University College of Medicine in Korea conducted a clinical study of 114 adults, twenty to sixty-five years old, who were overweight.[41] The participants received either 5 billion units of pure *L sakei* isolated from kimchi twice a day or a placebo capsule. All were encouraged by a research coordinator to eat a healthy diet and exercise for thirty minutes at least three times per week throughout the twelve-week study. At the end of the study, those who consumed the kimchi *L sakei* lost a little

---

* You can of course make your own kimchi to taste using the basic ingredients.

more than half a pound of body weight. By contrast, the placebo group gained 1.1 pounds. When fat mass was measured, L sakei caused almost half a pound reduction—meaning the lost weight was fat—compared to the placebo group, who gained 1.3 pounds of fat. Waist circumference also shrank slightly in the L sakei group.

Kimchi is also eaten when freshly made. Researchers at the Ajou University School of Medicine in Korea wanted to see if there was any difference between fresh and fermented kimchi when it comes to weight loss.[42] They recruited twenty-two adults with an average age of thirty-eight who were overweight or obese. They obtained fresh (one day old) or fermented (ten days old) kimchi, made by the same factory. Half of the group ate fermented kimchi for four weeks. Then they took a break for two weeks, during which they ate no kimchi. Then they ate fresh kimchi for the next four weeks. The other half did the opposite: first fresh kimchi, then no kimchi, then fermented kimchi. The dose was two cups of fermented or fresh kimchi per day. All the meals during the study were provided by clinical dieticians.

At the end of the study, fermented kimchi provided greater overall benefits. It reduced body fat percentage twice as much as fresh kimchi. Fermented kimchi also improved metabolic measures better than the fresh kind. Fasting blood glucose and fasting insulin are markers of metabolic health, and both decreased—by 6 percent and 26 percent, respectively—with fermented kimchi. Researchers also detected a more than 4-point beneficial drop in blood pressure after four weeks of eating the fermented version. By contrast, participants eating the fresh kimchi had no significant change in blood pressure. Total cholesterol declined by 5 percent with fermented kimchi, as did blood levels of leptin (by 23 percent) and inflammatory markers. All of the changes that resulted from eating fermented kimchi reflected an improvement of metabolism. When it came to weight loss, however, fresh kimchi actually performed better! It produced a 3.3-pound weight reduction, which was 25 percent more than the 2.65 pounds dropped for those eating fermented kimchi.

Ready to buy some kimchi? Keep store-bought, jarred kimchi unopened in a cool, dry location. After opening, make sure you screw on the cap tightly and place the jar in the refrigerator. At room temperature, opened kimchi might last only one week. In the refrigerator, it can last three to six months. Just be aware that bacterial fermentation will continue to go on even in the refrigerator. Here's a tip from someone who learned something the hard way (me): when reopening the jar, do it over a sink, as the buildup of fermentation gas will cause the liquid to bubble out of the jar.

Capers

You will find these little round green treasures in bottles near the pickles, packed in small jars with brine and vinegar, or dry-cured and packed with large speckles of sea salt. Capers are the tiny, handpicked flower buds of a wild bush that grows natively in dry, rocky, sunbaked areas across the Mediterranean. As an ingredient, they add life to any dish. Utilized across millennia in cooking and for health applications, capers were mentioned in the Roman cookbook *Apicius* (circa fourth century CE) and even described in the writings of the ancient Greeks and Romans for their ability to improve digestive health.

Today, capers are harvested on the Sicilian island of Pantelleria, from the volcanic soil of the Greek island Santorini, and from other locales in Turkey, Morocco, and Iberia. The flavor of a caper is bright, sharp, piquant, and lemony. Southern Italian and Greek recipes call for it in pastas, salads, and sauces to enhance the taste of already delicious dishes.

Capers contain extremely high levels of the bioactive quercetin, at a level sixty-six times that of an onion.* Recall from Chapter 4 that quercetin lowers body weight, creates beneficial brown fat cells to help burn down harmful white fat through thermogenesis, and lowers inflammation

---

* S. Bhagwat and D. B. Haytowitz, "USDA Database for the Flavonoid Content of Selected Foods," US Department of Agriculture, *Agricultural Research Service* Release 3.2 (2015): 1–173.

within fatty tissue itself. Capers also contain other health defense–activating bioactives such as rutin and sulforaphanes, which have antiobesity properties.[*]

Dry-cured capers have a more intense flavor and a crunchier texture than ones packed in liquid. If you use capers marinated in liquid, you'll need to do a thorough rinse to taste more caper and less salt or vinegar. You can throw whole capers into a salad or use them as a garnish on cooked fish or poultry or give them a coarse chop and integrate them into a salsa, tapenade, or cooked dish or sauce.

Cans

Tomato Paste and Canned Tomatoes

Look past the rows of jarred premade pasta sauce and find the canned tomato products (peeled whole, pureed, or crushed) and tomato paste. In my pantry, I always keep a stock of these two products. Traditionally, Italian and Greek villagers made tomato paste so that they would have tomatoes available during the winter months, but I use it all year long. Tomato paste is an ultraconcentrate of tomatoes, made by boiling away the water of fresh tomatoes. If you enjoy tomatoes, you'll love the paste ten times more because it amplifies the umami flavor.

Recall from Chapter 6 that the bioactive lycopene is found in tomatoes and is responsible for their fat-fighting properties. In clinical studies, eating tomatoes has been shown to lower body weight, decrease cholesterol and triglycerides, and lower inflammation. The lycopene in

---

[*] Y. Hashizume and M. Tandia, "The Reduction Impact of Monoglucosyl Rutin on Abdominal Visceral Fat: A Randomized, Placebo-Controlled, Double-Blind, Parallel-Group," *Journal of Food Science* 85, no. 10 (2020): 3577–3589; M. Yagi, Y. Nakatsuji, et al., "Phenethyl Isothiocyanate Activates Leptin Signaling and Decreases Food Intake," *PloS One* 13, no. 11 (2018): 1–19; Y. Liu, X. Fu, et al., "The Protective Effects of Sulforaphane on High-Fat Diet-Induced Obesity in Mice Through Browning of White Fat," *Frontiers in Pharmacology* 12 (2021): 1–13.

tomatoes is highly concentrated. Because tomatoes are cooked to make the paste, the preparation transforms the natural trans-lycopene (that is poorly absorbed by the gut) into cis-lycopene, which is readily absorbed by the gut and shuttled into your bloodstream.[43] Canned tomatoes, whole or pureed, are also good sources of lycopene. A comparative study of lycopene in tomato products was conducted by California State University, showing that tomato paste has three times the lycopene compared to tomato puree and twice as much as in commercial tomato juice.[44] So, if it's lycopene you want, go for the paste!

I like to use tomato paste that comes in a tube, which makes it convenient for cooking, and, once opened, the tube has a longer shelf life than an opened can of paste. You simply squeeze out the exact amount you need like toothpaste, recap the tube, and store it in the refrigerator. If the tube is sealed tightly, the tomato paste will last for several months.

When buying tomato paste or tomato puree, the key is to make sure the tube and the cans are not damaged. Air can spoil the product, and any leakage in the cans can lead to bacterial growth. Although you can buy premade tomato sauce in the middle aisle, I prefer to make my own sauce from canned tomatoes when I don't have fresh. This way, I can control the seasonings and know the identity of all the ingredients. I recommend you do the same. Although all tomato products have lycopene, I look for the products made with the San Marzano tomato varietal—they contain very high levels of this fat-fighting bioactive.

Spices

Cinnamon

The spice section in the middle aisles is a hunting ground for intense flavors and potent bioactive compounds. A familiar spice is cinnamon, which comes from the bark of a tree that originated in what is known today as Sri Lanka, formerly Ceylon. Cinnamon, used in China for more than four thousand years, was brought to Europe by explorers of East Asia via the Silk Road. From there, the spice made its way into the cuisines and traditional healing of cultures in India, Rome, North Africa, and the Middle East.

In the market, cinnamon is sold as both a powdered spice and as bundled sticks of curled tree bark, known as quills. This popular spice imparts a sophisticated, spicy, sweet, and citrusy flavor that is used for braising, steeping, baking, and marinating, and for sprinkling on foods and mulling for beverages.

Cinnamon contains more than twenty bioactives that can influence your metabolism.[45] Cinnamon extract causes white fat cells to become brown fat cells, and it increases the amount of uncoupling protein 1 (UPC1) in the cell, the trigger for fat-burning thermogenesis.[46] One bioactive in cinnamon is called cinnamaldehyde. This activates the TRPV1 receptor and triggers your brain to release catecholamines, the same stress hormone activated by eating chilis. As you learned earlier, this starts a chain reaction in brown fat leading to thermogenesis. Another cinnamon bioactive, eugenol, increases healthy gut bacteria in your microbiome, and this is protective against obesity.[47] In lab mice, cinnamon extracts reduce blood lipids and make it harder to gain weight.[48]

A human study of cinnamon was conducted by the Fortis-C-DOC Centre of Excellence for Diabetes, Metabolic Diseases and Endocrinology in India.[49] Researchers recruited 129 men and women, average age forty-five, who were obese and with metabolic syndrome (exhibiting at least three of the following: high blood pressure, high blood glucose, high triglycerides, low levels of good HDL cholesterol, and abdominal obesity). Half of the group were given the equivalent of one-half teaspoon (3 grams) of cinnamon to consume each day. The cinnamon was packed into capsules like a supplement so that the dosing could be precise and easy to swallow. The other half received a placebo capsule that had roasted wheat powder with cinnamon flavoring but no actual cinnamon.

For the four weeks before beginning the capsules, all the subjects were asked to begin a healthier diet that was compliant with the Dietary Guidelines for Asian Indians.[50] They were also instructed to take a forty-five-minute brisk walk each day for physical activity. They continued the healthy diet and exercise regimen while they consumed the cinnamon or placebo for sixteen weeks. Body measurements and blood tests were taken at the beginning and end of the study.

Subjects who ate cinnamon lost 7.7 pounds, which was ten times more than the amount lost by the placebo group (who lost 0.8 pounds). Cinnamon eaters also shrank their waist circumference by 2.2 inches, seven times more than the placebo group. Their elevated levels of fasting blood glucose and hemoglobin A1C improved by being lowered by 10 percent. Cinnamon also reduced the systolic blood pressure (top number) by 13 points, which was twice the reduction seen with the placebo group.

Overall, the cinnamon reduced the problems of metabolic syndrome by 35 percent, which was seven times greater than the placebo group, with no side effects reported from eating cinnamon.

You can find two main types of cinnamon in the market: Ceylon cinnamon, which is true cinnamon, and cassia cinnamon, which tastes exactly like cinnamon but is not from the cinnamon tree. Both types activate brown fat.[51] Cassia cinnamon contains a small amount of coumarin, a potent blood thinner that's only present in trace amounts in the Ceylon variety, so this can be an issue for people who are taking blood thinner for medical reasons.[52] It's wise to check the label to determine the exact type of cinnamon you are buying, and if you have any concerns about blood-thinning effects, check with your doctor. If you have any doubt, choose Ceylon cinnamon; it's the real deal.

Turmeric

While in the spice section, you'll also find turmeric. This yellow-orange spice is derived from a flowering plant related to ginger that is native to

India and Southeast Asia. The turmeric plant's stems from which the spice is extracted are rhizomes, which means they grow partially underground, just like the wasabi plant.

Turmeric has many uses. The fine yellow-orange powder is peppery and fragrant and is used in curry mixes. Turmeric is also sometimes found on ingredient lists as a natural food colorant. The brightly colored powder is used as a dye for paper, wood, textiles, and clothing, including the vibrant golden robes of Buddhist monks. What you need to know for our purposes is that turmeric is a revered medicinal herb in Ayurvedic and traditional Chinese medicine dating back more than five thousand years.[53]

A potent bioactive compound called curcumin is the star feature of turmeric. This polyphenol stimulates thermogenesis by increasing the secretion of norepinephrine to activate brown fat. Curcumin also prevents fat stem cells from developing new adipose tissue,[54] and it causes harmful white fat to transform into useful brown fat. Curcumin is also a well-documented anti-inflammatory substance, and this effect is amplified by its beneficial effect on the gut microbiome.[55] Lab studies have shown curcumin protects rats from weight gain.[56]

To see whether these metabolic effects translate to humans, a team from the University of Genoa in Italy recruited forty-four men and women, aged eighteen to seventy, who were overweight and diagnosed with metabolic syndrome.[57] The subjects were already part of a thirty-day weight-loss program, but they were considered weight-loss "nonresponders," since they were having difficulty losing weight. Despite being on a calorie-restricted diet (500 calories less per day than their usual), lifestyle interventions of seventy minutes of exercise three times per week, and counseling, they had lost less than 2 percent of their starting weight. The researchers wondered if adding curcumin to their program would activate weight loss in this group.

Half of these nonresponders received curcumin twice a day in an amount equivalent to one and one-third tablespoons of fresh turmeric.

To help the body absorb the curcumin, the subjects also received piperine, a bioactive from black pepper, in an amount equivalent to one-third of a teaspoon of pepper with each dose of curcumin.[58] Black pepper and turmeric are a natural combination in a spice mix. Clinical studies from St. John's Medical College in India showed that adding piperine can increase the blood levels of curcumin by 2,000 percent. The curcumin/piperine was taken twice a day. The other half of the nonresponder group received a placebo. They continued the same weight-loss program for another thirty days. Body measurements and blood tests were taken at the beginning and end of the study.

After thirty days, the curcumin/piperine combination caused the previous nonresponders to lose nine pounds, more than twice the weight of the group taking the placebo. The curcumin/piperine eaters also lost three times more body fat than the placebo group. The researchers estimated, in fact, that when the curcumin/piperine combination is added to calorie limitation, exercise, and nutrition counseling, it can cause a weight loss of 2.2 pounds every ten days!

The curcumin/piperine group also shrank their waistline by 1.6 inches, whereas the placebo group had no significant change. These results were in line with other clinical studies showing curcumin can lower body weight and shrink waist circumference.[59]

I suggest shopping for turmeric at your local Asian or Indian grocery store, where you'll likely find fresher batches due to faster turnover of the shelved product. A good test for the freshness of a spice is to smell it. For turmeric, the aroma should be musky and peppery. Store your turmeric powder in a dark, cool, dry place. It will last for a few years, though the aroma will fade over time. You also can find fresh turmeric rhizomes in the produce section of the market. Look for firm pieces with the skin intact. Similar to ginger, peel the skin before use, and grate or slice the yellow-orange interior. Store fresh turmeric in the refrigerator in an airtight container for a few weeks.

Dried Chili Peppers

I love trying different kinds of dried chili peppers that are classic ingredients in both Mediterranean and Asian food cultures. In the spice display, you'll find red chili pepper flakes, sometimes called crushed red pepper. This is the chili that local pizzerias keep in jars on the table for you to shake onto your slice. Crushed red pepper flakes are made from multiple cultivars such as Anaheim, serranos, and jalapeños. All contain capsaicin and capsinoids that turn on thermogenesis and cause weight loss.

In grocery stores, you'll also find dried whole peppers packaged in bags. In open-air markets or specialty shops, vendors may display them braided and hanging from the ceiling in dramatic displays. Ancho, chipotle, and Calabrian chilis are smoky-hot, while pasillas have a chocolate note, and bright-red árbol chilis are fiery-hot. The facing heaven chili (*chao tian jiao*) is a special variety featured in the spicy dishes of Sichuan Province in China. All are good sources of capsaicin and capsinoids.

How much chili spice is needed to reduce fat? Researchers at the University of Mary Hardin–Baylor in Texas added capsinoids extracted from dried red chili peppers, or a placebo, to the diet of seventy-five healthy adults, aged eighteen to fifty-six, who were overweight.[60] The dose of chili pepper was 4 milligrams per day for twelve weeks, which is comparable to one-third of a teaspoon of red pepper powder or a bit under one teaspoon of cayenne pepper powder. The subjects ate their normal diet, but those who had the chili pepper extract reported they felt less hungry, so they ate fewer calories. The chili eaters lost 0.5 pounds, while the placebo eaters *gained* 2.3 pounds.

Cacao

Dark Chocolate/Cacao

You may be surprised that I'm including chocolate in this chapter. After all, chocolate is technically a confection, and as a candy usually contains unhealthy fats, added sugar, and often artificial flavors, artificial colors, and preservatives. I'm highlighting *dark* chocolate because it is so beneficial for cardiovascular health that you can benefit from eating it (in moderation) to activate your body's health defenses. A body of lab and epidemiological evidence also demonstrates that it can combat obesity.

Cacao is a plant-based food and contains potent bioactives including proanthocyanidin, theobromine, and lycopene. It is also rich in gut microbiome–feeding dietary fiber, even in powder form.[61] Lab studies have also shown eating pure, unsweetened dark chocolate has a prebiotic benefit and can aid the growth of beneficial bacteria in the gut microbiome, an action that improves metabolism.[62] In the lab, cacao flavanols reduce the buildup of adipose tissue, and they can increase the production of UCP1, the trigger for thermogenesis in brown fat.[63] Cacao also reduces the inflammation within excess fatty tissue.[64] Another bioactive in cacao called theobromine can prevent the development of fat mass and weight gain in mice.[65]

Recall that high blood pressure is a sign of metabolic syndrome. Your arteries are normally elastic to help keep your blood flowing, but aging and obesity can stiffen them, interfering with circulation. Dark chocolate stimulates the production of nitric oxide in the body, which helps to dilate and repair stiffened blood vessels, which improves blood flow.[66]

A large study called the Healthy Lifestyle in Europe by Nutrition in Adolescence Cross-Sectional Study examined 1,458 teenagers aged twelve to eighteen from nine European countries.[67] The researchers compared the dietary intake of chocolate of these teens with their height, weight, body composition (measured by skinfold test and bioelectrical impedance of fat), and level of physical activity (measured by the accelerometry in their mobile devices). The analysis showed that teens who consumed the highest level of chocolate (42.6 grams per day)—about one standard-sized chocolate bar—had significantly lower amounts of total body fat and central abdominal fat and a smaller waist circumference, even adjusting for factors such as tea and coffee drinking and intake of other foods with fat-fighting powers.

Similar findings came from a study of 13,626 adults in their mid- to late forties living in the United States who are part of the National Health and Nutrition Examination Survey. Researchers from Anglia Ruskin University in England compared daily reported chocolate-eating habits with body composition and adiposity. They found that, regardless of the total number of calories eaten each day, people who ate any chocolate at all had a smaller waist circumference, indicating less visceral fat inside the belly. In this large epidemiological study, chocolate eating was also associated with a lower body mass.

Be aware, however, that other clinical studies have shown eating chocolate leads to weight gain.[68] That's because it is hard to control the type of chocolate people eat. Some of it is the pure, good dark stuff, but too often it's candy laden with added sugar, emulsifiers, preservatives, and fillers that are decidedly bad for your metabolism.

If you choose to eat chocolate, always look for the highest-quality dark chocolate you can find, the darker the better (I recommend chocolate with 80 percent cacao or higher), with the highest percentage of cacao and no refined sugar. Remember, the biological benefits of cacao against adipose tissue can be outgunned by the fat-fueling effects of the other ingredients. Don't wolf down the bar. Eat it slowly and savor the chocolate. Take the time to smell it. Inhaling chocolate aroma (85 percent cacao) has been shown to activate parts of your brain that stimulate satiety, or fullness,[69] so you will feel like eating less afterward.

Tree Nuts

The first nut harvests were from walnut forests in the mountains of Central Asia more than seven thousand years ago. Many types of nuts were traded along the Silk Road, from where they spread to distant lands by caravan. Today, you can usually find an entire section in the middle aisles of grocery stores devoted to different kinds of tree nuts—walnuts, almonds, pecans, macadamia, pine nuts, pistachio, and more—that you can buy in bulk.

Nuts have a trove of fat-fighting, health-boosting compounds, and epidemiological studies have shown eating tree nuts is associated with a lower risk of cancer, cardiovascular disease, diabetes, and obesity.[70] A major reason for these benefits is very likely because of the effect of nut fiber on the microbiome, which reduces inflammation, fortifies immunity, and streamlines metabolism.[71]

Tree nuts are great sources of protein, and they are energy-dense as well as high in beneficial fats. The fat in a walnut is a beneficial polyunsaturated fatty acid known as alpha-linolenic acid, which is converted in your body into omega-3 fats.

Walnuts can aid in weight loss. Researchers from the University of Wollongong in Australia[72] developed a twelve-month clinical study called HealthTrack lifestyle intervention trial, in which walnuts were one of the dietary interventions.[73] The study enrolled 175 subjects, mostly women in their early forties who were obese, and divided them into three groups. Group 1 was assigned a nurse who gave them only general dietary advice based on the Australian Guide to Healthy Eating, emphasizing more fruits, vegetables, whole grains, seafood, and lean meats, and less dairy.[74] Both Group 2 and Group 3 received highly individualized recommendations from a dietician based on daily energy targets for each individual. The dietician also provided advice on physical activity based on the National Physical Activity Guidelines of Australia. Participants of both groups also had a trained health coach speak with them every three months. The one difference: Group 3 also *added* one-quarter cup of walnuts (30 grams), which amounts to seven whole walnuts each day, to their diet. This group also received suggestions on different ways they could incorporate the walnuts in their food to keep things varied and interesting. Body weight was measured at the beginning, after three months, and at the end of one year.

The study results showed that everyone lost weight with dietary guidance. But significantly, at the three-month mark, the Group 3 walnut eaters lost 5.4 pounds, which was 23 percent more weight lost than just having personalized advice (Group 2), and 54 percent more than just receiving general advice on healthy eating (Group 1). The walnut eaters tended to eat more fruits and vegetables than the other two groups. They also ate less of the "discretionary (junk) foods" that were high in salt, saturated fat, or added sugar.

Asking people to eat seven walnuts a day without fail for one full year is a tall order. The HealthTrack subjects were extremely compliant for the first three months, leading to the weight loss I've just described. But by twelve months, only 32 percent in Group 3 were still compliant with the walnut intervention, so the weight-loss advantages were no longer seen by the end of the year.

The HealthTrack results are backed up by other studies of nuts and weight loss. The Nurses' Health Study included 51,188 women whose nut consumption habits were compared to their body weight.[75] The study concluded that those women who ate one-quarter cup (30 grams, or 1 ounce) of tree nuts two or more times per week gained 75 percent less weight, compared to women who rarely ate nuts. This was true whether the women were normal weight, overweight, or obese. Nut eaters tended to weigh less, and they were 23 percent less likely to become obese over an eight-year period.

The protective effect of nuts against obesity was also observed in a Spanish study involving 8,865 men and women. These individuals took part in the Seguimiento Universidad de Navarra follow-up project that was conducted by the University of Navarra.[76] This study, which began in 1999 and has since continued, examines whether nut consumption within the Mediterranean diet is associated with weight *gain*. Researchers sent subjects a dietary questionnaire that tracked their consumption of walnuts, almonds, hazelnuts, and peanuts. They also recorded each person's physical activity and their body weight.

The results showed that people who ate nuts at least two times per week (one-quarter cup each time) over a twenty-eight-month period had a 31 percent reduced risk of gaining weight (by more than eleven pounds), compared to people who rarely or never ate nuts. The risk of becoming obese associated with nut eating was reduced by 50 percent.

When you buy nuts, make sure you know what you are getting. Always read the ingredient label. Ideally, the nuts should not have any artificial additives that might harm your metabolism or health defenses. Whether you eat them as a snack, use them for cooking, or make trail mix with them, it's best to store tree nuts in an airtight container in a dark, cool location. They will last six months or so. After that, nuts become rancid because they contain high amounts of unsaturated fats. Keeping nuts in a sealed jar in the refrigerator will extend their life by a couple more months, and freezing tree nuts will keep them edible for about one year. If you buy commercially packaged nuts, make sure to take note of the expiration date on the label.

A final note on nuts: you can also find them in the middle aisles among cheap snack foods. Avoid the ones that have added sugar or those that have been sprayed with artificial flavorings and color.

Tinned Seafood

We are going to have an in-depth visit to the fresh seafood section in the next chapter, but the middle aisles will have stacks and stacks of canned and tinned ready-to-eat seafood tucked away. These are precious gems hidden in plain sight. Look past the generic cans of tuna that are doppelgängers for cat food (that's what I thought they were when I was a kid), and you will notice rectangular tins of sardines, mackerel, anchovies, mussels, squid, and octopus.

If you live in Europe, you will immediately recognize these as gastronomic delicacies. On their labels you often see the word *conservas* (which means "preserved")—these are carefully selected and artfully tinned seafoods from Spain, Portugal, and the South of France. If you're in one of these countries, you'll find even more exotic products in tins, such as sea urchin, cockles, razor clams, baby squid, and baby eels. These are sold in village markets, grocery stores, and specialty stores. You can now order them online. Even if you are not a seafood aficionado (yet), I recommend you take a close look at them—the packaging is usually beautiful, and the contents are metabolic health-in-a-tin.

To make these products shelf-stable, the seafood is cooked by steaming and then packed in seasoned liquid, or sometimes just brine or extra virgin olive oil. Different ingredients are then added: piquillo peppers, garlic, lemon, bay leaf, capers, or other herbs and spices that create inventive and sophisticated flavors in the final product. These are absolutely the easiest and one of the tastiest ways to eat seafood you might otherwise be a bit hesitant to buy fresh and cook, like anchovies and sardines.

The primary bioactives in seafood are omega-3 polyunsaturated fatty acids. I'm going to discuss these in detail in the next chapter, but suffice it to say, omega-3s are fat fighters that also activate all five of the body's health defense systems. They can help better your odds against the diseases people fear the most. A study of 7,142 individuals living in different regions of Italy, for example, showed that those who consumed the most tinned fish had up to a 34 percent lower risk of developing colorectal cancer.[77] A group at Hospital del Mar Medical Research Institute in Barcelona looked at people's omega-3 blood levels and found that those who regularly ate oily fish had higher levels of omega-3s, and this correlated with an increased life expectancy of almost five years—a benefit equivalent to quitting smoking—compared to those who had low omega-3 levels.[78]

From the clinical studies I'll describe in more detail in Chapter 8, eating seafood fights body fat and improves your metabolism. What's great is you don't need to eat much to receive the benefits. To help you pinpoint the amount of tinned or canned fish you need to eat, I've calculated the amount of healthy omega-3s in fresh fish that have shown fat-fighting efficacy and translated this into an equivalent amount of tinned and canned seafood you would need to eat to get the same amount of omega-3.[79] The magic number is 284 milligrams of omega-3 per serving, eaten three times a week for eight weeks. Clinical studies have shown that eating this amount of seafood can lead to almost four pounds of weight loss and a reduction in waist circumference of 1.3 inches.

I eat tinned seafood in two simple ways. For an easy lunch, I'll eat it right out of the tin along with a slice of fresh whole-grain bread and vegetables like zucchini, endive, celery, carrots, or broccoli. If I'm in the mood, I might combine these for a composed salad. Don't throw out the juice from the can; you can use it as the base for a delicious dip or dressing.

For an easy dinner, I might cook some whole wheat or squid-ink pasta and mix in the tinned seafood (sardines are one of my favorites), throw in some capers, squeeze a lemon, and sprinkle some toasted crunchy breadcrumbs on top.

Asian markets carry their own versions of packaged seafood. For a special treat, look for abalone, a marvelous mollusk. Abalone, both canned and dried, is a connoisseur's delight. In Asian culture, this pricy delicacy is often given as a gift during festive occasions. Abalone is delicious when slow-cooked in a braise with dried shiitake mushrooms and oyster sauce.

* * *

This completes our tour of the healthy finds in the middle aisle and sets the stage for our next step in our supermarket foraging: the fresh seafood section. You may already love this section, but whether you do or you don't, I predict that you will be amazed to learn what science has discovered about the benefits of eating many types of seafood. Even if you think you don't like the taste of fish or shellfish, I urge you to keep an open mind to the range of delightful flavors that exist. Many of them are not stereotypically "fishy," and all are beneficial for your metabolism. Let's go add more health to your shopping cart!

TABLE 7.1. FOOD DOSES

Food	Daily Doses
Apples (dried)	¾ cup
Barley	I cup (cooked)
Capers	3 ½ tablespoons
Chickpeas (cooked)	0.8 cup
Chili peppers (dried)	⅓ to I teaspoon
Chocolate (dark)	Standard size (41 grams) bar or less
Cinnamon	½ tablespoon
Extra virgin olive oil (EVOO)	2 tablespoons
Gochujang	2 ½ tablespoons
Kimchi	2 cups
Lentils (cooked)	¾ cup

Mushrooms:
  Oyster (dried)
  Porcini (dried)
  Shiitake (dried)
	
	I ½ cups
	3 cups
	I cup

Navy beans (cooked)	¾ cup
Peas (cooked)	¾ cup
Prunes	6 dried
Tomato paste	I heaping tablespoon

Tinned or canned fish (3 x per week):
  Anchovies
  Sardines
  Salmon
  Tuna
	
	Approx. ½ tin or can
	0.2 can (I forkful)
	¼ tin or can
	I can

Tree nuts:
  Almonds
  Cashews
  Macadamias
  Pecans
  Pistachios
  Walnuts
	
	¼ cup (23 almonds)
	¼ cup (18 cashews)
	¼ cup (12 macadamias)
	¼ cup (19 pecans)
	¼ cup (49 pistachios)
	¼ cup (14 walnut halves)

Turmeric	2 ⅔ tablespoons (plus ⅔ teaspoon freshly cracked black pepper)
Vinegar	2 tablespoons

CHAPTER 8

The Daily Catch

Yes, I know: many people have strong feelings about seafood, but regardless of your current outlook, I invite you to get to know the fish market. Beyond health, one good reason why seafood is so central to both Mediterranean and Asian cuisines is that it can be really delicious, so you might just be surprised and delighted.

What makes seafood so beneficial? Primarily, it's the omega-3s: long-chain omega-3 polyunsaturated fatty acids found in the flesh, skin, and eggs of seafood. Specifically, they are eicosapentaenoic acid (EPA) and docosahexaenoic acid (DHA). These two bioactives are made by phytoplankton (microalgae) eaten by the small fish, like anchovies and sardines, and shellfish that are low on the totem pole of the ocean's food chain.[1] The smaller fish and shellfish are eaten by larger fish, which become prey to even larger fish, and so on. Omega-3s keep building up in the flesh of larger and larger fish higher up on the food chain.

Researchers have measured the amount of omega-3s in a wide variety of seafood, and in this chapter, I'm going to tell you how much (the dose) of each of these seafood selections to eat. The dosing information was calculated by identifying the actual amount of omega-3s in each species, then calculating how much of a serving would generate the same omega-3 dose that's found to be effective for fighting fat and improving metabolism in clinical studies involving codfish. I have done all the math (it was no mean feat) for you. All you have to do is pick the seafood you enjoy, look at the food dose, and get cooking!

Seafood and Body Fat

When it comes to helping you fight body fat, omega-3s in seafood are like a Swiss Army knife: they have multiple biological uses. Omega-3s cause harmful white fat to undergo browning and become useful brown fat. Omega-3s trigger brown fat cells to start thermogenesis, which increases your metabolism by burning down harmful white fat.[2]

Researchers have learned of a clever way that omega-3s reduce the inflammation associated with excess fat.[3] Omega-3s get absorbed into fat cells and are metabolized, which creates proteins that are released like cellular firefighters into the surrounding fat mass to extinguish the inflammation caused by fat.[4,*]

Eating fish containing omega-3s can also help you *lose* body fat. Researchers from the University of Iceland studied 324 people from Iceland, Ireland, and Spain, aged twenty to forty, who were overweight or obese.[5] They were divided into four groups and assigned to eat cod, salmon, a fish oil capsule (1,300 milligrams of omega-3), or no fish or fish oil three times per week for a total of eight weeks. The researchers had everyone on a 30 percent calorie-restricted diet with a specific macronutrient composition. The caloric restriction helped ensure no one was overeating and leveled the playing field for this type of weight-loss research.

---

* Ideally, you want to counter the buildup of body fat *before* it becomes a major problem. Scientists from the University of Southampton in England, working with colleagues in Australia and the Czech Republic, studied the protective mechanism of the proteins (called specialized pro-resolving mediators, or SPM) in fifty people who were obese. They found that the existing fat in obesity is not able to generate as much SPM. This means people who are obese have a harder time battling fat inflammation. As with most things concerning your health, prevention and early intervention are more effective than waiting until disease has set in—and eating seafood can help.

After the eight-week trial, cod eaters and fish oil capsule eaters lost 23 percent more weight—a total of 10 pounds in women—compared to the no-fish eaters. The salmon eaters lost even more weight, 32 percent more, or a total of 15.4 pounds. If you are a salmon lover and want to fight body fat, dig in!

But the salmon results were not surprising. What was eye-opening in this study was that cod was also effective for weight loss. The prevailing wisdom is that you need to eat oily, fatty fish to get the benefits from omega-3s. But cod is not considered to be an oily fish—it has much less omega-3s than salmon. Cod has only 284 milligrams of omega-3 poly-unsaturated fatty acids in the serving size (5.3 ounces) that each person in the study received. Compared to an oily fish like salmon (1,565 milli-grams), cod is considered a lean fish, with 5.5 times lower omega-3 levels.

To further explore the power of cod, researchers from the same university ran another study with 126 individuals from Reykjavik, Iceland, aged twenty to forty, who were overweight or obese.[6] The same 30 percent daily caloric restriction was used for everyone to kick-start the process of weight loss. The question was, does adding cod accelerate the process? No one ate any seafood other than what the researchers gave them.

The study group was divided into thirds. One group was given no fish or seafood. The second group received cod to eat three times a week. The serving size was 5.3 ounces, a little smaller than the size of two decks of playing cards. To study the effects of more frequent food dosing, the third group was told to eat the cod five times per week. Everyone was provided specific instructions on how to prepare their meals (healthy methods of preparation, no deep-frying). Everyone's body measurements were taken at the beginning and end of the study, which lasted eight weeks.

By the end of the study, everyone lost weight, as was expected. The individuals who ate cod five times per week, however, lost 3.8 more pounds than the no-fish group. They also lost 1.3 additional inches from their waistlines. And, remarkably, those who had elevated blood pressure—a cardinal sign of metabolic syndrome—saw a beneficial drop.

This data upends the popular wisdom that only a few kinds of fish contain enough oil to be beneficial to your metabolism. Sure, oily fish, like anchovies, sardines, and salmon, have omega-3s, but they are far from being the only beneficial seafood.

This discovery means seafood with much lower amounts of omega-3s is also beneficial, and it opens the door to many other nonfatty fish and seafoods that contain "cod-level" omega-3s. As it turns out, many of these lower omega-3-level seafoods are found in the cuisine of the Mediterranean and Asia. Shellfish like clams and mussels have omega-3s, too, as do lobster, shrimp, crab, squid, and even octopus. If you are a vegan, fear not. All of the omega-3s in seafood ultimately come from algae. So you can also get your omega-3s by eating tasty seaweed, a traditional food that is prized by food cultures from Asia to Europe.

I need to point out a few facts about these Icelandic studies. First, they involved lowering daily calorie intake, which can cause weight loss by itself. Participants did not eat more food; they ate less. But adding fish as the sole intervention can *increase* the amount of weight lost. The second point is that the subjects cooked the fish in healthy ways. They did not eat deep-fried fish (sorry, fish-and-chips lovers!), nor did they cook their fish in unhealthy oils.[7] Always remember that how you cook food matters. The cooking method can turn a healthy food into an unhealthy one—or, better, make it even healthier. Baking, broiling, roasting, sautéing, steaming, and stewing are all healthy ways to cook seafood. Third, the subjects kept up with their normal levels of activity and did not become couch potatoes. You do need to stay active in order to burn calories.

Now that the gate is wide open, let's dive right in to find other seafoods that can fight fat. I want to intrigue you with the sheer variety of tasty choices, so I'll start with some of the more exotic items enjoyed by seafood enthusiasts—and save the more familiar fish until the end.

Roe

If you are exploring unique tastes, you must try the roe (eggs) of certain seafoods. Roe is naturally packed with healthy fats, so it takes remarkably little to get a major dose of omega-3s.[8]

Tarama

The dried and salted eggs of cod or other whitefish are used for a delicious traditional Greek appetizer spread called taramasalata. You can find these eggs at the seafood counter, but some stores may have premade taramasalata available. The roe is pureed with three other fat-fighting ingredients—extra virgin olive oil, lemon juice, onion—and bread, then seasoned with more lemon (it may include a touch of vinegar, which would raise the antiadipose ante). This is a heart-healthy dish packed with mouthwatering umami and a taste of the sea. Taramasalata can be used as a spread or dip for vegetables or pita. Watch out for bright-pink colors in factory-made taramosalata. Cod eggs are naturally beige in color, and the pink hue is usually from artificial food colorants that are added.

Cod eggs have slightly more omega-3s than cod meat, so you only need to eat 1.5 tablespoons of tarama to match the omega-3s in the cod serving shown to be effective in the human weight-loss studies—that's only two bites of taramasalata spread on pita bread if you eat it as an appetizer like they do in Greece.

Salmon Roe

A delicacy in Japan, salmon roe is a visual and taste delight—the eggs resemble red-orange, translucent pearls. Each egg bursts in your mouth with a delicate, briny, and slightly sweet taste. Salmon roe is used for sushi, as a topping for rice or noodles, and to make a healthy mousse.

A little-known fact is that the red color of salmon roe is from a marine carotenoid called astaxanthin. This bioactive itself can reduce inflammation within adipose tissue, and it protects the normal healthy function of preadipocytes and healthy fat cells.[9] In the lab, astaxanthin also has prebiotic effects and is beneficial for gut health.[10] It can also stimulate angiogenesis defenses to improve healthy circulation, and it protects stem cells against oxidative stress.[11]

To achieve the same amount of omega-3 from salmon roe as in the cod studies, you would need to eat only one tablespoon—the same amount that would be used to top *ikura* (salmon roe) sushi that could be eaten in a single bite.

Sea Urchin

You will know all about sea urchin roe if you are from Sardinia or Sicily, where it is called *ricci*; or Greece, where you would know it as *achinós*; or Japan, where it is called *uni*. The five orange lines of eggs lining the interior shell of fertilized sea urchins are a highly prized delicacy. They melt in your mouth and have a fresh, creamy, slightly tropical and sweet flavor that is almost aphrodisiacal. In the Mediterranean, sea urchin roe is eaten right out of the shell of a live urchin with a spoon, or it is scooped out and whipped raw into a pasta or risotto, baked as a gratin, used as a rich topping, or simply spread on toast. In Japan the roe is assembled into sushi, and it is eaten raw as street food in China.

Not only does sea urchin roe contain abundant omega-3s; it has also been found to have antibiotic activity against common bacteria.[12] Researchers have found potent antioxidant activity, which is thought to be due to the bioactive astaxanthin that, just as with salmon roe, gives the urchin roe its lovely orange color.[13]

If you are lucky, you can sometimes find live urchins the size of tennis balls in a seafood market. To get the same amount of omega-3 from eating urchin roe as in the cod studies, you'd need to eat the eggs of two medium-sized sea urchins. Each urchin has five lines of eggs inside its shell, so that would be a total of ten lines of urchin roe. More commonly, you'll see this roe sold in wooden boxes prepacked in rows of orange slivers. In this case, the dose is ten slivers out of the box.

Caviar

Author Ian Fleming first described James Bond's fondness for caviar in the 1953 novel *Casino Royale*, but the ancient Greeks wrote about these delicate fish eggs from sturgeon fish thousands of years before. The name comes from the Persian *khâvyâr*, which means "egg bearer." Originally harvested from wild sturgeon, an ancient and now endangered fish that swims in the Caspian and Black Seas, caviar became the food of noblemen and aristocrats during the Byzantine Empire more than five hundred years ago.

There are twenty-eight surviving species of sturgeon, but traditionally only three—the Beluga, Ossetra, and Sevruga—are used to produce caviar. Their roe ranges in color from dark green and gray to jet-black and has a buttery, nutty, slightly salty flavor.

Today, sturgeon aquaculture is used to provide a sustainable source of roe. Nonlethal ways of harvesting the eggs have been developed, including performing a cesarian section on the fish to retrieve the eggs, then allowing them to heal and make more. The eggs are harvested, rinsed, salted, and packed.

The cost of caviar is astronomical, so I'm certainly not recommending it as a routine way to get your healthy omega-3s, but caviar *is* famously delicious and it does contain healthy fat-fighting fats. Lab research has shown that an extract from caviar stimulates fat cells to release adiponectin, the hormone needed for a healthy metabolism.

To match the cod dose of omega-3s, you'd need to eat two tablespoons of caviar, or about 35 grams. The cost of this would be the equivalent, at this writing, of USD $100, making this an extravagant way to get your omega-3s. But it could be a luxurious treat.

Bottarga

This delicacy of the Mediterranean, a favorite of mine, is made from the edible egg pouch of the gray mullet or tuna, removed by fishermen from their day's catch. The entire pouch, eggs intact, is salted and cured, resulting in a slim, elongated solid orange block of dried roe. You can find this in a specialty food store or a seafood market, or it can be ordered online. The bottarga from Sicily and Sardinia is often considered the highest quality, but it is also found in France, Spain, Greece, Egypt, and Tunisia—all Mediterranean countries.

The flavor of bottarga is intense and briny. Connoisseurs grate it like Parmesan cheese on top of pasta or vegetables or almost any dish to impart a salty, tangy flavor. Bottarga can also be simply sliced and eaten alone as an appetizer. You can even find bottarga powder online as a salty, rich seasoning.

Bottarga does contain omega-3s, but at a level almost forty times lower than in salmon roe and twenty times lower than in tarama (cod roe). You will not be getting a full dose of omega-3s from bottarga, but by grating some onto a salad or pasta as if it were cheese, you'd get to enjoy it with the knowledge that it contributes a little bit to your omega-3 quota.

Shells and Claws

Atlantic and European Lobster

The lobster is without a doubt one of the kings of seafood. Its tender meat, which has a sweet and slightly briny flavor, is pricy, so this is a dish often reserved for special occasions. There are two types of lobsters you should know about: the American lobster (*Homarus americanus*) is from the Atlantic Ocean. The other lives in the waters from Norway all the way down to the Mediterranean. It is called *Homarus gammeris*, or the European lobster.

With a hard exoskeleton, large front claws, and eight walking legs, both the Atlantic and European lobsters are armored like tanks and live on the rocky bottom of the ocean. Lobsters can live a long time and can grow to forty or more pounds (each pound equates to about seven years of age). The ones you find in the seafood market, on ice, or sometimes alive in a tank are usually between one and three pounds. The claw and tail sections contain the treasured meat. Large lobsters over two pounds, however, have a substantial amount of leg meat worth the effort to excavate using a lobster pick.

In China, lobster is cooked by hacking it into segments and stir-frying the meat in its shell over high heat in a wok with ginger, scallions, and soy sauce. Japanese recipes call for marinating and grilling halved lobsters. American and European traditionalists boil or steam the lobster to enjoy the meat in its elemental form, dipped in vinegar (healthy and fat fighting) or butter (tasty, but not so healthy). Fancier preparations parcook the lobster, remove the meat from the shell, and combine it with a rich sauce. Lobster shells and parts can be boiled with aromatics to make an intensely flavored stock for a lobster bisque. The shells also contain the bioactive astaxanthin—the same anti-inflammatory, antioxidant, and prometabolism hormone found in the roe of salmon and in the sea urchin.

The astaxanthin explains the color of a cooked lobster. When alive, lobsters have a dark shell. This hue is the result of a substance called "crustacyanin," a cluster of pigment molecules that take on a bluish-green and brown shade when clumped together. At high cooking temperatures (boiling water, steam, hot oil), the crustacyanin molecule falls apart and the pigments are released. Astaxanthin, which is red, is one of those pigments, which is why lobster shells turn bright red-orange when cooked. Lobster stock and bisque are made by cooking down the shells. These have a reddish color due to the astaxanthin.

In addition to the meat and shell, lobsters contain two other delicacy elements, but only one that I recommend. Tomalley, a dark-green material found in the main body (thorax) of the lobster, is the hepatopancreas, a part of the lobster's digestive system. It is equivalent to the liver and pancreas of birds and mammals but combined into one organ. When cooked, the material turns light green. It has an intense, creamy, sweet lobstery flavor akin to chicken or duck pâté (since they are all liver). While connoisseurs love its taste, it does come with a serious health warning: because of the toxins in the ocean, tomalley can contain high levels of carcinogens called polychlorinated biphenyls (PCBs) as well as other toxic chemicals.[14] Even if you love the taste (which I do), I don't recommend eating lobster tomalley.

The other special food item found in female lobsters are the eggs, or roe, known as "coral." Lobster eggs are jet-black when raw, but they turn a vibrant red color when cooked. Just like the lobster shell, the roe contains astaxanthin. This alone makes lobster coral worthy of eating.[15] Chefs use the roe to make rich, lobster-flavored sauces. If you buy a female lobster to cook, you might be delighted to find some coral when you open its shell.

Both Atlantic and European lobsters have omega-3s in their meat. Researchers from Wellesley College have shown these fats actually play a role in the lobster's health by regenerating their nerves.[16] To get the same amount of omega-3 from lobster as cod, you'd need to eat the meat from one large or three smaller-sized (one-pound so-called chix) lobsters.

Spiny Lobster

It looks like a prickly lobster without claws, but the spiny lobster isn't actually a true lobster. They are their own genus with more than sixty different species. Living in the warm waters of the Caribbean and the Mediterranean and off the coasts of Australia and South Africa, spiny lobsters (also called rock lobsters) are a culinary treat. They are caught by divers or in traps and shipped to the market. Although they live in rocky holes in shallow waters, large groups of spiny lobster migrate during the winter months by touching antennae to tail and marching like soldiers in single-file groups of fifty or so, heading to warmer waters. Unlike true lobsters that are green-black when alive, spiny lobsters are naturally red-brown. Among the other traits that distinguish it from true lobsters, the spiny lobster has characteristic forward-facing protective spines on its shell, and two oversized antennae.*

The best part of a spiny lobster for eating is its tail. About a third of its body weight is tail meat. The meat is firm and sweet, and it can be cooked by grilling, sautéing, steaming, or boiling. Spiny lobster tails are often sold frozen—look for ones that are vacuum-packed to seal in the freshness. If you can find live spiny lobsters, you'll receive the addition of edible leg meat. Like true lobsters, spiny lobsters have tomalley, which is very flavorful but best avoided because of the heavy metals it can contain.[17] Tip: handle live spiny lobsters by holding their sturdy antennae, as the spines on their carapace, or body shell, can puncture your skin.

Spiny lobster tail meat is a rich source of omega-3s. You only need to eat a little more than half of an average spiny lobster tail to get the same effective dose of omega-3 for weight loss found in cod—perfect for a shared meal.

Langoustine

One of the main edible crustaceans of Europe, the langoustine, also called the Dublin Bay prawn, is a type of small lobster that only grows to about ten inches long. Its other name, the Norway lobster, is more accurate because it's neither a shrimp nor a prawn. The langoustine has large distinctive black eyes shaped like kidney beans, hence the Latin genus name *Nephrops* (*nephros* means "kidney"). Alive, their bodies are bright orange and pink. Although they do have claws, there is not much meat in them. The tail meat is the prize. This is what is traditionally used to cook "scampi" when you see the genuine article on a restaurant's menu. Shrimp is not scampi; langoustine is scampi.

---

* When threatened by predators, to repel the enemy, spiny lobsters rub the base of their antennae against a file-like organ, which makes a rasping noise that can be heard up to two miles away underwater.

If you are lucky to have a major seafood wet market nearby, you might find live langoustines, but they are difficult to keep alive after capture. Boiling, roasting, or grilling are the easiest ways to cook whole langoustines. The tail meat is harvested by commercial fishers and flash-frozen. The taste of scampi is mild and sweet, making it highly versatile for cooking and delicious to eat.

To get the same amount of omega-3s in langoustine as in cod, you'd need to eat six langoustines, just enough to fill a dinner plate. When eating a whole langoustine, don't forget to suck the head, which contains healthy fats, of which 23 percent are omega-3s.[18]

King Crab

An enormous eight-legged creature that lives on the seafloor in the cold waters of the Bering Sea between Alaska and Russia, the king crab is the largest edible crab on Earth. King crabs are a colorful species varying from red to gold, blue, and brown, and they generally weigh up to ten pounds. The largest one was reported to be twenty-four pounds. Their body is like a round armored vehicle bristling with spikes. Their leg span can be as wide as six feet. Divers report an eerie but awesome sight when they witness throngs of king crabs walking across the seabed, as they migrate from shallow water in the spring to deep-water feeding grounds.

King crabmeat is a delicacy, flaky and sweet, with just a hint of brine. Although some Chinese restaurants feature fresh Alaskan king crab, which you can select live from a wall of tanks on dramatic display, king crab is usually sold as precooked legs and frozen—and they are delicious. Live or frozen, king crab can be steamed, stir-fried with ginger and scallion, or cooked with spicy salt and pepper.

To get the same amount of omega-3 as the effective dose of cod, you would need to eat just half of one leg segment of the Alaskan king crab. Tip: to get the best part of the king crab, ask your fishmonger for the premium part called the "merus." This is the fleshiest part of the leg, the equivalent of the crab's tenderloin.

Blue Crab

Often referred to as Maryland crab or Chesapeake crab, the blue crab has blue-tinged claws with a greenish body and a white underside. The hard-shell version of these crabs is caught by the bushel and sold live in seafood markets. Part of the commercial catch of blue crabs is steamed, and the meat is carefully picked out by hand in a factory, then packed for sale.

During the early summer months, the crabs are harvested as "soft-shells," as they have just molted their hard shells. Once removed from the water, their newly forming shells will not harden, so you can eat the whole crab, shell and all. Soft-shell crabs are kept alive on ice at the seafood market. When you buy them, ask the fishmonger to clean them for you by removing their mouthparts, gills, and tail cover. Soft-shell crabs are one of my favorite seafoods. Unlike the hard-shells, you can eat the entire plump, juicy body and get all of the meat.

To get the cod equivalent of omega-3s from blue crab, you would need to eat the meat of three blue crabs.

Stone Crab

The Florida stone crab has a hard brown shell and a roundish body that makes it look like a stone, but it is famous for only one thing: its claw. Each fall, more than 2 million stone crabs are caught with traps in the shallow waters of the Gulf of Mexico and the Atlantic Coast of Florida. The crabbers measure the size of the claw—it must be a minimum of 2 ⅞ inches from the tip to the first knuckle—and if it meets the specification, it is twisted off and the crab itself is pitched back into the water, where it will regenerate its claw in a year or two. The claws are cooked and sold according to their size. Stone crab claws contain a firm, sweet meat. Crab aficionados know it as the reward for breaking open the hard claw with a hammer or a nutcracker.

There is a lot of omega-3 in a stone crab claw. To get the same effective dose as in cod, you'd only need to eat one medium-sized claw. One and done—and delicious!

Chinese Mitten Crab

Also known as the Shanghai hairy crab, the Chinese mitten crab is one of the top delicacies of China. These crabs start their life in freshwater, then migrate to saltwater as they mature, finally returning to freshwater when breeding is done. The crab is about the size of your fist, with a dark olive green-brown shell. Its defining feature is its claws, which are covered in brown fur, making them look very much like the crab is wearing hairy mittens. The "fur" is actually made of fine bristles (called "setae") whose function biologists have not yet deciphered.

"Hairy crab season" is celebrated between October and November in the region around Shanghai, when family and friends come together to dine on crabs. Stacks of live green crab, with claws and legs neatly bound in twine, are piled in crates at every fish market. They are even sold from vending machines and in subway stations. Nearly every local restaurant advertises its special hairy crab menu. When I visited my relatives in the city of Changshu during hairy crab season, I was amazed by the festive energy sparked by this crustacean. The enthusiasm was warranted, I must say—the crab is delicious, with fragrant, sweet meat.

Traditionally, mitten crab is boiled, and then the shells are cracked with a mallet. The meat is carefully picked out and dipped into a tasty sauce made from vinegar and ginger. The tomalley, or hepatopancreas, of the crab is rich in omega-3s. Perhaps because they spend much of their lives in freshwater, the tomalley of mitten crabs is safer to eat than that of lobsters. An analysis by scientists from Jiangsu University concluded that eating the tomalley did not pose a dietary health risk.[19] If you'd like to try this, look for tomalley that is yellow-colored, which contains more healthy fat.[20] Female mitten crabs are prized for their roe, which is rich, creamy, and laden with omega-3s.

The most highly prized wild mitten crabs are harvested from Lake Yangcheng in Jiangsu Province in China. But the crabs are also sustainably pond-reared for the annual celebration. The mitten crab is native to the Yellow Sea between China and Korea but somehow found its way to North America—including the Hudson River and San Francisco Bay—and to Europe in the waters of Denmark, Germany, Finland, Sweden, and Russia. Outside of Asia, these crabs are considered an invasive species because they prey on local crustaceans and overtake their territory. To enjoy them as I have—they are truly a delicious delicacy that is culturally revered—you have to travel to Asia.

The mitten crab has abundant omega-3s in its meat and eggs.[21] To get the same amount as the effective dose of cod, you'd need to eat two and a third crabs—a dose easily accomplished during hairy crab festival season.

Shrimp

One of the most popular seafoods in the world, shrimp have ten legs, a meaty tail, and long antennae. The terms "prawn" and "shrimp" are often used interchangeably, but they are not the same. Some people believe "prawn" refers to large shrimp, but there is no such distinction.

Thousands of species of shrimp populate our planet in both saltwater and freshwater. Farmed shrimp is a major industry in the seafood world. Commercial shrimpers harvest their catch in large nets and bring some of it alive to wet markets. A large portion of the catch is frozen or cooked, shelled, and then processed for shipping. The shrimp you see displayed on ice in the seafood section of a supermarket was most likely previously frozen and thawed. You can also go to the freezer section and buy frozen shrimp by the bag.

Shrimp is also a feature of many Mediterranean and Asian recipes and can be prepared in a multitude of ways—steamed, boiled, grilled, sautéed, wok-seared, and deep-fried (not recommended for health). They can be eaten plain or with a sauce, with vegetables or pasta, or in a rice dish like risotto. Shrimp can also be stuffed into the center of a piece of tofu, which is a classic Cantonese dish you'll find on some Chinese restaurant menus.

Most often shrimp is sold with just the tail still attached. You can find head-on shrimp in fresh markets, and in Asia shrimp is often cooked with the head on. Food connoisseurs know that when whole shrimps are cooked, you can suck the head section and get an intensely flavored shot of shrimp liquid that multiplies the taste of the tail by a factor of ten.

A number of useful bioactives have been found in shrimp. They contain the fat fighter astaxanthin in the head and shell. Bioactive peptides with antioxidant activity are present in fermented shrimp pastes.[22] They are also decent sources of omega-3s. To get the same amount as was found effective in the clinical studies of cod, you would need to eat four medium-sized shrimp—perfect for a meal.

Mantis Shrimp

Beautiful and bizarre, this tasty crustacean looks like a cross between a praying mantis, a shrimp, and a colorful caterpillar.* The mantis shrimp is found in waters throughout the world, and they are commonly sold live in the wet markets of the Mediterranean (especially Venice and Barcelona) and in Hong Kong and other seaport cities of China, Vietnam, and Japan. I've rarely seen them in the United States, although they do live in Maryland's Chesapeake Bay and off the coast of South Carolina. They are beautiful specimens for marine aquarists, and they can grow as long as ten inches or more.

All available mantis shrimp in the market is brought to you by fishing trawlers or from artisanal fishers who specialize in catching mantis shrimp for seafood wet markets.[23] The live mantis shrimp can be boiled, grilled, pan-roasted, stir-fried, or sautéed with a variety of sauces. Mantis

---

* Marine biologists will tell you that the mantis shrimp is an underwater martial artist. It uses its foreclaws to stun its prey by punching them like a boxer whose fists fly at fifty miles per hour. They strike with the force of a bullet. So powerful is each blow that a cavitation bubble forms in front of the claw, producing a shock wave like a torpedo hitting a battleship. When a mantis shrimp goes after a crab for dinner, its strikes literally remove the claws of the crab as it delivers a knockout blow.

shrimp is eaten as sushi and sometimes appears on the menus of fine dining restaurants. In Taiwan, Thailand, or Vietnam, you can find them as street food. The tail section contains all the meat, which is sweet and tender. Preparing mantis shrimp involves cutting into the shell of the tail before cooking to make removing the meat easier.

Like other crustaceans, mantis shrimp contain omega-3s.[24] To get the amount equivalent to the cod dose, you would need to eat three mantis shrimp—a nice dinner portion.

Just the Shell

Oysters

Oysters have been a prized seafood since ancient times. Their shells have been found by archaeologists in middens, ancient kitchen trash piles dating back thousands of years. Oysters are flat shellfish found in brackish waters and are cultivated today in many parts of the world. Certain species are farmed for food, while others are raised to create pearls. The United Kingdom, coastal Europe, the Pacific Northwest, Australia, and Japan are among the best-known regions for farming oysters for seafood markets.

Your idea of eating oysters may be slurping them raw off a half-shell accompanied by a mignonette dipping sauce. But there are many cooking methods for oysters, including grilling, broiling, steaming, or sautéing the meat out of the shell. Smoking and frying are popular and tasty ways to cook oysters, but not recommended for health. Oysters are also used as ingredients in stews and soups.

It is a fair amount of work to buy fresh oysters and to shuck (open their shells) them at home. But the effort is worth it. You'll get soft, creamy meat bathed in a briny juice. Pro tip: use an oyster knife and wear a glove to protect your hand from the blade and shells. Discard any oysters with a broken or crushed shell. If you are cooking the oysters, take care not to overcook them, since the meat can become tough and chewy. If shucking is too much work, don't worry; preshucked oysters in containers are often for sale in the seafood section. Oysters can also be found in the middle aisles, cooked, smoked, and tinned.

Oysters contain a number of bioactives, including polysaccharides, peptides, and omega-3s. They obtain their healthy fats from the plankton they feed on. Bioactive extracts from oysters stimulate the immune system and have potent antioxidant and antitumor effects.[25] When it comes to omega-3s, you only need to eat three medium-sized oysters to get the same amount as the dose in the weight loss studies using cod. What a nice appetizer!

Mussels

Another prized seafood that has an eight-thousand-year culinary history is the mussel. Mussels have an oval shell that is thicker on one end, and they are jet-black with tinges of blue or orange and green, depending on their species. You will find them in markets along coastal Europe, from Scotland to Spain to Italy, and along the coastlines of North America. Mussels have been cultivated since at least the thirteenth century. They are grown on wooden poles to which they become attached in clumps.*

Mussels in the seafood market are sold alive on ice, sometimes packed in burlap or mesh bags. They cook very quickly and can be steamed, pan-roasted, or sautéed. When preparing mussels, examine their shells carefully. Discard any with cracked or smashed shells. When you bring them home, look for any mussels with open shells and tap the shell lightly. It should snap shut, indicating the mussel is still alive. If the shells do not close, the mussel is dead and should be discarded.

To prepare mussels, simply soak them for fifteen minutes in a bowl filled with cold water. This allows them to expel any sand or debris that might be trapped inside their shells. During cooking, the mussel shells

---

* Mussels anchor themselves to surfaces using unique threads that project from their shells. The threads are called the "byssus," which chefs refer to as the "beard."

will open, releasing their tasty juices. There's a myth that mussels that don't open during cooking should be discarded. That is incorrect! Those that have not opened simply haven't fully relaxed the shell muscle that holds them closed during cooking. Just take a sharp knife and insert the point between the shells to twist them open. The meat will be perfectly cooked and safe to eat.

Mussels feed on omega-3-rich plankton floating in the sea, so they are loaded with healthy fats—so much so that pet foods are made with mussels to provide dogs with healthy omega-3s that reduce joint inflammation. Lab researchers have also discovered that the meat of mussels has antioxidant properties.[26]

If you want to enjoy a bowl of ten to twelve mussels, you would get the same amount of omega-3s as the cod studies—enough for a satisfying meal.

Razor Clams

The razor clam was named for its unique shape: it resembles an old-fashioned straight razor. These six- to nine-inch-long clams are harvested individually by raking the sand in the intertidal zones of the Atlantic and Pacific Oceans, European coast, and Asia. Razor clams are remarkable diggers. They hide in the sand, and, to escape predators, they can bury themselves vertically at a rate of half an inch per second by jetting a stream of water from the bottom end of their vertically held shell to essentially create quicksand below it. The clam then extends its foot through the loosened sand and contracts its body to descend more deeply.[27]

You'll never forget the delicious meaty and sweet flavor of a razor clam. You can find live ones in a wet market. To clean them, just rinse to remove any sand. The best way to cook a razor clam is also simple. Place them on a griddle or in a pan with some extra virgin olive oil or steam them for about five minutes until their shells pop open and release their juices, which can be used as a natural sauce.

Razor clams have abundant omega-3s. To get the same amount as the effective dose in cod, you'd need to eat only three—so tasty!

Sea Scallops

With colorful radially patterned flat shells the size of a coffee saucer or even bigger, sea scallops are among the largest shellfish in the seafood market. Their edible meat is called the "nut" and is firm and sweet. Sea scallops can be broiled, roasted, steamed, or pan-seared. Unlike mussels, sea scallops are not anchored to rocks. Instead, a scallop moves about by opening and closing its shell quickly, using a form of jet propulsion to propel itself forward in the water.

Commercial scallopers dredge the seafloor to harvest them, but this damages the seafloor and its ecosystem, so a more sustainable approach is for divers to harvest them by hand. This is why you see the name "diver scallop" in the seafood market or on restaurant menus—it signals that the scallop was caught manually.

In a seafood market, you might find live sea scallops in their shells on ice. The shells may be cracked open slightly, but, like mussels, tapping them will cause them to snap shut in defense. When you find sea scallop meat already separated from the shells, it usually indicates that they were thawed from a catch that was frozen at sea. The process of removing the nut and flash-freezing it is called dry packing. This is the best form of frozen scallop.

Scallops can also be "wet-packed." This means that, before freezing, the nut is soaked in a chemical solution called sodium triphosphate that helps the color of the meat remain bright white and preserves the flesh to extend its shelf life. The treatment also helps the meat absorb 30 percent more water, making the scallops heavier. Wet-packed scallops can have a slightly soapy taste, and the retained water is released when they are cooked, which effectively steams the scallop meat rather than allowing them to form a brown crust. For this reason, I recommend dry-pack scallops as the best choice for cooking.

Off the coast of Japan, the giant Ezo scallop (also called the Yesso scallop) is used by master chefs for sashimi, ceviche, or seared scallop dishes. They are prized for their orange roe, in which researchers from Hokkaido University have discovered a new marine carotenoid called pectenovarin.[28] Since carotenoids such as astaxanthin have potent anti-obesity and other biological effects, you can add pectenovarin to the list of Mother Nature's "farmacy."

Sea scallops nuts are large, about 1 ½–2 inches around, and are not to be confused with the tiny marble-sized nuts of bay scallops that come from the cold, shallow water of the Atlantic. All scallops feed on plankton, so they imbibe healthy omega-3s that accumulate in their flesh.[29] To get the same amount of omega-3 as the effective dose of cod in clinical studies, you'd need to eat only four sea scallops.

Tubes and Tentacles

Sea Cucumber

Sea cucumbers get their name because they are shaped like their namesake—except they have a soft, leathery body. Populating the floor of every ocean at great depths, they are a relative of the starfish and sea urchin.* There are more than one thousand species of sea cucumber, and they play an important role in maintaining the health of the seafloor. By digesting the detritus from marine life that sinks to the bottom and expelling it as nutrients, sea cucumbers are the ocean's recyclers.

Traditionally, they are collected singly in shallower waters by divers from boats, but sea cucumber farms have sprung up in China, Indonesia, Australia, and the Maldives in the Indian Ocean. In Asia, you will find live sea cucumbers in plastic buckets of seawater at the wet markets. They are fascinating to see when you are visiting the market, and I've

---

* The sea cucumber is an echinoderm, which in Greek means "hedgehog skin," referring to the texture of their outer layer.

also seen them on the sandy bottom while swimming in the Mediterranean Sea.

Eaten as part of traditional Chinese medicine for thousands of years, sea cucumbers have surprised modern scientific researchers, who discovered some attention-worthy properties in this seafood.[30] An extract from the bodies of ten different kinds of sea cucumbers can reduce body weight and improve blood lipids in lab mice fed a high-fat diet.[31] Yet another bioactive, called a triterpenoid saponin, can reduce the size of harmful visceral fat cells.[32]

To cook sea cucumbers, boil them for as long as an hour to soften the flesh. Then chop the meat into pieces and slowly braise until they are fork-tender with a jellylike consistency. Be sure to include other ingredients such as shiitake mushrooms, garlic, and oyster sauce because the meat of the sea cucumber is bland, but it readily absorbs the delicious flavors of the braise.

Sea cucumbers contain omega-3s. To get the same amount as the effective dose of cod, you would need to eat an amount of sea cucumber the size of two decks of playing cards, which would be a generous helping at dinner.

Squid

If you enjoy calamari, then you have eaten squid. A popular item on Mediterranean and Asian menus, squid is cooked in many different ways: grilled, stir-fried, or deep-fried. Squid have soft tubelike bodies, large eyes, eight arms, two tentacles, and a hard internal cartilage shaped like a knife blade, called the gladius, which resembles a medieval feather quill pen (the gladius is also known as the "pen"). They also have a small sac that contains jet-black ink that the animal squirts into the water to create a dark cloud as it escapes predators. The name "calamari," in fact, comes from the Latin calamarium, which means "inkpot" or "reed pen."

Although giant squids really do exist (inspiring the legendary Kraken, a mythical ship-sinking Nordic sea monster), the squid you are most likely to encounter in the seafood market is the longfin species, a mere seven to ten inches in length. For cooking, their entire body can be cut into rings or strips. The arms and tentacles are tasty parts that are sometimes cooked separately. One of my favorite squid recipes is a stir-fry with garlic, pepper, onions, and a black bean sauce. I also enjoy calamari stuffed with pine nuts, raisins, parsley, chopped tentacles, and breadcrumbs. Go beyond ordering deep-fried squid (delicious but unfortunately not healthy), and you'll find there are many ways to enjoy it MediterAsian style.

Squid ink is rarely used for cooking (the sac is tiny, and it would take a lot of squid to yield much ink), but it stimulates all five of the body's health defense systems, yielding antiangiogenic, pro-regenerative, and anti-inflammatory properties.[33] The substance called "squid ink" on restaurant menus is usually ink from the cuttlefish, not squid (see following discussion).

Squid bodies and tentacles contain healthy omega-3s. For a cod-equivalent dose of squid, you'd need to eat ten average-sized squid tubes (because they are thin) or just three squids' worth of tentacles (which are meaty and dense, packed with omega-3s).[*]

Cuttlefish

This cousin of the squid is known as the "chameleon of the sea" for its ability to change color. In fact, the cuttlefish is better at blending into a background than a true chameleon.[**] Within one second it can transform its skin colors into fourteen different complex patterns to express its emotions (fear, anger) or to camouflage itself from predators. Cuttlefish have tentacles and a body similar to a squid, but cuttlefish are squatter and wider.

---

[*] Squid tentacles are denser and are solid meat, compared with the tubes, which are hollow, so you get more omega-3s. They are also not technically all tentacles—they are called appendages. Each squid has eight arms and two true tentacles, giving each squid ten total appendages.

[**] True chameleons can change their colors only in a limited manner, and they cannot truly mimic the exact patterns of their surrounding environment. Cuttlefish can.

Cuttlefish are popular in Mediterranean cuisine. You'll see them prominently displayed in the famous Rialto Fish Market in Venice, Italy, and the Mercado de la Boqueria in Barcelona, Spain, where their ink sacs are as prized as their flesh. The black ink, when cooked, delivers a briny and rich umami flavor that colors anything you cook it with a dramatic jet-black.

Seppie al nero is a delicious Venetian dish made with cuttlefish cooked in its own ink. In fact, the "squid ink" used for pasta, risotto nero, or black paella is actually cuttlefish ink! In the lab, cuttlefish ink has powerful antioxidant and anticancer properties against breast cancer cells.[34] Interesting fact: fossils of giant prehistoric cuttlefish from 160 million years ago revealed that the ink from the past is exactly the same as it is today, making this one of the world's oldest healthy ingredients.[35]

Dried cuttlefish is shredded and sold as a popular snack food in Asian markets. A different preparation is a popular Cantonese dish of marinated orange-colored braised cuttlefish. The entire cuttlefish is hung from hooks in food stalls and sliced at home. A stir-fry recipe for cuttlefish uses ginger, garlic scapes, chili bean paste, and vinegar, making it a quintet of fat-fighting ingredients.

Cuttlefish eat crab and shrimp, so they accumulate the omega-3s from their prey and this builds up in their body and tentacles.[36] To get the same amount of omega-3 as the effective dose of cod in clinical studies, you would need to eat 4.7 ounces of cuttlefish, an amount roughly the size of one and a half decks of playing cards.

Octopus

The octopus is the defining traditional seafood dish of Greece, one of my favorite Mediterranean countries when it comes to simple, healthy eating. Octopus salad or a grilled tentacle with extra virgin olive oil, a splash of red wine vinegar, oregano, and lemon—these are what I associate with seaside cafés on the Greek islands. I have even twice caught octopus myself in the sea. The first time, in Crete, after it was tenderized in the traditional way, the chef at a local taverna cooked it by simmering it gently then grilling it. Delicious. The second time, in Sardinia, I handled the octopus gently in order to observe its remarkable behavior before letting it swim back into its rocky hole in the sea.

Octopus is highly perishable, so unless you live by the sea, what you find for sale in the seafood market is most likely frozen and then thawed for display. Although the entire body is edible, most recipes just call for the tentacles. The flesh of octopus is firm and has a mild, slightly meaty flavor. Besides grilling, you can braise octopus. Its tentacles become tender, and the meat absorbs the flavors of the braise.

If you are a true food adventurist, you can dare to try a Korean dish called *san-nakji*. This is octopus sashimi but with a twist: the tentacles are cut into pieces while the octopus is still alive, and the pieces keep wiggling vigorously as they are dipped in sesame oil. The nerve fibers in the tentacles will continue to fire for quite a long time, creating a spectacle at the table. When you eat the octopus's bits, you are supposed to chew quickly to break them down or risk having the suction cups stick in your throat and become a choking hazard.* I was once a guest of honor at a lunch in Busan, Korea, where *san-nakji* was served. Was it a bit shocking? Yes. Was it delicious? I have to say, it had a wonderful briny taste—like the freshest sashimi you can imagine.

Korean researchers discovered in the lab that natural chemicals extracted from octopus meat have potent antioxidant effects.[37] They are a good source of omega-3s.[38] For a cod-like dose, you'd eat a three-ounce portion of octopus, which is equivalent to one large portion of a cooked tentacle, which could be an entrée. Combined with tomato, red onion,

---

* Although this has been reported in the news, it's uncommon to be choked by a writhing tentacle, and this likely is more urban legend intended to heighten the theater and fear factor of eating *san-nakji*.

sliced jalapeño, extra virgin olive oil, and vinegar, a fresh octopus salad makes a sextet of fat-fighting ingredients.

Fins

Halibut

You will see only its precut steaks and fillets in the seafood market, but the halibut is the largest flatfish in the Atlantic and Pacific Oceans. It can grow to be eight feet long and weigh over five hundred pounds. Halibut is fished for sport as well as commercially. The flesh is tender, white, and flaky. It has a delicious, mild flavor when baked, roasted, and grilled. Halibut is also used for making fish chowders.

You would not need to eat much halibut to get the same amount of omega-3 as in the cod studies, only a piece about half the size of a deck of playing cards. Besides its omega-3s, halibut is a good source of vitamin D.

Sea Bass

You'll see the term "sea bass" in markets and menus, but this is a generic name that refers to several types of fish. The European, or Mediterranean, sea bass, also called branzino, is one of the most popular fish in Europe and North America. The ones you'll find in the supermarket usually come from fish farms in Greece, Turkey, and Egypt. Black sea bass is another species entirely, related to the grouper, that is caught in the Atlantic Ocean. Its meat is firm and sweet, making it popular in Chinese cooking. The striped bass is a completely different species found off the Atlantic Coast of North America. It has dark lines resembling racing stripes running along its sides, hence its nickname "striper." These fish are farm-raised as well as line-caught in the wild and brought to the market by fishers.

The Chilean sea bass is not a true bass at all (the name was invented by Lee Lantz, a clever marketer and fish wholesaler in 1977 to make it

sound appealing to American consumers). Its real name is the Patagonian toothfish, and it is fished in deep waters off the Patagonian Conti-
nental Shelf. You'll find it in seafood markets as thick cuts of white-fleshed
fish that tastes buttery because it is loaded with omega-3s.[39]

All of these "sea bass" species are delicious because of their firm,
white flesh and sweet taste. They can be grilled, roasted, pan-seared,
baked, broiled, steamed, or eaten as sashimi. Sea bass are highly versatile for cooking, and any one of them pairs well with lemon, orange,
tarragon, thyme, fennel, dill, paprika, ginger, and garlic.

Researchers have discovered bioactives in both the skin and meat of
sea bass.* To get the same amount of omega-3 from sea bass as the cod
studies, you'd need to eat a piece the size of one and one-third decks of
playing cards.[40]

Hake

The hake is a deep-water fish whose flesh has a milder and sweeter taste
than its relative, the cod. A popular fish on Mediterranean menus, it is
known in France as *merlu* (its Latin name is *Merluccius*) and in Spain as
merluza. In England, hake fillets are battered and fried for the classic pub
dish known as fish-and-chips. In Asia, hake is ground into a fish paste,
which is then fashioned into sticks of imitation crabmeat known as
surimi (Japanese for "ground meat").** You can pan-fry, poach, or roast
hake, or cook it as part of a stew, using either a Mediterranean- or Asian-
style recipe.

Researchers from the Instituto de Investigaciones Marinas in Spain
examined the skin and bones of the European hake and found peptides

---

* In the lab, sea bass skin peptides have been shown to speed wound healing, reduce inflammation, and beneficially change gene expression for repair of injured cells. Studies conducted at the China Medical University in Taiwan showed that sea bass peptides can
stimulate angiogenesis defenses to help accelerate wound closure in mice.
** Surimi is just processed fish molded into a shape, like meat used in a meatball. I recommend checking the ingredients to make sure there are no artificial colors or flavor enhancers
added.

with potent antioxidant properties.[41] Hake flesh is also rich in omega-3, which comes from its diet of smaller fish.

To get the same amount of omega-3 as the effective dose of cod in clinical studies, you would need to eat a serving of hake about the size of a deck of playing cards.

Sea Bream

The sea bream is a popular eating fish, especially the gilt-head bream, which is recognized by a bright-gold band between its eyes that resembles the nose bridge of eyeglasses. In Italy, it is known as *orata*; in France, as *daurade*; and in Spain, as *dorada*. The sea bream's flesh is firm and has a rich taste with no trace of fishiness, making it a good choice for fish first-timers.

Most of the gilt-head breams you'll find in the fish market come from fish farms in Greece and Turkey, although sometimes they are wild-caught. Black sea bream is another species with a delicate, sweet taste you will find on restaurant menus.

When you buy a whole bream, it should be firm, with clear eyes and pink gills. Ask the fishmonger to scale and gut the fish for you. The whole fish can be baked with lemon and garlic or grilled. A Cantonese way of cooking a whole bream is to steam it with rice wine, soy sauce, sesame oil, ginger, and scallions.

You can also have the bream filleted. If you cook with fillets, however, you will first need to remove the "pin bones" (they are actually small, calcified ligaments, not bones) from the flesh. Use a pair of tweezers to pick out the ligaments. To cook a fillet, score it on the skin side, then pan-fry the bream with some extra virgin olive oil for a delicious, crisp skin, or you can poach it for a more delicate flavor. You can make a sauce of tomatoes, garlic, olives, herbs, and capers to accompany it.

Sea bream acquire their omega-3s from their diet of small fish and crustaceans. Farmed breams are sometimes fed seaweed to enhance their omega-3 content, and their feed is sometimes even enhanced with olive oil extracts to increase their overall bioactive levels.[42]

To get the same amount of omega-3 in sea bream as the effective dose of cod, you'd need to eat a serving just over half the size of a deck of playing cards. A light meal.

Dover Sole

Featured on the menu of many traditional fine dining restaurants, the Dover sole is a cousin of the flounder. Its name comes from the town of Dover, England, which was in the nineteenth century the biggest market supplier of this fish to Londoners. The white flesh has a mild, sweet flavor. Dover sole is often cooked whole, bone in, and filleted just before serving, often with a delicate sauce. Try ordering it at a restaurant to taste how a chef would prepare it, but don't be afraid to cook it yourself at home—its mild flavor and easy handling makes it a delicious crowd-pleaser, even for people who don't normally love fish.

With roughly the same amount of omega-3 as the sea bream, you would eat a serving half the size of a deck of playing cards to get the effective dose as in the cod studies.

Turbot

Shaped like a diamond, the turbot is a prized fish with flaky, white meat that is perfect for baking, poaching, or sautéing. It is a type of flounder that produces large fillets as well as "kernels" of tasty fatty meat where the fins meet its body. Wild-caught turbot flesh has a firm texture, and it has an even nicer flavor than farmed turbot, which is also delicious. Check the origin of the fish with your fishmonger. Frozen fillets may be labeled "European turbot," but it is sometimes another species of flounder and not the real deal. Fresh turbot is the best choice, so ask your fishmonger if it is available.

To obtain the cod dose of omega-3 from turbot, you'd want a serving the size of one and one-third decks of playing cards.

Mackerel

The mackerel is an open-ocean fish that migrates in large schools. Its distinctive vertical black stripes on an iridescent upper body give it the appearance of sporting war paint. The stripes play a role in its swimming—they provide visual cues to fellow mackerel as they swim together in fast-moving schools. The position and movement of the stripes tell the mackerels when to make adjustments in their swimming speed and direction based on what is happening with their neighbor.

Mackerel flesh is dark-colored and rich-tasting. It's similar to tuna but more buttery and sweeter. Despite what you might believe, mackerel can taste less fishy than salmon. It is prized by chefs because its big flavor allows it to pair well with other ingredients and sauces. Fresh mackerel must reach the market quickly because its high oil (omega-3) content quickly spoils the fish. Try some tinned mackerel for a quick, convenient, and tasty way to eat this fish—this is considered a delicacy in the Mediterranean region (look for it in the middle aisles).

There are more than thirty different species of mackerel, but the ones most commonly seen in fish markets are the Atlantic mackerel, Spanish mackerel, and king mackerel. Be aware that king mackerel is known to contain high levels of mercury, so I recommend avoiding this species.[43]

Scientists have discovered eye-opening bioactivity in mackerel. The meat of the Pacific mackerel contains bioactive peptides that are powerful antioxidants.[44] Researchers from Laval University in Canada have also discovered antibacterial peptides in the Atlantic mackerel.[45] Other researchers working in the lab have studied mackerel skin and found a protein that has blood pressure–lowering and blood-thinning properties.

If you can find fresh mackerel, try pan-frying its fillets or grill or poach the whole fish. Pacific mackerel is popular in China, Japan, Thailand, and Korea, where it is prepared in many different ways. You can find it as street food or as a more elaborate dish braised with ginger and soy.

Mackerel is a true metabolic powerhouse. It is so chock-full of healthy fat that to get the same amount of omega-3 as in the cod studies, you'd only need to eat one flavor-packed forkful!

Sardine

Also known as pilchard, the sardine is a time-honored seafood of the Mediterranean. Caught at night by drawing schools of the fish into a wide, encircling net, commercially caught sardines are sold fresh for the market as well as packed into tins with olive oil and herbs.

Sardines have tender and oily meat with a strong, slightly salty flavor. When cooked properly—they are excellent grilled, roasted, or poached and dressed with extra virgin olive oil, garlic, lemon, and herbs—a sardine will make you appreciate why this fish is considered a delicacy in Portugal and Spain and why it is so appreciated by food connoisseurs.

Sardines contain bioactive peptides that can improve metabolism.* In the lab, these peptides lower blood cholesterol, decrease the fat hormone leptin, and reduce weight gain when fed to laboratory rats.[46] Low on the ocean's food chain, sardines feed on omega-3-producing plankton. As a result, their bodies are rich in these healthy fats.

To get the same amount of omega-3 as the effective dose of cod in clinical studies, you would only need to eat one quarter of a sardine—another fish that delivers its benefit in a single forkful.

Anchovy

These small blue-green fish caught along the coasts of Mediterranean countries are featured in seafood markets throughout Europe.** They are a star ingredient in many Italian and Spanish recipes. In addition to

---

* Sardines are also a good source of vitamin D.

** In ancient Greece and Rome, anchovies were once used to make a rich umami sauce called *garum*. Garum was created by fermenting anchovy guts, which yielded a mouthwatering rich, savory paste used to flavor meats, fish, vegetables, and other dishes. Garum factories once populated the lands known today as Portugal, Spain, France, and Italy.

being available fresh, anchovies are sold in tins and jars, cured with salt and brine, or packed in olive oil.

Fresh anchovies can be pan-fried whole, or they can be scaled and filleted, then marinated with olive oil and lemon. Tinned anchovies can be cooked into a pasta dish, made into a paste, added to a salad, or used as a pizza topping. A traditional Provençal dish called *pissaladiere* is a pastry crust topped with caramelized onions, olives, garlic, and anchovy fillets. Chinese recipes use anchovies in stir-fries with onion, ginger, and garlic.* Tiny dried anchovies are added to sautéed bok choy with garlic and soy sauce to give the vegetable an umami twist. A Korean side dish called *banchan* is made by stir-frying dried baby anchovies with chili sauce and sesame seeds. Anchovies are also used to make Vietnamese fish sauce. In whatever form you eat them, anchovies deliver a potent dose of healthy fat-fighting omega-3s.

Another delicious anchovy product is *colatura di alici*, made in the fishing village of Cetara on Italy's Amalfi Coast. This amber-colored liquid is the Mediterranean equivalent of Vietnamese fish sauce; it is the dripping from salted anchovies that are aged in brine for up to three years. Colatura di alici can be used to make a potent salad dressing, a sauce for braised green vegetables, or as a wonderful baste for roast chicken. A simple spaghetti made with only three ingredients—colatura di alici, garlic, and pasta—is one of the tastiest Italian dishes you'll ever have, and a delicious way to obtain your omega-3s.

Anchovies are at the bottom of the food chain, and they feed directly on omega-3-producing plankton. Their flesh is thus naturally oily. You would need to eat only three anchovies, hardly one bite, to get the cod-equivalent dose.

---

* Researchers from Zhejiang Ocean University in China have discovered that anchovies produce a bioactive protein in their meat. This peptide has antibacterial properties that can kill the bacteria E. *coli*. Other researchers have discovered anchovy proteins that lower blood cholesterol and reduce inflammation when fed to lab mice. Anchovies are also a good dietary source of vitamin D.

Seaweed

If you want to obtain some marine omega-3s from a meatless source, seaweed is an excellent choice. Seaweed has a rich umami flavor and is a wonderful complement to fish and shellfish dishes. Certain seaweeds are able to synthesize their own omega-3s, but they also contain other bioactives that can boost your metabolism and health defenses.

Seaweed is very much a part of the traditional cuisine of Asia and some parts of Europe. Sea farmers grow different species in floating nets as an important food source. Adding seaweed to your diet is a nutritious and tasty way to top off your dose of healthy marine fats. The various types of edible seaweeds are also good sources of iodine, vitamins, minerals, and a fat-fighting bioactive known as fucoxanthin.

Wakame

You will have eaten wakame if you've ever ordered seaweed salad in a Japanese restaurant. In the salad, wakame is mixed with sesame seeds. It has a slightly sweet flavor and a silky texture. Wakame is also used as a sea vegetable in miso soup.

Research from the Centre for Environmental and Marine Studies at the University of Aveiro in Portugal has shown that wakame has one of the highest concentrations of omega-3s among all the edible seaweeds.[47] It also contains the bioactive fucoxanthin, a carotenoid that gives the seaweed its distinctive brown color.

Scientists at Hokkaido University in Japan discovered that fucoxanthin causes fat cells to increase their production of uncoupling protein 1 (UCP1), the trigger for thermogenesis that increases metabolism.[48] When lab animals are fed fucoxanthin from wakame, the thermogenesis shrinks white adipose tissue.*

---

* Fucoxanthin performs other health duties as well. It boosts the angiogenesis defenses with cancer-starving properties. It causes tumor cells to undergo self-destruction, a process called apoptosis, or programmed cell death. Remarkably, lab studies show that fucoxanthin also

You can buy fresh or prepared wakame in the seafood section or an Asian market, and you'll find packages of dried wakame in the international section of many grocery stores. To get the same amount of omega-3 as the effective dose of cod in clinical studies, you'd only need to eat one-tenth of a cup of wakame. That's about two bites of a seaweed salad in a sushi bar.

Kelp (Kombu)

One of the largest seaweeds in the ocean, kelp forms underwater forests from the bottom of the seabed, with long, twisting blades extending up toward the surface. Also known as "kombu," kelp has been eaten in Asia for centuries. Kombu is an umami-packed food that adds flavor to soups, and it is also eaten as a dried snack.*

Researchers from Guangdong, China, discovered that kelp has anti-obesity effects.[49] In the lab, they fed kelp to obese mice eating a high-fat diet and found it suppressed the development of adipose cells and improved their metabolism. Kelp lowered the mice's appetite and reduced their food intake by causing their gut and brain to release more glucagon-like peptide-1 (GLP-1). This is a metabolic hormone that diminishes hunger and prompts the body to secrete more insulin, making metabolism more efficient.

Kelp is a good seaweed source of omega-3s, and you can find it fresh in many Asian markets and seafood markets, and the dried form can be ordered online. To get the cod equivalent, you would only need to eat one-third of a cup of kelp.

---

prevents the growth of colon cancer stem cells. Some of this bioactive's anticancer effects appear to result from its ability to modify the gut microbiome by increasing the presence of beneficial bacteria. Korean scientists from Dongguk University also discovered that fucoxanthin has potent anti-inflammatory activity.

* Commercially, kelp is also the source of alginate, a material used by the food industry as a thickener, a coating, and an additive for ultraprocessed foods. Europeans burned kelp to make ash for making glass and soaps in the 1800s.

Dulse

Dulse is a branched seaweed with red and purple fronds and a single stem (stipe) that anchors it to rocks on the seafloor. Its culinary roots lie in Ireland, Scotland, and England. Traditionally, dulse was collected at low tide, cleaned of any attached snails, then dried on rocks.

Dulse has a unique savory, smoky umami flavor that is likened to bacon. One of its natural compounds is glutamic acid, which is a potent natural flavor enhancer. Although this is the same substance found in monosodium glutamate (MSG), in its natural form, glutamic acid does not cause headaches or other effects some people experience with MSG. Dulse is eaten fresh or dried and can be found in seafood markets that carry fresh seaweed. It can be steamed or pan-fried, used in chowders and stews, or baked into a traditional white soda bread or scones. You can also buy dulse as flakes and as a powder.

Dulse contains fucoxanthin, antioxidant peptides, and omega-3s.[50] To get the same amount of omega-3 as the effective dose of cod, you would need to eat an easily achievable one-fifth of a cup of dulse.

Porphyra

If you love sushi and have eaten maki rolls, then you already love the dark-green wrapping—a dried edible seaweed called porphyra. The seaweed has been shredded and re-formed using a Japanese papermaking process. You'll also find it packaged as a stand-alone seaweed snack, in addition to being sold as a Japanese-food ingredient in the international section of the supermarket. In England, Ireland, and Wales, porphyra is called "laver." It is boiled and pureed to make laverbread, a seaweed product used as a traditional ingredient for soups or sauces, or mixed with oatmeal. Researchers from the University of Maine have shown that porphyra seaweed contains omega-3s, though in smaller amounts than the other seaweeds I've described, so just enjoy it (don't worry about the dose), knowing you'll get a little in each bite.[51]

TABLE 8.1. SEAFOOD DOSES

Seafood	Dose Equivalent of Effective Omega-3 Dose of Cod (150 grams)
Roe	
Caviar	2 tablespoons
Salmon	1 tablespoon
Sea urchin	2 sea urchins' roe
Tarama	1 1/2 tablespoons
Shells and Claws	
Blue crab	3
Gulf shrimp	4 medium
King crab	1/2 leg segment
Langoustine	6
Lobster (American and European)	1 large or 3 small (chix)
Mantis shrimp	3
Mitten crab	2 1/3
Spiny lobster	1/2 medium tail
Stone crab	1 medium claw
Just the Shell	
Mussels	12
Oysters	3 medium
Razor clams	3
Sea scallops	4
Tubes and Tentacles	
Cuttlefish	1 1/2 servings the size of a deck of playing cards
Octopus	1 large tentacle
Sea cucumber	2 servings, each the size of a deck of playing cards
Squid	10 medium tubes or 3 squid tentacles
Fins	
Anchovies	3
Dover sole	1/2 playing card deck–size serving
Hake	1 serving the size of a deck of playing cards
Halibut	1/2 playing card deck–size serving
Mackerel	1 bite-sized forkful
Sardine	1 bite-sized forkful
Sea bass	1/2 playing card deck–size serving
Turbot	1 1/3 playing card deck–size serving
Seaweed	
Dulse	1/5 cup
Kelp (Kombu)	1/3 cup
Wakame	1/10 cup

* * *

I hope I've succeeded in expanding your interest in exploring the seafood section of the market. If you are already a fan, dive in with gusto and keep exploring new types of seafood. But if you are new to this section, my recommendation is that you pick one item that you find interesting to start, then look up a recipe that you can easily make at home. If you feel gun-shy about cooking seafood, then first order it at a restaurant to see how the pros do it. As with all food, you will enjoy seafood even more when you are knowledgeable about what you buy, cook, and eat. Do your research, check with your fishmonger, know where your seafood comes from, and prepare it in healthful ways—and, as with everything, savor what you eat and stop before you feel full.

Now let's continue through the market to find something healthy and satisfying to drink with your delicious meal.

CHAPTER 9

Liquid Gold

On your journey through the supermarket, you've encountered delicious, health-promoting foods to eat during your meals, but let's not forget the importance of what you drink. Scientific research shows that what we drink, and how much, strongly influences our health. Specific beverages can also help us fight body fat. You are what you eat, but it's also accurate to say, "You are what you drink." Let's go find the beverages that are liquid gold for your metabolism.

An average adult human body is made up of 60 percent water. If you weigh 150 pounds, 90 pounds of you—11 gallons—is liquid. That's the equivalent of twenty 2-liter bottles of your favorite drink! You expel half a gallon every day through urine, stool, and sweat—more if you are outdoors in the heat and physically active. What's more, you lose at least another quarter of a gallon invisibly through the humidified air you exhale from your lungs and from evaporation off your skin.[1] This kind of fluid loss is called "insensible" because you usually don't feel it or see it, and it is difficult to measure.

That's a lot of liquid for you to replenish, three-quarters of a gallon every day, which is why we need to drink liquid. Some water is naturally present in our food, like the juice of an apple, the liquid in tomato sauce, or water naturally present in fish or chicken, but this is not nearly enough to keep up with the amount the body expels. This deficit must be filled by the beverages you drink each day.* Not all drinks are created equal, and some do a better job keeping you hydrated and healthy than others. And some beverages are harmful.

The simplest way to hydrate is to drink water. The word "hydrate" literally means "to combine with water." But drinking just water isn't all that interesting, and the beverage options you find in the supermarket are legion. Unless you have something specific in mind, the choices of what to drink can seem overwhelming.

The first step in cutting through the clutter is to steer away from beverages that are not beneficial for your health. These are sodas and other "sugar-sweetened beverages," a category that includes sports drinks, energy drinks, and many bottled teas and coffee drinks. A Harvard study of 14,971 men showed that even moderate consumption of soda and sugar-sweetened beverages can lead to significant weight gain and increased risk of obesity.[2] This is because regular soda contains an astonishing amount of added sugar. One twelve-ounce serving contains 39 grams of it, the equivalent of nine teaspoons' worth! Add to that the artificial flavors, artificial coloring, preservatives, and other additives

---

* The reason the urge to drink is so compelling lies in our biology. The behavior is hardwired into our brain and connected to the mouth and esophagus. Thirst neurons in the brain sense when fluid levels are low. These specialized neurons are located in the subfornical organ, a small mass of tissue near the base of the brain, about a finger's length deep behind your nose. As your body loses fluid throughout the day, your blood becomes more concentrated. This triggers your thirst neurons like the warning on your car's fuel gauge signaling you are low on gas. The subfornical organ neurons make you feel thirsty, and you will instinctively begin to look for something to drink. When you start to quench your thirst, the fluid activates special sensors in your mouth and esophagus as liquid runs down your throat. These sensors tell your brain to tone down the feeling of thirst *within one minute* of drinking. Your brain quickly calculates how much liquid you need to hydrate properly and resets the fuel alarm before the liquid you swallowed even reaches your bloodstream, which takes about ten minutes. A cold drink quenches thirst faster than a warm one because the subfornical organ is more sensitive to cooler temperatures. This is why a glass of cold water after exercise is so much more appealing than a warm one. After a few greedy gulps, you put the glass down because your brain automatically tells you to stop when it reaches homeostasis.

found in most sodas, and you have a liquid that's not only packed with empty calories; it is laden with chemicals that have the potential over time to degrade your metabolism and health defenses.

Juices may seem like a healthier option, but many commercial juices have sugar added to make them more appealing to your taste buds. Just read the ingredient label. These pumped-up juices beguile your brain to crave them, but they lack the valuable components of the whole fruit, like pulp, fiber, and fat-fighting bioactives. Even if you juice fresh fruit yourself, you can get a caloric overload if you drink too much in one sitting. It takes three to four medium-sized oranges, for example, to make one cup of fresh-squeezed orange juice. A tall glass contains two cups, or eight oranges' worth. Since a single orange has around 9 grams of sugar, a tall glass of juice contains 72 grams of sugar—equivalent to seventeen teaspoons, or almost twice the amount of sugar in a can of soda! So, even if you include the good stuff—the fruit pulp—in your fresh juice, that's a *whole* lot of sugar.

Think of how easy it is to guzzle down a glass of orange juice. All those calories you'd be pouring in—about 240 calories in that tall glass, even if it has zero *added* sugar—can tax your metabolism. On the other hand, if you sat down to enjoy a ripe orange, you might eat one whole fruit including some of its fibrous, good-for-gut-health white pith, but it's unlikely you'd eat eight oranges at a time.[3] Whenever you have a craving for juice, eat the whole fruit if you can.

Diet sodas contain sugar substitutes that reduce the number of calories but pose a whole other set of potential health risks. Lab studies of nonnutritive sweeteners like aspartame, sucralose, and even stevia show they can cause dysbiosis, knocking your gut microbiome off-balance, which has harmful implications for your metabolism, immunity, inflammation, and other key determinants of health.[4] A study out of the University of Texas Health Sciences Center in Houston of 6,814 adults aged forty-five to eighty-four found that drinking even one diet soda per day was associated with a 36 percent increase in the risk of developing metabolic syndrome, and a 67 percent greater risk of type 2 diabetes, compared to individuals who did not drink any diet soda.[5,*]

Wine, beer, and distilled spirits are also sold in some supermarkets. In addition to the usual cautions about alcohol and health risks, these beverages also disrupt your metabolism. A study of 1,869 people from the UK Biobank, led by researchers from Iowa State University, found that people who drank more beer and hard liquor had greater amounts of visceral fat and more insulin resistance.[6]

The good news is that there are beverages that are beneficial to your metabolism. As with the foods I've described, I'm going to tell you about useful beverages based on clinical studies. You'll see the doses of the beverages studied. These doses are useful as a reference and not as a rule. The best way to gauge how much liquid you should drink is to listen to your body, since it is always seeking to be well hydrated. Also, keep in mind that the beverages I'm about to describe are choices—you do not need to drink them daily.

Water

H_2O

The world's first and most popular beverage is not only a requirement for your health; it can also aid your enjoyment of eating. I prefer to drink water with my meals because it's flavorless: water quenches my thirst but doesn't change the taste of my food. When I was a kid, I remember attending the annual city folk festival in Pittsburgh, sitting at a long picnic-style table surrounded by an array of delicious home-cooked foods from Greece, Italy, the Philippines, Slovakia, Ireland, and other countries. I purchased fruit punch from one of the stands as my beverage, and every time I sipped it, the aftertaste of the punch overwhelmed the

---

* This study was part of the Multi-Ethnic Study of Atherosclerosis, and the subjects were white, African American, Hispanic, and Chinese adults.

flavor of each bite of my food so much that it ruined the taste. I switched to water on the spot, so I could enjoy the rest, and I've never looked back.

When it comes to your metabolism, drinking water is *far* superior to drinking a zero-calorie diet beverage.[7] It doesn't matter if the water is still or carbonated. Researchers from the University of Nottingham in the United Kingdom and the Tehran University of Medical Sciences in Iran wanted to know what would happen if people on a weight-loss program who drink diet beverages switched to water. They recruited seventy-one Iranian women who were obese and already in a weight-loss program. The women regularly consumed diet beverages. The subjects were divided into two groups. One group replaced drinking their regular diet beverage with one cup of water, seven days a week. The second group continued to drink diet beverages five days per week after their lunch, then water after lunch for the remaining two days of the week. Their body weight, blood glucose, and insulin levels were assessed at six months and twelve months.

By the end of the study, at twelve months, the women who drank water lost seventeen times more weight than those who drank the diet beverage (3.74 pounds versus 0.2 pounds). They also had lower levels of fasting glucose and less insulin resistance, both signs of a better metabolism. The water drinkers also had more stable blood glucose after eating. All three results show that water improved metabolism compared to diet beverages.

Drinking water at a meal stretches the walls of your stomach and tricks your brain into thinking you are full, so your eating pace slows down. It also triggers your body to start thermogenesis and to burn more energy. Researchers from Humboldt University in Berlin, Germany, studied this effect in fourteen healthy, normal-weight men and women.[8] They instructed each subject to fast for 12.5 hours overnight. In the morning, they gave each person two cups of water to drink in a lab where their metabolism (energy expenditure) was measured through a technique called whole-room indirect calorimetry.[9] Within ten minutes after drinking water, the subjects' metabolisms started to increase. By sixty minutes after drinking water, their energy expenditure increased by 30 percent.

The reason for water's metabolic effect is not precisely known, but it's surmised that the body needs to warm up water in the stomach, and this energy expenditure somehow triggers the β3-adrenergic receptors on fat cells, turning on thermogenesis.[10] Another possible mechanism is that the stomach detects a difference in concentration of particles in water compared to blood through special sensors called osmoreceptors.[11] Once the sensors are activated, they command the body to start thermogenesis. Based on these results, the researchers calculated that drinking six cups of water per day would burn 17,400 calories a year, which is the energy content of about five pounds of body fat.

On average, Americans consume five and a half cups of water each day, according to the US Centers for Disease Control and Prevention.[12] That's a lot less than the ten to fifteen cups per day recommended by the Institute of Medicine, but it's still 126 gallons per year. Roughly a third of that is bottled water, which you may be drinking at the gym, while bicycling, or while traveling.[13] In the United States alone, consumers drank 15 billion gallons of bottled water in 2020. My recommendation is to save your money and drink well water or filtered water. Bottled water has three problems. First, it is expensive. Second, the bottles generate mountains of plastic waste that damage our environment. And third, the bottles shed microplastics in the water, which we swallow. One analysis of eleven different brands of bottled water found as many as twenty-five hundred particles in a single cup of water.[14] The health effects of ingesting microplastics aren't yet known, but sometimes you don't need to wait for research to know that something is not good for you.[15]

Beverage dose: *Drink as much water as your body tells you*
This advice might seem obvious, but many people ignore their body's own signals. Better than counting the glasses of water you drink each

day—from a medical perspective, there is actually no magic number that is correct for everyone—here are two simple ways to make sure you are keeping up with your fluids. First, check your urine. It should be pale or slightly yellow. If it's dark yellow or brownish, you need more fluid. Second, check in from time to time and ask yourself if you feel thirsty. If you do, this is your body sending a signal that you should drink more water.

Tea

Tea is one of the world's most popular beverages, second only to water. I grew up drinking tea, and I often sip cups of it all day long. With so many types of tea enjoyed around the world, I'm still learning about them and exploring different varieties that can be found in grocery stores, specialty tea shops, and online.

Green Tea

The origin story of green tea dates back at least five thousand years to Emperor Shennong in China, who is said to have sipped a cup of hot water into which a few tea leaves had accidentally blown in from a nearby shrub. The emperor found the tea leaf–infused hot water to be calming and enjoyable, so he ordered his men to prepare it for everyone. Whether or not this tale is true, green tea did originate in China, and from there it spread to India and Japan to become a cultural legacy of Asia.

Green tea is made from the leaves of the shrub *Camellia sinensis*. Leaves and buds are picked by hand twice a year, in the early spring and early summer. The leaves are processed in ways that produce different types of tea. After picking, they are wilted on mats to dry and wither, then rolled or twisted to break down the cell walls of the leaves, and then sometimes oxidized to turn the green leaves brown (in the case of darker teas), then dried. Green tea is the least processed of all the teas.

Tea leaves contain bioactive compounds that dissolve into the beverage when steeped. Two bioactives in tea, epigallocatechin-3-gallate (ECGC) and chlorogenic acid, increase body metabolism and help to burn fat.[16] Researchers from Isfahan University of Medical Sciences in Iran studied the effect of green tea on metabolism and body fat. They recruited seventy women from a diabetes clinic who were diagnosed with metabolic syndrome. The subjects were divided into two groups. One group was given seven ounces (four-fifths of a cup) of green tea to drink three times a day for eight weeks. A placebo group received the same amount of lukewarm water to drink. Body measurements and blood tests were taken at the beginning and end of the study.

At the end of eight weeks, the study showed tea drinkers lost more weight (two pounds) and had a smaller waist size (by three-fourths of an inch) than those who drank lukewarm water. Green tea also improved systolic blood pressure (top number), fasting blood glucose, and blood lipid levels. Bad (LDL) cholesterol declined by 9 percent.

A similar study was performed at the Tehran University of Medical Sciences examining the benefits of different daily doses of green tea.[17] Researchers recruited sixty-three men and women aged thirty-five to sixty-five who were slightly overweight and had type 2 diabetes. The subjects were divided into three groups, with one drinking four cups of green tea per day, another two cups per day, and a third group had no green tea as a beverage for two months before the study. The green tea was made using tea bags that were steeped in boiled water for five minutes.

At the end of the two months, the subjects who drank the greatest amount of green tea—four cups per day—lost almost three pounds and saw their waist circumference shrink by 1.7 inches. Their systolic blood pressure (top number) declined by 6 percent. Those who drank two cups of green tea daily saw their waist size shrink by 1.4 inches.

The supermarket has an entire section devoted to a variety of teas. You may have a tea shop nearby that is dedicated to selling teas from around the world. But if you are looking for a special tea, do a search and find online sellers that can ship the tea to your home. You can buy loose-leaf tea you sprinkle into a cup with your fingers or tea bags for dunking. I personally prefer pure teas, not flavored ones. If you enjoy flavored teas, with fruit, spices, or flowers, check the ingredient label to make sure the flavoring and any additives are natural.

Beverage dose: *two to four cups of green tea per day*
This might seem like a lot of tea to someone who isn't a regular tea drinker, but it's easy to make it part of your daily routine. Just keep a mug with you during the day and periodically fill it with more hot water or add some more tea leaves. Many people in Asia sip tea all day long, consuming as many as six to ten cups by the time they go to bed.

Matcha

Many people who enjoy sushi at Japanese restaurants are familiar with matcha, a green tea made from an intensely green-colored powder. In fact, powdered tea was a tradition in China brought to Kyoto, Japan, by a Zen Buddhist monk named Myoan Eisai who visited the country in 1191. The production of matcha begins with the tea shrub, whose leaves are grown under shade for around twenty days before harvest. The blocking of sunlight stresses the tea leaves, making them produce more polyphenols, such as EGCG and L-theanine. Like EGCG, L-theanine has antiadipose effects. Lab studies from Fudan University show that this bioactive causes white fat cells to undergo browning to result in useful brown fat.[18]

The matcha leaves are picked and allowed to dry, and the stems and veins are removed. Then the dried tea is slowly ground into a fine powder by a mill. Unlike other brewed teas, matcha tea includes the entire tea leaf. As a result, it contains more EGCG than typical green tea. According to one analysis by the University of Colorado, matcha has 137 times more EGCG than a typical commercial green tea.[19] Want to get the most out of this form of green tea? Researchers from Pomeranian University in Poland showed that brewing matcha at 90 degrees Celsius and steeping for ten minutes extracts the highest levels of polyphenols.[20]

A study led by researchers from the University of Chichester in the United Kingdom studied the effect of matcha on metabolism in thirteen women of normal weight, aged nineteen to thirty-five.[21] They were given the equivalent of four cups of matcha over a twenty-four-hour period before being asked to perform a brisk thirty-minute walk on a treadmill. During this time, the researchers found that matcha increased whole-body fat oxidation, a marker of metabolism, in subjects by 35 percent. Thus, drinking matcha within a short period before exercise can help to burn even more body fat.

Matcha also can counter the metabolic effects of a high-fat diet. This has been studied in mice by researchers from Zhejiang University in Hangzhou, China. They added matcha to the mouse diet and found it lowered serum total cholesterol and triglycerides, while it increased levels of beneficial high-density lipoprotein-cholesterol.[22] Matcha also suppressed levels of harmful low-density lipoprotein-cholesterol (LDL).

Beverage dose: *four cups of matcha per day*
This is an easily achievable amount of matcha to drink. Think of it as ordering a cup at a sushi bar when you're seated at your table and having a few refills before you finish the meal.

Oolong Tea

A semi-oxidized version of green tea, oolong is a traditional Chinese tea that originated in Fijian Province. Today, it is cultivated in both mainland China and Taiwan. After being withered and oxidized, the tea leaves are rolled into long, curling leaves or shaped into small beads. The degree of oxidation influences its distinctive flavor, which is prized by tea aficionados. It is more complex than green tea but not as strong in flavor as a black tea.

In addition to EGCG and L-theanine, oolong tea contains a bioactive called oolong tea polysaccharide that suppresses the growth of fat cells by turning off their gene expression.[23] In the lab, oolong is one of the most potent teas for preventing weight gain in lab animals.[24] The antiobesity effects of oolong tea were studied by researchers from Jinan University in Guangzhou, China, and their colleagues. They recruited 102 subjects aged eighteen to sixty-five from the city of Fuzhou, the capital of Fijian Province. The subjects were overweight or obese. Oolong tea (2 grams) was steeped for five minutes in one and one-quarter cups of boiling water. They drank two servings each in the morning and afternoon, for a total daily dose of four cups of oolong tea for six weeks. Body measurements and blood samples were taken at the beginning and end of the study.

At six weeks, the subjects had lost an average of 6.4 pounds, and their waist circumference shrank by one inch. When the group was analyzed further, 70 percent of the severely obese subjects had lost 2.2 pounds, and 20 percent lost 6 pounds, with four cups of oolong tea per day as their only intervention. Most (65 percent) of the overweight and obese subjects lost more than 2.2 pounds. Blood tests also showed that drinking oolong tea decreased the level of triglycerides, as a sign of improved metabolism.

A study by US Department of Agriculture researchers showed that drinking six cups of oolong tea every day for three days resulted in a 3 percent improvement in overall metabolism.[25] When it came to fat oxidation, the oolong drinkers experienced a 12 percent increase in fat burning. Besides EGCG, L-theanine, and oolong polysaccharides, the caffeine in tea directly stimulates thermogenesis and burns down body fat.

Beverage dose: *five to six cups of oolong tea per day*

Pu'er Tea

This smoky, fermented black tea is named after the market town of Puer in which it originated in Yunnan Province, Southwestern China, more than two thousand years ago. Some of today's source trees in Yunnan are hundreds of years old.

Pu'er tea leaves come from a varietal of the *Camellia sinensis* tree that has broader leaves. After picking, the leaves are withered, dried, hand-rolled, and piled to undergo natural fermentation by bacteria in the air for forty-five days. The tea is then sorted, dried, and pressed into cakes. The processing was originally intended to preserve the tea on its long journey along the Silk Road trading routes to Tibet. Pu'er has a dark, earthy, smoky taste that is like a rich black tea. It is considered a digestif, and I especially enjoy it after a meal.

Pu'er has the same fat-fighting bioactives found in other teas, including EGCG and L-theanine. But what makes pu'er highly unusual is that it is a probiotic. In 2018, a new species of bacteria named *Pueribacillus* was discovered growing in the tea leaves.[26] While the role of these bacteria hasn't been defined, like other fermented foods, pu'er contributes to gut health and supports the microbiome. Another bioactive called strictinin found in pu'er tea reduces harmful cavity-causing bacteria in the oral microbiome.[27] Lab studies in mice show that extracts from pu'er can prevent weight gain, even if the animals are fed a high-fat diet.[28]

Researchers from Chung Shan Medical University in Taiwan studied the effect of daily pu'er tea on body weight and metabolism.[29] They enrolled seventy subjects and divided them into two groups. One group received tea made from an extract of pu'er tea leaves three times each day, while the other group received a placebo tea. The study ran for three months and, at the end, showed a 5.6-fold increase in weight loss in the pu'er drinkers, compared to placebo drinkers, who lost only 1.5 pounds over the same period.

Another clinical study from Beijing Medical University in China studied a pu'er tea extract for its effect on metabolism.[30] The researchers recruited ninety men and women who were overweight and had metabolic syndrome. The subjects were divided into two groups and given either four capsules of pu'er extract to take twice a day just before meals for three months or a placebo. The calculated dose of the tea was one-half teaspoon of pu'er powder in each cup. At the end of three months, the subjects who had pu'er extract saw a 77 percent greater reduction in their body mass index, compared to the control. Blood levels of total cholesterol, harmful LDL cholesterol, and triglycerides were also lower in the pu'er group.

You can find pu'er tea at most tea shops, and it is available from a number of sources online. If you have an Asian market nearby, check for pu'er on its tea shelves.

Beverage dose: *two cups of pu'er tea per day*

Coffee

I love drinking coffee, lots of it, every day. I enjoy its taste and have ever since I lived in Italy (where I was introduced to espresso) during my gap year after college, and in Greece (where I discovered Turkish/Greek coffee). I was drawn in both by the flavor and the stimulating effects of the caffeine. In medical school, I guzzled coffee while memorizing textbooks, and, later, during my residency training years, I drank lots of coffee to help me stay awake during long on-call evenings. Today, science shows that the benefits of coffee extend well beyond its ability to keep you alert. Coffee is beneficial to your metabolism and helps you fight body fat.

Remarkably, for such a widely consumed beverage, the exact origin story of coffee is unknown. It came from Ethiopia where coffee shrubs are indigenous, but how it became popularized and when it began spreading to other countries is unclear. We do know that coffee was traded from Africa to Arabia, and then to the Mediterranean. The coffee shrub was also brought to India, and from there transported and grown in other Southeast Asian countries like Vietnam, Cambodia, Burma (now Myanmar), and Thailand. Regardless of the location where it's grown, most commercial coffee comes from two different varietals of the plant: Arabica and Robusta.

Throughout history, coffee has been both embraced and rejected because of its stimulating effects on the brain. When I was a kid, I was told coffee was an "adult" beverage for this reason. But caffeine is only one component of the brew.

Coffee beans contain chlorogenic acid, which, as you learned in Chapter 4, has potent antiobesity effects. This bioactive prompts fat stem cells to create more useful brown fat, and it increases metabolism by triggering thermogenesis. A clinical study of coffee and body fat involving 504 men and women living in Indonesia showed that drinking coffee was linked to lower fat, even when the caffeine was removed from the equation, highlighting the power of chlorogenic acid.[31] The caffeine that is found in the coffee most people drink, however, does itself increase metabolism.[32] What's more, coffee's effect on brown fat thermogenesis is more pronounced in people who have a lean build than in people who are obese.[33]

Researchers from the Harvard School of Public Health along with collaborators in Singapore and Switzerland studied the effect of coffee on metabolism. They recruited twenty-six men and women, aged thirty-five to sixty-nine, who were overweight with insulin resistance. The subjects were of Chinese, Malaysian, and East Indian descent. Of the two groups, one was given four cups of coffee (made with Robusta coffee beans) to drink each day for six months. The other group had a placebo beverage that was designed to look, smell, and taste like coffee but had no coffee in it. All the subjects were prohibited from drinking other coffee during the study. The subjects drank one cup of their beverage at breakfast, at midmorning, at lunch, and after lunch. They were not allowed to drink coffee after 8 p.m. to prevent interference with their sleep. No other dietary change was made.

At the end of the study, the body fat of the coffee drinkers, which was measured by a body composition analyzer, shrank by 4.6 pounds. In contrast, the group who drank the placebo beverage actually gained 4.4 pounds of body fat.

You have probably heard that the caffeine in coffee (and tea) is a diuretic that can dehydrate you. As a medical student, I heard the same thing from my professors and wondered whether it causes weight loss by making you urinate more and lose fluid weight. A carefully designed clinical study was conducted by the University of Birmingham in England to examine coffee and dehydration. The study showed that moderate coffee drinking does *not* cause you to lose more body fluid than drinking water.[34] So you can enjoy your coffee without worrying that it is drying you out.

Beverage dose: *four cups of coffee per day*

Cocoa Beverages

The cacao bean was used to make an ancient Mayan beverage called *xocolatl*. This was considered one of the foods of the gods. According to archaeologists, *xocolatl* was not sweetened with sugar. Instead, it was served bitter, sometimes flavored with chili or a hint of vanilla.[35] In Mesoamerica, a cocoa beverage was consumed daily by the masses, like we do with coffee today, and it was also used in rituals and ceremonies.

When the Aztecs conquered the Mayans, however, they made chocolate a food of the privileged. The common thread was a recognition of the healing properties of the cacao bean and the cocoa powder made from it. When the conquistadors brought cocoa to Europe, Spanish confectioners added sugar to cocoa powder to create something more like the chocolate drinks and bars we know today.

The cacao bean, as you saw in Chapter 7, has antiadipose effects. Although dark chocolate does have many health benefits, eating chocolate bars is not a wise approach for fighting body fat because they usually contain sugar and other additives. But what about drinking pure cocoa powder, xocolatl style?

Researchers from the National Polytechnic Institute of Mexico studied the effect of a cocoa drink on metabolism and body composition.[36] They recruited fifteen men and women who were overweight and diagnosed with metabolic syndrome. One group received a beverage made with cocoa powder dissolved in three-quarters of a cup of water to drink each day for four weeks.* The other group was given a placebo beverage with no cocoa.

At four weeks, the cocoa beverage drinkers had lost 5.3 pounds, which is 40 percent more weight than the placebo drinkers. Cocoa drinkers also saw their waist size shrink by 1.4 inches, twice the amount of change as in the placebo group. The cocoa beverage also caused improvements in metabolism, leading to a 58 percent greater reduction in total cholesterol levels. Subjects' beneficial HDL cholesterol levels increased, while their harmful LDL cholesterol was lowered by 17 percent. Blood glucose levels improved, and there was a 2.4-fold greater lowering of triacylglycerol, a marker of fat deposition, in the cocoa drinkers, compared to the placebo drinkers. If you enjoy the earthy

---

* To design your own high-flavanol cocoa beverage like the one in this study, you would need to have 80 milligrams of cocoa flavanols per cup. My research reveals this is about two tablespoons of typical cocoa powder, but there is a wide range of flavanol levels in powder based on the quality of the cacao bean and how it was processed. Another useful thing to know is cocoa powder is not "hot chocolate," which contains sugar and many other additives.

flavor of pure cocoa, you can tap into some meaningful benefits for your metabolism.

You can find unsweetened cocoa powder in the middle aisles usually near the baking goods. Check the ingredients to make sure there are no added sugars, artificial flavorings or colors, or hydrogenated fats in the powder. You can add natural spices and flavorings on your own. You'll find it easier to dissolve cocoa powder in hot water, but you can get its health benefits hot or cold. To drink it cold, just make it the night before and chill in the refrigerator overnight.

Beverage dose: *three-quarters of a cup of cocoa beverage per day (average of two tablespoons of high-quality cocoa powder dissolved in water)*

Plant Milk

Many people are interested in alternatives to dairy milk. Plant-based milk (sometimes called "mylk" to avoid confusion) is made from nuts and legumes, does not contain lactose, and is low in saturated fat and cholesterol. The nut or bean is soaked in water and then ground up, and the liquid is strained. Plant-based milks are a great alternative for those who are lactose intolerant or are avoiding dairy for health, religious, or ethical reasons. Be sure to read the label of any commercial beverage, however, to make sure there are no undesirable additives.

Soy Milk

It may seem like a modern invention, but soy milk was developed more than two thousand years ago in China. It's the liquid that comes from boiling and mashing soybeans and is one of the precursors to making tofu. Soy milk can be served cold or hot, salty or sweetened, plain or savory. It is used as a dairy substitute by coffee drinkers who are lactose intolerant. A soup made from soy milk is a popular traditional offering for dim sum, the brunch-like meal of small, tasty treats. And just like soybeans, soy milk has been shown to have an antiobesity effect.

Researchers at Universiti Tunku Abdul Rahman in Selangor, Malaysia, conducted a study of 258 Malaysian Chinese residents, aged twenty-one to sixty, on the effects of soy milk. The subjects had their metabolism measured through blood tests, physical activity questionnaires, and a dietary survey of their meals and snacks.[37] The study found that 21 percent were overweight and 40 percent were obese, with more obesity in younger subjects aged twenty to thirty-three. Remarkably, drinking soy milk was one of only three factors that predicted less obesity. In fact, there was a 55 percent lower risk of obesity in people who drank soy milk.

Soy milk can have a beneficial effect on your waist size, when compared to cow's milk, as found in a study by researchers from the Tehran University of Medical Sciences.[38] The clinical trial recruited twenty-four overweight and obese women aged twenty to fifty from Tehran. The subjects were divided into two groups, both of which were on calorie-restricted diets. One group received one cup of soy milk to drink every day for four weeks. The other group received one cup of cow's milk each day. After this initial period, they took a two-week break to "wash out" any effects of their beverage. Then each group switched to the other beverage and drank this daily for another four weeks. The results showed that soy milk but not cow's milk led the women to achieve a 7 percent greater decrease in waist circumference.

You'll find soy milk in the dairy section of the supermarket, along with other plant-based milks. While other milks, like almond milk and oat milk, are also good substitutes, I prefer soy milk because its traditional heritage makes it a classic MediterAsian beverage.[39] It is a great substitute for dairy if you like milk but want to be dairy-free or reduce your intake of saturated fat. If you are looking for a healthy swap-out of cream for your coffee (or cocoa beverage), try soy milk.

Beverage dose: *one cup of soy milk per day*

Fruit Juices

"Is juice good for my health?" I am often asked. I always reply that the whole food is much more beneficial than just the juice. Drinking juice doesn't count toward your intake of vegetables or fruits because the pulp, the pith, and the peel—all parts that contain useful bioactives—are usually removed. Moreover, many of the commercial juices you find in the grocery store are highly processed, made from concentrated extracts, and contain added sugar and other additives, while most of the beneficial pulp and bioactives have been removed.

That said, some juices are worth knowing about because clinical studies have shown that drinking them can benefit your metabolism.

Tomato Juice

I've loved tomato juice since I was a kid and had always assumed that it was invented in South America, where tomatoes originated, or by the Italians or Spaniards who brought them to Europe centuries ago. Contemporary lore, however, says otherwise. Tomato juice was apparently invented by Louis Perrin, a hotel chef, in 1917 as a breakfast juice at the French Lick Resort, in French Lick, Indiana. Whether or not there were earlier iterations (I suspect there must have been), tomato juice deserves its modern reputation as a healthful beverage. It contains the bioactive lycopene found in whole tomatoes, which, as you learned in Chapter 6, has antiadipose power.

Researchers from China Medical University in Taichung, Taiwan, studied the metabolic effects of drinking tomato juice in a group of healthy people.[40] They recruited twenty-five women aged twenty to thirty, who were all normal weight. The subjects were given 1.2 cups of 100 percent pure tomato juice to drink each day for eight weeks. They were told to otherwise maintain their normal diet and exercise routines. Body measurements and blood tests were taken at the beginning and end of the study.

At the end of the eight weeks, everyone was weighed and measured, and their before-and-after blood tests were compared. The results showed that daily drinking of tomato juice led to a little more than one pound of weight loss over eight weeks, and it caused a little more than 0.5 percent of their body fat to be shed. The waist circumference of tomato juice drinkers decreased by just over one-half inch. Cholesterol and blood levels of an inflammatory marker called MCP-1 also declined.* There was one marker that *increased* by 25 percent after drinking tomato juice, and that was adiponectin, the fat hormone whose role is to sensitize your cells to insulin and optimize your metabolism.

There are many commercial types of tomato juice, including some made by adding other vegetables and spices that have their own metabolic benefits. As with any product, check the ingredient label so you know what else is included besides tomato. Avoid packaged juices that contain added sugar. And remember that you can easily make your own homemade tomato juice with fresh garden tomatoes. (Tip: adding some fresh lemon juice to tomato juice will enhance and brighten the flavor.) As with any juice, drinking tomato juice in moderation is key, so limit your intake and don't guzzle it for hydration. Tomato juice has about the same number of calories as orange juice, but it also contains five times as much dietary fiber that is beneficial for gut health. Sip it slowly to enjoy its lovely umami taste!

Beverage dose: *1.2 cups of pure tomato juice per day*

Watermelon Juice

As an alternative to tomato juice for obtaining lycopene, you can consider watermelon juice. Once the rind is sliced away, pureeing chunks of

---

* MCP-1 is monocyte chemoattractant protein-1, a protein that attracts cells called macrophages to participate in inflammation.

the fruit in a blender creates a sweet pink juice that is loaded with lycopene. Researchers from the US Department of Agriculture conducted a clinical study of watermelon juice in healthy individuals. They blended watermelon chunks to make three and a half cups of juice (containing 780 grams of lycopene) and found that drinking it daily for three weeks could double the lycopene levels in the blood, at levels equivalent to drinking tomato juice (although tomato juice contains more beneficial dietary fiber than watermelon juice).[41] This dose of watermelon juice seems to top off your body's lycopene levels because when the researchers doubled the amount of watermelon juice the subjects drank, it did not further increase their lycopene blood levels.

One benefit watermelons have compared with tomatoes is the presence of citrulline. This is an amino acid that the body metabolizes to create nitric oxide, the chemical signal used in your body to control many life-supporting cellular processes. Lab studies have shown that nitric oxide helps to create more brown fat for thermogenesis, and it can protect the health of blood vessels and lower blood pressure as a countermeasure for metabolic syndrome.[42] Nitric oxide also promotes the activity of stem cells in your body to help regenerate tissues and organs that are damaged by metabolic diseases.

You can make your own watermelon juice with a ripe melon, which will have a fresher taste than commercial juices. Be aware that processed bottled watermelon juice is often sugar-sweetened and sometimes contains artificial coloring and flavoring to enhance its appearance and flavor. Eating chunks or slices of fresh watermelon is very MediterAsian and will give you all the benefits of the juice, and some fiber.

When you enjoy this sweet beverage, keep in mind that a cup of watermelon juice has 2.2 times the amount of sugar in tomato juice. It's best not to make it a daily beverage but rather to consider it a drink that can add variety for your palate while getting the benefits of lycopene and citrulline in your body.

Akkermansia-Generating Beverages

There are a few prebiotic beverages in the middle aisles that deserve a place in your MediterAsian approach to eating. In Chapter 4, I told you that a healthy gut bacterium called *Akkermansia mucinophila* protects against obesity, metabolic syndrome, and diabetes and that this bacterium declines in number as you age.[43] Cancer researchers have also found that patients with *Akkermansia* in their gut have better immune responses when they are treated using immunotherapy.[44] *Akkermansia* can be very easily killed off by commonly prescribed antibiotics, so it's worth knowing about the beverages that can help it grow back.

The *Akkermansia* drinks are pomegranate juice, cranberry juice, and Concord grape juice.[45] Each is loaded with polyphenols that stimulate the gut to produce healthy mucus, which is the environment in which *Akkermansia* thrives. These juices have undergone human studies for their metabolic effects. Let's look at the evidence.

Pomegranate Juice

Pomegranate has been a popular fruit in Mediterranean, Asian, and Middle Eastern cultures for thousands of years. Its juice is used to make syrups, glazes, and beverages. Researchers from Nanjing University and Zhejiang University in China discovered that the ruby-colored pulp around the seeds from which juice is pressed has metabolic effects. When the pulp was fed to mice eating a high-fat diet, it reduced their body weight gain by 35 percent, compared to those who did not have pomegranate.[46] The pulp also improved their insulin sensitivity by 43 percent. When the researchers examined the gut microbiome, they found eating pomegranate increased the population of *Akkermansia*.

Pomegranate's fat-fighting abilities were verified by researchers from the West National Medical Center in Guadalajara, Mexico, in twenty obese adult volunteers.[47] One group received one-half cup of 100 percent organic pomegranate juice each day for thirty days. The other group was given a placebo for thirty days. At the end of the study, the pomegranate drinkers lost 1.1 pounds and reduced their body fat by 1.4 percent. In contrast, the placebo drinkers actually *gained* 2.2 pounds and increased their body fat by 1.1 percent.

I recommend that you consume pomegranate juice modestly because of its high sugar content, which is 25 percent higher than a soda. But the 100 percent juice will give you the useful bioactives as well as the prebiotic dietary fiber of the whole fruit.

Beverage dose: *one-half cup of pomegranate juice per day*

Concord Grape Juice

Do you remember the grape flavor of purple-colored candy when you were a kid? That is the exact replica of the actual flavor of the Concord grape and its juice. The taste brings back my childhood memories. Real whole grapes are much better for you, of course! Concord grapes are rich in anthocyanins. In the lab, the anthocyanins and other bioactives in grape juice prevented weight gain and the ability of fat to grow, and they reduced inflammation in mice fed a high-fat diet.[48]

A clinical study of Concord grape juice was led by researchers at Purdue University. They examined its effects on metabolism in thirty-four men and women who were overweight. One group of subjects was given one and one-half cups of Concord grape juice to drink every morning for one week. The other group drank a grape-flavored beverage that contained no polyphenols as a placebo.* The researchers checked the subjects' blood glucose after eating and surveyed their appetite levels.

At the end of one week, the Concord grape juice drinkers experienced reduced hunger and less desire to eat, and they consumed fewer

---

* The juice used in the study was Welch's 100% Grape Juice Concord Grape.

calories. A separate Purdue study showed that drinking Concord grape juice, despite its similar sugar content to pomegranate juice, did not cause weight gain.[49]

Beverage dose: *one and one-half cups Concord grape juice per day*

Cranberry Juice

Cranberries are small bright-red berries that arise from low, creeping shrubs in the United States, Canada, and South America. They are consumed in many forms, including juice, dried like raisins, and cooked as a sauce. Cranberries contain bioactives like anthocyanins, procyanidins, and other polyphenols.

In lab studies, cranberry extracts fed to mice eating a high-fat diet resulted in 22 percent less weight gain, compared to those not consuming any cranberry.[50] Researchers found that cranberry extracts activate metabolism by increasing the uncoupling protein 1 (UCP1) and by turning on thermogenesis.

The effect of cranberry juice on human metabolism was studied by researchers from the University of Londrina in Brazil.[51] They recruited fifty-six men and women who had been diagnosed with metabolic syndrome. Of the two groups, one was given three cups of cranberry juice per day, with half consumed at lunch and the other half at dinner for two months.* The other group just maintained their usual diet and lifestyle.

At the end of the sixty-day study, results showed that cranberry juice drinkers had a 20 percent increase in their blood levels of adiponectin, the fat hormone that helps cells better utilize blood glucose. Adiponectin's anti-inflammatory effects also help counter the damage caused by excess fat. The cranberry juice drinkers also had 30 percent lower blood levels of homocysteine. Homocysteine is an amino acid that is known to

---

* The juice used in this study was Juxx Cranberry manufactured by the Brazilian company Juxx.

be elevated in metabolic syndrome. A high level is a cardiovascular risk factor and is associated with adipose tissue growing like a rind around the outside of the heart.[52]

Pure cranberry juice has about 15 percent less sugar than pomegranate or Concord grape juice but it can be quite sour. Be aware that commercial cranberry juices are often mixed with other juices and may contain added sugar and artificial colorants and flavoring. I recommend looking for pure cranberry juice that you can dilute and adjust its flavor to taste at home. You can also get the benefit of cranberry bioactives and their dietary fiber by eating dried cranberries.

Beverage dose: *three cups of cranberry juice per day*

Citrus Juice

The orange fruit had its origins in Southeast Asia dating back more than two thousand years. Originally small and bitter, the orange was cultivated to be sweet and tangy by the Chinese. From there, it was introduced to Europe, where it achieved such acclaim that King Louis XIV of France dedicated grounds in the Palace of Versailles—named the Orangerie—to grow orange trees.

When I was growing up, "OJ" was considered to be one of the core elements of a healthy breakfast. It contains not only vitamin C, I was told, but also calcium and vitamin D. This perception was the result of effective marketing designed to sell citrus juice to every household. At the beginning of this chapter, I mentioned how eating the whole fruit is more beneficial than guzzling down its juice. I called out oranges especially for their high sugar content because a tall glass of OJ has more sugar than a can of soda. So, a question I am often asked is whether or not orange juice is really beneficial to your health.

Orange juice does not necessarily cause you to gain weight, as long as you drink it in moderation to limit the sugar you ingest. Whole oranges contain dietary fiber that is good for the microbiome as well as the fat-fighting bioactive hesperidin.[*] Among citrus fruits, the Valencia orange contains the highest levels of hesperidin.[53]

Hesperidin has been shown to help people who are normal weight slim down while building muscle. A clinical trial was conducted at the University of Murcia in Spain on forty healthy amateur competitive male cyclists, eighteen to fifty-five years old.[54] They were all within normal weight and very physically fit, cycling six to twelve hours per week.

Half of the cyclists were given an orange extract high in hesperidin, equivalent to four and one-half cups of orange juice (this was equivalent to thirteen Valencia oranges or eighteen navel oranges, but without the sugar). The other half were given a placebo capsule.[**] At the end of the eight-week study, the cyclists taking hesperidin showed a significant improvement in their already fit body composition. They lost 18 percent of their total body fat and dropped 15.5 percent of the fat mass of their lower leg. The hesperidin group also gained 2 percent more total muscle mass, reflecting a resculpting of the body. There were no changes to fat or muscle in the group taking the placebo

For these cyclists, the real measure of benefit was exercise performance. The subjects were taken to a performance lab and asked to ride a stationary bike.[55] The hesperidin group had a 2 percent improvement in the maximum power they could generate, compared to what they were capable of before the study. The placebo group exhibited no change in their performance. Two percent improvement might not seem like much to most people, but for a competitive athlete, every little bit of edge counts toward a victory.

Other citrus, like lemons and limes, also contain hesperidin, but only about half as much as the Valencia orange. Nonetheless, it's another reason to consider using fresh and fragrant lemons and limes in your kitchen. Lemons remind me of the Mediterranean flavors on Italy's

---

[*] While citrus juice contains hesperidin, the majority is in the fruit solids, including the pulp, rind, and skin.

[**] The authors report 1 liter of orange juice = 444 mg hesperidin.

Amalfi Coast and the Greek islands. Limes are used as condiments in Thai and Vietnamese cuisines. In addition to hesperidin, citrus fruits contain fat-fighting bioactives like naringenin, limonene, and nobiletin, which can activate brown fat and stimulate thermogenesis, helping to elevate your metabolism. These are some of the benefits you can gain by exploring delicious citrus fruits, such as pomelos, satsuma mandarins, clementines, tangerines, Sumo oranges, blood oranges, and kumquats and adding them to your diet.[56]

The bottom line, it's fine to drink the freshly squeezed juice of oranges or other citrus fruits but do it in moderation. They have potent bioactives and fiber, but also a lot of sugar.

* * *

A Final Note on Beverages

As you move through the supermarket, keep in mind that water is the very best beverage you can consume, followed closely by tea and coffee. These three should be the primary beverages you reach for when it comes to metabolic health. Any other beverage I've mentioned should be consumed in moderation—and always avoid those with added sugars. (Also see Table 9.1.)

When you have a glass of any beverage, don't feel like you have to drink every last drop. Don't just quit the "clean plate club"; you can quit the "empty cup club," too. Your brain's thirst nerve centers will tell you when you've had enough to drink to fulfill your body's fluid needs. Listen to it, so you don't overindulge in any beverage. Drinking too much of anything, even water, can be dangerous. Gulping down a whole gallon jug of water within a few hours can cause water intoxication, which can lead to dangerous brain swelling.

Drink fruit juices sparingly and focus on the ones that contain the most health-promoting compounds. Most beverages can be made at

TABLE 9.1. BEVERAGE DOSES

Beverage	Daily Doses
Water	1–2 cups
Tea:	
Green tea	2–4 cups
Matcha	2 cups
Oolong	5–6 cups
Pu'er	2 cups
Coffee	4 cups
Cocoa beverage	¾ cup
Soy milk	1 cup
Fruit juices:	
Concord grape	1 ½ cups
Cranberry	3 cups
Pomegranate	½ cup
Tomato	1.2 cups

home with a juicer or blender, and, of course, coffee and tea are simple to brew using hot water. You can keep a jug of cold tea or coffee in the refrigerator for a few days. Use a glass or metal container to avoid the shedding of microparticles from a plastic container. During the summer, you can even freeze these beverages as ice cubes and use them for cooling down on a hot day while giving your metabolism and health a boost at the same time. Expanding your kitchen skills to prepare your own beverages will not only impress your family and friends—it will reward you with better health.

Now that you understand the science behind foods in the middle aisles and the produce, seafood, and beverage sections of the supermarket, you are ready to begin an exciting metabolic health journey using the MediterAsian Way of eating. It's time to put these ingredients into action and propel yourself—and your metabolism—to a higher level of health.

PART 3

A PLAN FOR LIFE

It doesn't matter where you start. What matters is what
you do.
—*David Baltimore, 1975 Nobel Laureate*

CHAPTER 10

Find Your Own Way

The variety of food and beverage options available in the market offers you so many possibilities for healthy, joyous eating. But all that abundance can be overwhelming, especially since we are bombarded by advice from all corners about what and how to eat. Perhaps that's what inspired you to pick up this book—beyond the supermarket of foods, you need help navigating the ideas about what to do with them. There are so many different diet plans out there, all claiming to help you become healthier and more fit. Each one is different, and sometimes they conflict—but all claim to be the "right" way.

Here's the truth when it comes to food and health: the goal you want to aim for is to improve your metabolism. Losing weight is only one part of that goal. And as long as the approach is scientifically and medically sound, any plan for weight loss can work . . . if you stick to it. But the hardest part of shedding unwanted body fat—and keeping it off, which is needed for metabolic health—is sticking to the plan. As perhaps you may have already experienced, being "on a diet" poses challenges (from boredom to feeling deprived) that make failure seem inevitable. From the moment you start the diet for the sole purpose of losing weight, you already know there will come a time when you go off it. That is, unless your plan is uniquely your own.

Let's get real. Out of all the experts writing books about how to eat to lose fat, including me, there is only *one* expert on the foods you like best, *one* expert on how your body feels after you eat, and *one* expert on which foods bring you joy and which ones you detest. That expert is *you*. If you want to change your eating habits with the goal of losing unhealthy body fat to heal your metabolism once and for all, then knowing the relationship between your body and food is paramount. So is enjoying what you eat.

I can't emphasize this point enough: you need to find the approach that works best for you. Most diets have rigid rules and sound like a lot of hard work, a mindset reinforced by many doctors who take a scolding approach when they talk to their patients about diets and weight loss. Those messages make eating (especially healthy eating) sound like anything but fun. I know from my own experience and that of my patients that it's almost impossible to stick to behaviors that feel restrictive and impersonal. Human nature seeks freedom and connection, and we're more inclined to stick with things that make us happy and that we enjoy. Strict diets also make you feel like you have to live up to other people's standards, not your own.

The MediterAsian approach is both flexible and personal. It embodies time-honored traditions in its approach to ingredients. Both Mediterranean and Asian cultures emphasize fresh, seasonal, whole foods prepared using recipes that date back generations and, often, many centuries. Their dishes have great flavor that values the quality of the ingredients. The way they combine ingredients yields a final result that is far more complex and delicious than the sum of its parts. Just think about the complex flavors of a gazpacho, the cold soup from southern Spain, or a vegetable stir-fry with oyster sauce, compared to their starting components.

There's another reason I favor the MediterAsian Way. For millennia, these cultures have known that food and health are intertwined. Many of the ingredients used in Mediterranean and Asian cooking and traditional healing are the exact foods I described in Part 2—the ones validated by scientific evidence to improve your metabolism while activating the five health defense systems. Long before pharmaceuticals existed, home cooks in all the civilizations along the Silk Road used food as medicine. Rosemary, olive oil, and licorice were known in the Mediterranean to be healthful.[1] The ancient playbook for medicine— *De materia medica*—was written by first-century Greek physician Dioscorides, who included sage, fennel, and chamomile among his list of more than two hundred plant-based remedies. Traditional Chinese medicine is also based on food. In fact, the way you say "take your medicine" in China is *chī yào*; literally, "eat your medicine." Ginger, garlic, onion, and mushrooms are just a few examples of Chinese healing foods. Food as medicine is ingrained in nearly every MediterAsian dish.

MediterAsian eating is also grounded in the tradition of sharing, which enhances both its pleasures and its health benefits. I've said it before but it bears repeating: eating together provides social connection, which is known to be key for health and longevity, and the opportunity to savor food and eat more slowly, which is better for your metabolism.[2] Family-sized platters give everyone a chance to sample a variety of foods and eat to their own personal level of satisfaction, contrary to the typical style of serving each person their own pre-plated meal, with everyone getting the exact same items and (large) portions. Food variety not only prevents boredom for your palate; studies have also shown that better health results when your gut bacteria are fed a diversity of foods.[3] A healthy, well-fueled microbiome promotes gut health and, hence, improves metabolic as well as brain and immune functions.

But what if—despite reading all this—MediterAsian isn't right for you? Maybe you're not a fan of the cuisines or cooking methods. That's totally okay, even though I encourage you to be open-minded and explore them. You can use the ingredients in this book and find ways to use the foods in virtually any cuisine or genre of cooking. The recipes are less important than the strategy (and science) of using these foods in a way that fits with your personal preferences and lifestyle.

Suit yourself and your own preferences. By being true to yourself and finding your own way, you will be able to tailor your approach to healthy eating so you can stick with it. What you do need is to develop an eating strategy this is uniquely your own, make sure it works for you, and reinforce it until it becomes a natural, habitual way of living.

I can help here, too, because I do not believe there is only one way to approach eating to beat your diet. You need to find the best path for yourself. That's the way that will let you win the fight against excess body fat. For inspiration about how to develop a sustainable strategy that can last your lifetime, and how to do it in a powerful, personal, and thrilling way, I'd like to share lessons I learned from a seemingly unlikely source: a childhood hero of mine, the legendary martial artist Bruce Lee.

The Way of Bruce Lee

At five feet, eight inches tall and 130 pounds, Bruce Lee had a lean, cut physique that he kept in perfect shape through relentless training and careful nutrition. He had very little body fat. Lee was a fitness icon as well as an iconic martial artist. You only need to watch one of his films to be awed by his physical prowess.* Decades after his untimely death in 1973, Bruce Lee continues to inspire generations of people around the world to study martial arts.** He was one of its original global ambassadors. What most people do not know is that Bruce Lee developed a strong philosophy for adapting to and overcoming obstacles—including health challenges—and winning. His philosophy continues to influence many people, including today's top athletes. And me.

As a teenager, I was a huge Bruce Lee fan. His lightning-quick fighting moves were hypnotizing, and his ripped physique was so defined, his

---

* Bruce Lee's best-known martial arts films are The Big Boss, Fist of Fury (also released as The Chinese Connection), The Way of the Dragon, Enter the Dragon, and The Game of Death, which he did not complete before his death.

** Bruce Lee's untimely death at age thirty-two was attributed to an allergic reaction he had to a medication he had been given that caused lethal brain swelling.

muscles looked like they'd been drawn by a comic book artist. In my youth, I related to Bruce Lee's identity because we are both Asian Americans, and the themes of his movies hit home for me—overcoming injustice, racism, and bullying. The idea of achieving victory against great odds inspired me. Bruce Lee fought his opponents with speed, skill, grace, and efficacy. As a teen, I aspired to have his physical abilities.

While part of me still hopes one day to gain those remarkable physical skills, I've had a lot more success incorporating the other themes that Bruce Lee espoused, ones that made me appreciate him even more as an adult. His writings and films contain lessons that come from Lee's own background as an athlete who studied philosophy. He taught the importance of learning new skills and adapting them to your own unique physical abilities and limitations. He exemplified how one can respect traditional ways without being beholden to traditional rules, and how not to be afraid to solve problems by creating your own solutions. Lee said, "Research your own experience. Absorb what is useful, reject what is useless, add what is essentially your own."[4]

I've employed many of these principles throughout my life and career. They helped me at every point in my journey—to balance work and play during my years as a medical student, to have the confidence to develop my own approach to patients as a young doctor entering into an authoritative medical establishment, to succeed as a scientist pursuing new ideas within a conservative research community, and as a physician, to continually seek effective solutions at the frontiers of science that can help individuals overcome life- and limb-threatening diseases. Many of my successes have hinged on my willingness to think beyond conventional wisdom and to overcome obstacles by refusing to be constrained by the limitations that others try to impose. These principles helped me establish my own path in studying food as medicine. They can help you, too.

I had to teach myself nutrition because I had no education about it during my formal medical training. I also had to dodge and weave to avoid attacks on my interest in food healing from "superiors" who believed that pharmaceuticals are the only solution to health. To bring deeper science to the study of food, I also had to convince my research colleagues to test food using the systems traditionally reserved for testing pharmaceuticals. To establish myself in a crowded universe of health influencers, I had to stick to the science and boldly challenge the myths and urban legends of healthy eating that propagate on stages, television, podcasts, and social media. My own path has also been to practice what I preach—which is aligning my appreciation for good food with my commitment to good health.

So when it comes to finding your own way to fight body fat, Bruce Lee's wisdom is gold. That may sound like a stretch, so let me explain. Lee used combat training as a metaphor for solving problems and achieving success in life. Don't waste time debating the merits of different approaches—be direct, deal with the situation, and get results!

Lee created a new form of martial arts called *Jeet Kune Do*, or JKD, which translates to "Way of the Intercepting Fist." It was more of an approach to fighting than a specific style like the revered traditional martial arts of kung fu, karate, jujitsu, aikido, or Thai kick boxing. Lee believed that these traditional arts, while beautiful for exhibition, were way too rigid to be useful in a real-life fight. After all, the strict patterns of punches and kicks taught by those styles don't match the unpredictable nature of a real encounter with an assailant on the street.

Lee's book *Tao of Jeet Kune Do* describes his approach. It offers philosophical strategies that have been adopted not only by the martial arts community but by life coaches and business consultants as well. Those strategies apply directly to how you can use food to improve your health.

Lee described techniques that enabled each person to recognize their own unique strengths (and limitations) based on their body type, their physical capabilities, and their skills. He believed that the best approach is to borrow from the best of *every* style of combat, so he urged his students to learn a multitude of fighting techniques. In Bruce Lee's world, there were heated debates over which fighting style was superior: kung fu, karate, tae kwon do, savate, or judo. He viewed these arguments as parochial and self-limiting.

I believe the same philosophy applies when it comes to debates over which diet is superior. To win, Lee said, you borrow from whatever works for you in any given situation. When you set your mind to a goal and apply these principles to your eating, you can maximize your body's ability to optimize its metabolism and fuel your health. There's no need to limit yourself to a single approach because there is no ultimate "right" approach.

Learning to apply different techniques to use food as medicine to heal and optimize your metabolism not only broadens your abilities; it also helps you break out of the mindset of any single school of thought and throws rigid diet rules and philosophies out the window—this frees you from the yoke of strict diets. You will become a more adaptive and flexible individual when it comes to food and health. If you've been frustrated with past efforts at weight loss or feel that dieting seems like an impossible mountain to climb, what I'm about to share with you will make it possible for you to accomplish your goals for a better metabolism and health while enjoying the process.

So here is my response to the "diet doctors" and other lifestyle gurus who promote inflexible rules and soulless eating programs. I've drawn five important principles from Bruce Lee's philosophy that can help you make your life better by charting your own path and eating to beat your diet.

Principle #1: Clear Your Mind of Assumptions

Bruce Lee believed people should be open-minded and aim to be free of rigid thoughts and preconceived notions. One of his most famous quotes is "Be formless. Shapeless, like water. If you put water into a cup, it becomes the cup. You put water into a bottle, and it becomes the bottle.

You put it in a teapot, it becomes the teapot. Now, water can flow, or it can crash. Be water."* His point was to be fluid and accepting.

Applied to eating, this means letting go of the rigidities in any past popular doctrines you may have embraced on how and why to "fight fat." If you've believed there is a "right way" or "wrong way" for losing weight and being healthy, now is the time to open your mind to what works for you.

You do not need to enslave yourself to strict diets that dictate your food choices. Be broad-minded, inquisitive, and flexible so you can remain open to new ideas as the evolving science of molecular nutrition and fat reveals new information and opens the door to new options. Closing your mind to new ideas offered by science stifles your ability to harness new discoveries to your advantage. By first emptying your mind, you will approach new ideas and new data differently. Allowing new facts in will help you to clarify and perhaps even redefine your goals.

You must also empty your mind of your own self-perceived limitations. Everyone has these, including me. Some of them are real limits, but if you hold on to the belief that you simply cannot achieve something that you truly desire, you will prevent yourself from accomplishing what you really want. Being "like water" means you can fill any space if you give yourself the chance to take action.

Principle #2: Understand Yourself and How You React

Acquiring self-knowledge is important for achieving success in life, according to Bruce Lee.[5] Rather than being distracted by the expectations of others, he believed in the power of understanding the truest essence of himself. As an actor arriving in Hollywood, Lee found himself

---

* This oft-cited quote was recited by Bruce Lee during an interview with Canadian journalist Pierre Berton. It originally came from a 1971 episode of the television show *Longstreet*, in which he was the guest star. In that episode, aptly titled "The Way of the Intercepting Fist," Lee played an antiques dealer teaching the show's blind protagonist, James Longstreet, how to prepare for a fight. His advice was given to help Longstreet overcome his fears and lack of confidence.

at first obeying the television producers who had stereotypes in mind for him to portray. While he initially conformed to those expectations, he later broke out of the mold by acting true to his character, which led to the iconic roles he played in his martial arts films. His self-reckoning also guided his actions as a practitioner and teacher of the martial arts, and in his personal life. Bruce Lee undertook a lifelong quest to understand his own true motivations so he could live an authentic life.

Bruce Lee said, "Learn your inner nature in order to control it."[6] When it comes to personalizing your diet to fight fat and unleash your optimal metabolism, understanding your inner nature is extremely helpful. Some questions to consider:

- What makes me choose the foods that I like to eat?
- Why do I sometimes choose unhealthy and fattening foods?
- Why do I want to make healthy food choices?
- When I eat with others, what do I naturally choose to eat?
- What is the most important thing to me when it comes to food?

By examining these questions and answering authentically, you can study your own motivations and know what drives your behavior when you sit down to eat. This self-inquiry will help you understand your own needs, which will enable you to make more conscious decisions that are aligned with your goals.

Each person's body experiences food differently from anyone else's, even your closest relatives. Your tongue and its taste bud distribution are unique and different from any other person's.[7] The tongue's taste buds are molecular receptors for the flavors of fat, umami, sweet, bitter, and salt. People who love spicy foods, for example, may have fewer taste buds on their tongue, so they are not as bothered by the burning sensation. Others who find spicy food intolerable may be "super-tasters" whose taste buds are so densely packed, even a small amount of spice causes a sensory overload.

When it comes to food and health, you'll hear many voices telling you what to do and how to do it. But the truth is, no single formula fits everyone or affects everyone in the same way. What might work for one person might fail for you. Your genetics, family culture, childhood experiences, personal psychology, social community, and moral compass combine to shape your food preferences and the choices you make. All of this is unique to you! Personalizing your nutrition means you need to first understand who you are at multiple levels. That is how you match your needs with nutritional therapy.[8]

Here are some more questions you can ask yourself in the quest for self-knowledge when it comes to food:

- What do I value when it comes to food?
- What life experiences shaped my food preferences (likes, dislikes)?
- Which foods bring me joy?
- Which foods do I truly dislike? Why do I dislike them?
- What are my weaknesses when it comes to food selection?
- What do I enjoy eating that makes me feel physically lousy afterward?
- Which foods do I enjoy eating that make me feel great?
- What makes me want to try a new food?
- Which foods that I enjoy are known to be beneficial to health?
- Which foods do I enjoy that are known to be detrimental to my health?
- How do I know when I have eaten just enough and eating more will make me uncomfortably full?

There are no wrong answers because each one comes from your unique body and personal experience. Write down the ways of eating you've experienced that improve how you feel—and make them part of your life. Also make note of which ways of eating make you feel lousy, unfit, and unhealthy—and don't repeat them, or at least keep them to a minimum.

The better you understand yourself, the easier it will be to act and react in ways that move you toward your goals. Self-knowledge is an ongoing pursuit because you change over time as new experiences shape who you are.

Principle #3: Keep Learning in Order to Achieve Mastery

Bruce Lee believed that mastering new skills for combat requires a series of progressive steps. He said there are three stages of learning: in the first stage, a "punch is just a punch."[9] You just do it without fully understanding what is involved. In the second stage of learning, "a punch is no longer just a punch." This is the stage of dissecting each aspect of the punch: how to make a fist, getting the right physical stance to deliver the punch, and how to deliver the blow with the most effective force. As you analyze and break down the movement, you practice and repeat it over and over. The third stage of learning is where "a punch is just a punch" again. By this last stage, you have dissected and understood the punch, practiced it over and over again, and integrated each component until the entire action becomes automatic and instinctive. This same process can be applied to learning any skill, including how to incorporate foods that streamline your metabolism and improve your health.

In relation to fighting body fat and improving your metabolism, I've developed a protocol that will help you achieve your fitness and fat loss goals. It contains a series of steps, each of which has a scientific rationale. Following the Bruce Lee model for mastery, I recommend that you first read the directions to see what needs to be done. Then break the entire protocol into its parts and make sure you understand why each component is important. Practice each step to become familiar with it. Once you have done it over and over, it will become second nature. You'll find you're naturally fighting your body fat without having to think about it.

But don't stop there.

Continual learning is vital so that you can keep up with new discoveries from science. Nutrition, fat loss, and health are fast-moving areas of research. Between 2020 and 2021, 614,495 research articles were published on "metabolism" alone. Scientific discoveries build upon one another with new data that leads to even more discoveries, and so on. Once a critical threshold is met, the science can be put into practice.

Bottom line: always be open to new information and keep learning. I'm an information junkie when it comes to the science of health. That's why I've made it my mission to help translate all the complicated findings for you as simply and accurately as possible—so you can get a head start in learning about the new science of fighting body fat.

Principle #4: Adapt to Whatever Life Throws at You

In his film *The Game of Death*, Bruce Lee ascends a stairwell to the top of a pagoda, where he is confronted by an unusual opponent played by basketball legend Kareem Abdul-Jabbar . . . the adversary is seven feet, two inches tall! The much taller, bigger, and stronger Abdul-Jabbar uses his elongated reach and rangy legs to pummel the shorter and slighter five-foot-eight-inches-tall Lee. To counter, Lee adapts by using flying kicks to reach the taller man's head, and he delivers rapid body blows while ducking under Abdul-Jabbar's long, lashing arms. When Lee discovers his opponent's eyes are ultrasensitive to light, he punches holes in the pagoda's rice paper windows to let in blinding sunlight, which allows Lee to overcome the giant. It's just a movie, of course, but the underlying lesson is to achieve victory by adapting and changing tactics to respond to unforeseen circumstances. This was a key component of what Lee taught his students in real life. He stated, "The inability to adapt brings destruction."[10]

When life's circumstances—a holiday, a wedding, travel, a change in employment—take you away from your usual pattern, don't give up on eating for your health. Improvise! You may be on a disciplined path of eating, but suddenly you're required to take a day trip to an area where you cannot easily find healthy food. Pivot and adapt by bringing food with you or by skipping a meal—fasting not only won't hurt you; it can heal you, as you will learn in Chapter 11. When you are invited to dinner at a friend's home, choose only the healthiest offerings. If you feel comfortable doing so, tell your hosts about your eating preferences ahead of time so they can accommodate you.

How we adapt to life's ever-changing circumstances is an important part of our character. Finding success sometimes means not giving in to the easiest solution but finding a new path that could be hidden in plain sight. Follow Bruce Lee's advice of "not being tense, but ready . . . not being rigidly set, but flexible. Aware and alert, ready for whatever may come."[11]

Principle #5: Be Mindful of What You Eat

As a teen, Bruce Lee was skinny and not particularly fit. When he began to study martial arts, he started to condition his body and mind. When it came to his diet, Lee ate nutrient-dense foods. He urged mindfulness in eating: "Eat what your body requires, and don't get carried away with foods that don't benefit you."[12] This means avoid overeating and choose foods that are beneficial to your metabolism over those that are detrimental.

Lee observed that a healthy person has a good balance between sensing what is around them and taking the proper action. He encouraged the cultivation of awareness—of self and of the world around us. Said Lee, "A mind that is in a state of awareness can concentrate."[13]

For Bruce Lee, this approach led him to have a lean, sinewy, muscular frame with very little body fat. The result was a perfect balance of strength combined with speed and agility. You can search for photos of him online to see what physical and mental conditioning plus a healthy diet can do for the human body. When he was thirty-two, Lee's doctors proclaimed that he had the body of an eighteen-year-old.

You have control of everything you feed your body, so it's vital that you are present and deliberate whenever you are planning meals, shopping for groceries, cooking, serving, and eating.[14] Self-awareness saves you from harmful self-indulgences and lets you find a healthier and more agreeable path of *moderation*. Notice I didn't say *deprivation*. Being intentional and mindful will help you make every decision count when it comes to your food and your health. This level of awareness has been shown to reduce binge eating and eating on impulse.[15] Researchers from the University of California, San Francisco showed in a clinical study of 194 adults that deliberate eating and coaching on mindfulness helps people lose weight, improve their blood sugar, and rightsize their overall metabolic health.[16]

Here are some easy ways to be mindful when you eat:

- Focus on the moment when you sit down to eat, and before beginning, acknowledge your thoughts and how you are feeling—in body and mind.
- Consider the health benefits (or harms) of every item on your plate.
- Take small portions when you serve yourself.
- Quit the "clean plate club." If you are being served, note how much you've been given and do not feel responsible for eating everything on the plate.
- Take your time to eat and savor. Don't wolf food down faster than your brain can sense when you've had enough. It takes about twenty minutes for your gut to send the hormonal signals that tell your brain, "You are full. Stop eating." Studies have shown that slower eating also tends to suppress hunger longer after the meal, which leads to less snacking.[17]
- Avoid reaching for food when you are feeling stressed, upset, or depressed. Stress often leads to emotional eating, which often leads to overeating as well as choosing less healthy foods.[18]

- If you can, eat with people who care about their food and health. Talking with others about your enjoyment of the food makes you more mindful of the sensations you are experiencing and puts you in touch with your body's responses.

* * *

Finding your own way to fight fat and improve your metabolism requires a commitment to more than just eating healthy foods and cutting out junky ones. It needs to become a new habit, a second nature in your life. My tips in Part 2 for navigating the supermarket will help you get the right ingredients. The principles of finding your own way (with a little guidance from Bruce Lee) will help you commit to a sustainable and agreeable strategy.

Now I'm going to share with you a detailed protocol that will help you use those ingredients and get cooking so you can combat body fat, improve your metabolism, and enjoy your meals all at the same time.

Are you ready to eat to beat your diet?

CHAPTER 11

The Eat to Beat Protocol

If your doctor has ever suggested you could lose a few pounds, your response was probably something along the lines of "Okay, what do you recommend that I do?" Perhaps the answer you received was vague or, worse, condescending, or not informed by science. You can put that all behind you. In this chapter, I'm going to give you a step-by-step plan that will help you accomplish four goals—fight body fat, improve your metabolism, activate your health defenses, and elevate your overall health—all using one approach. Every recommendation here is based on scientific research as well as my direct experience as a physician and scientist who has been studying food and health for decades.

The program unfolds in three stages.

- **Stage 1 (Weeks 1–2): MediterAsian Swaps.** Swap out the foods that slow your metabolism and start eating from a selection of 150 MediterAsian foods that actually fight fat.

- **Stage 2 (Weeks 3–6): MediterAsian Intermittent Fasting.** Intermittent fasting is a powerful way to reboot your metabolism—and it's not as hard to incorporate into your life as you might think. I will provide tools and guidelines to help you begin eating this way and still allow you to enjoy satisfying and delicious meals.

- **Stage 3 (Week 7 and beyond): Maintenance.** In this maintenance phase, you will set yourself up for long-term success. Make your new eating habits personal so that they become an automatic, permanent, and flexible part of your new, healthier lifestyle.

In the first stage, **MediterAsian Swaps**, I'll show you how easy it can be to start eating foods that will help you reach your metabolism. Rather than simply tell you what not to eat, I will show you how to identify the foods that are working against your metabolism and swap them for foods drawn from the healthy and delicious traditions of the Mediterranean and Asia—foods that will satisfy your cravings and appetite. During these first two weeks, I recommend you begin a food journaling practice to identify your current habits around food and eating so you know what to change and what to keep. You will record what you eat every day and how you *feel* before, during, and afterward.

The second stage is a four-week guide to **MediterAsian Intermittent Fasting**. Intermittent fasting is an especially powerful tool for fighting harmful fat and improving your metabolism. It's also a natural part of human behavior.

You might think intermittent fasting is hard, but I urge you to think of it as finding an eating window that works for you, a method that allows pretty much everyone to feel full and satisfied. Contrary to some practices, you can reap the benefits of intermittent fasting and still eat during as many as twelve hours of the day, which is not difficult for most people's schedules.

This stage includes four weeks' worth of recipes and a meal-planning calendar. These recipes are delicious and easy to prepare, so you get to *enjoy* eating while you fire up your body's fat-burning mechanisms. These recipes are meant to inspire you, but you can easily create your own meal plan.

The third stage, and the key to long-term success, is **Maintenance** tailored to fit your own preferences and real-life circumstances while fine-tuning your metabolism. This stage is missing from most diets, which is one reason people have trouble maintaining results. Knowing how to adapt and pivot your personal plan to meet life's ever-changing conditions can be the key to keeping your metabolism in optimal shape long term. The practices you learn in this part will help you develop good habits that can last a lifetime.

I'll describe each stage and start with an At-a-Glance flowchart (Figure 11.1) so you can get the big picture of each element of each stage before you get the details.

Ready? Let's go.

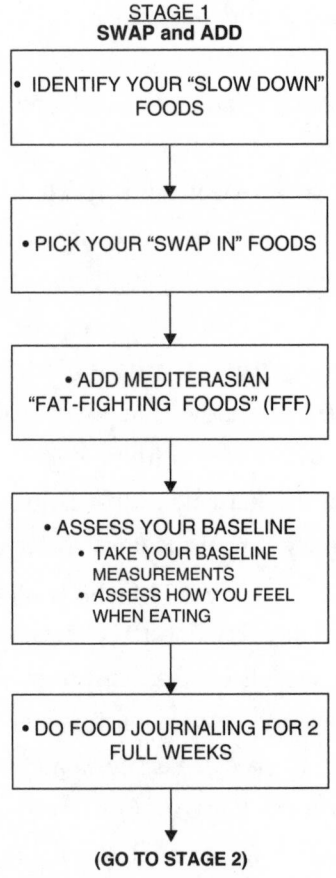

STAGE 1
SWAP and ADD

- IDENTIFY YOUR "SLOW DOWN" FOODS

- PICK YOUR "SWAP IN" FOODS

- ADD MEDITERASIAN "FAT-FIGHTING FOODS" (FFF)

- ASSESS YOUR BASELINE
  - TAKE YOUR BASELINE MEASUREMENTS
  - ASSESS HOW YOU FEEL WHEN EATING

- DO FOOD JOURNALING FOR 2 FULL WEEKS

(GO TO STAGE 2)

Figure 11.1 At–a–Glance: Swap and add.

Stage 1: MediterAsian Swaps (Two Weeks)

Identify Your "Slow Down Foods" and Pick Your "Swap In Foods"

Let's take stock of what you currently eat and how that is affecting your metabolic health. You'll begin by identifying the foods in your diet that are slowing down your metabolism. This is very important, so don't skip this step. To help you identify these foods, I've provided a list.

Take a look at Table 11.1. In the left column are the Slow Down Foods. These are the foods that, if eaten regularly and over time, *will* slow your metabolism, grow your fat, and interfere with your health defenses. Check the box of each Slow Down Food that you eat as a part of your diet, even if you only eat it occasionally.

How many Slow Down Foods did you check? Now go back to the top of the list and look at the right column. These are metabolically healthier Swap In Foods that you can use to replace the Slow Down Foods; many are inspired by the foods from the Mediterranean and Asia. For every major category of Slow Down Food on the left side, find at least one food in the right column (Swap In) that you can have as a substitute, and check the box next to it. Feel free to pick as many Swap In Foods as you like. The more variety, the better!

TABLE 11.1. SLOW DOWN AND SWAP IN FOODS
Check the box of each Slow Down Food (left-hand column) that you eat regularly. Then, for every major category, choose one or more Swap In Foods (right-hand column) that you like already or want to explore. You will avoid eating all foods from the Slow Down Foods list. For each food you avoid, you will substitute at least one from the Swap In Foods list.

Slow Down Foods	Swap In Foods
Refined Grains	*Swap In*
☐ Bread made with enriched or bleached flour	☐ Whole wheat bread
☐ Cream of wheat	☐ Brown or wild rice or quinoa
☐ Oyster crackers	☐ Cauliflower rice
☐ Prepackaged cheese crackers	☐ Carrots, celery, or cucumbers
☐ Prepackaged granola (in moderation)	☐ Foods with whole wheat, rye, or almond flour
☐ Prepackaged pastries	☐ Homemade nut and seed granola
	☐ Sourdough bread
	☐ Steel-cut oats

TABLE 11.1. SLOW DOWN AND SWAP IN FOODS (cont.)

Slow Down Foods	Swap In Foods
Refined Grains (cont.)	*Swap In (cont.)*
☐ Prepackaged peanut butter crackers ☐ Vegetable crackers and dip ☐ White crackers ☐ White flour ☐ White pasta ☐ White rice	☐ Vegetable crudité and guacamole ☐ Whole wheat, chickpea, or lentil pasta ☐ Zucchini noodles
Frozen Ultraprocessed Foods	*Swap In*
☐ Frozen entrées ☐ Frozen fried foods ☐ Frozen mac and cheese ☐ Frozen patties, fries, nuggets/ tenders ☐ Frozen pizza ☐ Frozen sandwiches and burritos ☐ Frozen waffles, pancakes, french toast ☐ Ice cream/frozen desserts	☐ Frozen fruits (mangos, berries, etc.) ☐ Frozen vegetables
Unfrozen Ultraprocessed Foods	*Swap In*
☐ Boxed or canned mac and cheese ☐ Buttermilk-based dressings ☐ Cream-based sauces ☐ Cream-based soups and bisques ☐ Fast food items, beverages, desserts ☐ Jarred or canned queso ☐ Mayonnaise-based dips and sauces	☐ Homemade dressing with yogurt, herbs, spices ☐ Homemade guacamole, salsa, pesto, tzatziki, hummus, tahini, baba ghanoush ☐ Homemade olive oil–based dressing ☐ Homemade vegan dressing ☐ Mustard ☐ Olive oil, tomato, or various plant-based sauces ☐ Vegetable-based soups and bisques
Fried Foods	*Swap In*
☐ Chips (potato and corn) ☐ Corn dogs ☐ Crab cakes ☐ Croquettes ☐ Doughnuts ☐ Falafel (fried) ☐ French fries ☐ Fried dough/funnel cake ☐ Fritters ☐ Mozzarella sticks ☐ Onion rings ☐ Samosas ☐ Tater tots and hash browns ☐ Wontons	☐ Air-fried or oven-baked vegetables ☐ Air-popped popcorn ☐ Roasted vegetables ☐ Unbreaded and air-fried falafel balls

TABLE II.I. SLOW DOWN AND SWAP IN FOODS (cont.)

Slow Down Foods	Swap In Foods
Dairy	*Swap In*
☐ Cheese (all kinds) ☐ Coffee creamer (all types) ☐ Cream (plain or flavored) ☐ Cream cheese ☐ Sour cream ☐ Whipped cream	☐ Coconut, almond, soy, or oat milk ☐ Kefir ☐ Plain Greek yogurt
Processed Meats	*Swap In*
☐ Bacon ☐ Beef jerky ☐ Chorizo ☐ Deli meat (bologna, ham, turkey, roast beef) ☐ Fast-food proteins (burgers, chicken, etc.) ☐ Hotdogs and sausages ☐ Pastrami ☐ Pepperoni ☐ Prepackaged/seasoned meats, chicken, fish ☐ Salami	☐ Burrito with beans and salsa ☐ Canned fish and other seafood ☐ Homemade patties made with beans, quinoa, herbs, spices ☐ Nut butters ☐ Tofu ☐ Tomato bread (Spanish style)
Meat	*Swap In*
☐ Beef/steak (any cut) ☐ Fried or with-skin poultry (chicken, duck, turkey) ☐ Lamb (tenderloin, leg, loin, rib) ☐ Pork (shoulder, leg, loin, belly)	☐ Legumes (beans, lentils, chickpeas) ☐ Mushrooms (all types) ☐ Poultry (chicken, duck, turkey), without skin, trimmed of fat ☐ Seafood (fish, shellfish), not fried ☐ Tofu
Foods with Added Sugar	*Swap In*
☐ Aspartame- and/or sucralose-based powders/additives ☐ Aspartame- and/or sucralose-based sweeteners ☐ Aspartame- and/or sucralose-sweetened foods ☐ Boxed cereals (esp. dessert/sweet-flavored) ☐ Candy ☐ Cream-filled cookies and cakes ☐ Energy bars ☐ Frosting ☐ Marshmallows	☐ Dark chocolate (80% or darker) ☐ Dried fruit (cranberries, blueberries, apricots, etc.) ☐ Homemade granola ☐ Homemade nut and seed granola (no sugar) ☐ Homemade trail mix (nuts, seeds, dried fruit) ☐ Natural sweeteners (monk fruit, honey) ☐ Pomegranate seeds ☐ Real fruit sorbet (no added sugar)

TABLE 11.1. SLOW DOWN AND SWAP IN FOODS (cont.)

Slow Down Foods	Swap In Foods
Foods with Added Sugar (cont.)	*Swap In*
☐ Milk or white chocolate ☐ Prepackaged cakes, pies, cookies, brownies, doughnuts ☐ Prepackaged granola (in moderation) ☐ Prepackaged ice cream and ice cream bars ☐ Sweetened peanut butter ☐ Trail mix (esp. ones high in chocolate or candies)	
Fats and Processed Oils	*Swap In*
☐ Avocado oil ☐ Beef tallow ☐ Butter (all kinds) ☐ Canola oil ☐ Coconut oil ☐ Corn oil ☐ Duck fat ☐ Flaxseed oil ☐ Grapeseed oil ☐ Lard (meat fat) ☐ Margarine ☐ Palm oil ☐ Partially hydrogenated oils ☐ Peanut oil ☐ Plant-based butter ☐ Safflower oil ☐ Sesame oil ☐ Sunflower oil ☐ Vegetable oil	☐ Olive oil
Beverages and Condiments with Added Sugar	*Swap In*
☐ Alcohol mixers/bases ☐ Aspartame- or sucralose-based sweeteners ☐ Aspartame- or sucralose-sweetened beverages ☐ Flavored or sweetened coffees and teas ☐ "Fruit" drinks (with added sugar and/or artificially sweetened)	☐ Coffee (hot or cold, no sugar) ☐ Fruit smoothie (can add greens) ☐ Kombucha ☐ Soy milk ☐ Tea (hot or cold, no sugar) ☐ Water (still or sparkling)

TABLE 11.1. SLOW DOWN AND SWAP IN FOODS (cont.)

Slow Down Foods	Swap In Foods
Beverages and Condiments with Added Sugar (cont.)	*Swap In*
☐ Milkshakes, sweetened/flavored milk ☐ Sodas (regular and aspartame/sucralose based) ☐ Sugar sauces (ketchup, chili sauces, caramel, BBQ) ☐ Syrups	
Alcohol	*Swap In*
☐ Beer and seltzers ☐ Bourbon ☐ Brandy ☐ Champagne ☐ Gin ☐ Rum ☐ Scotch ☐ Vodka ☐ Whiskey ☐ Wine	☐ Seltzer

Add Your MediterAsian Fat-Fighting Foods

As I explained in Part 2, science has identified many foods that *actually help you burn fat and improve your metabolism*. There are more than 150 fat-fighting foods, and the list I provide here is the first-ever published compilation of those with human evidence. These foods are very much a part of the culinary traditions of the Mediterranean and Asian countries.

Now you have the fun task of identifying which of these foods you already enjoy and which ones you'd most like to try so you can add them to your Swaps and incorporate even more metabolism-improving ingredients into your meal planning. Take a look at the list in Table 11.2 and check off all the foods that you like already and the ones you want to explore. You'll notice that there are no meats listed because they do not have fat-fighting properties. Also, be sure to check out the Sample Meal Guide (found in Chapter 12) for ideas on what to eat for these first two weeks.

TABLE 11.2. MEDITERASIAN FAT-FIGHTING FOODS

Check off the foods that you like already and the ones you want to explore.

Produce

Fruits

☐ Açai berries
☐ Apples, dried
☐ Apples, fresh
☐ Avocado
☐ Blackberries
☐ Black currants
☐ Blueberries
☐ Cherries
☐ Chokeberry
☐ Grapefruit
☐ Lemon
☐ Lime
☐ Lingonberries
☐ Oranges
☐ Pears (Anjou, Bartlett)
☐ Red and black raspberries
☐ Strawberries
☐ Tomatoes
☐ Watermelon

Vegetables

☐ Bok choy
☐ Broccoli
☐ Broccoli rabe/rapini
☐ Broccoli sprouts
☐ Broccolini
☐ Brussels sprouts
☐ Cabbage
☐ Carrots
☐ Chili peppers
☐ Chinese kale
☐ Choy sum
☐ Gai choy
☐ Garlic
☐ Mushrooms (chanterelle, cremini, enoki, oyster, porcini, portobello, shiitake, white button)
☐ Mustard greens
☐ Napa cabbage
☐ Onions (red, yellow)
☐ Ramps
☐ Romanesco
☐ Scallions

TABLE 11.2. MEDITERASIAN FAT-FIGHTING FOODS (cont.)

Produce (cont.)
Vegetables (cont.)
- ☐ Scapes
- ☐ Shallots
- ☐ Soybean (edamame, tofu)
- ☐ Wasabi
- ☐ Watercress

Middle Aisle Foods
Dried
- ☐ Buckwheat
- ☐ Cacao/dark chocolate
- ☐ Chickpeas
- ☐ Cinnamon
- ☐ Lentils
- ☐ Mushrooms (chanterelle, oyster, porcini, shiitake)
- ☐ Navy beans
- ☐ Nuts (almonds, cashews, hazelnuts, macadamias, pecans, pistachios, walnuts)
- ☐ Pearl barley
- ☐ Prune
- ☐ Red chili peppers
- ☐ Turmeric
- ☐ Yellow split peas

Bottled
- ☐ Extra virgin olive oil
- ☐ Vinegar (apple cider, balsamic, black)

Jarred
- ☐ Capers
- ☐ Gochujiang
- ☐ Kimchi
- ☐ Tomato sauce

Tubed
- ☐ Anchovy paste
- ☐ Garlic paste
- ☐ Tomato paste

Canned
- ☐ Tinned seafood (anchovies, shellfish, tuna)
- ☐ Tomatoes (whole, peeled, pureed)

TABLE 11.2. MEDITERASIAN FAT-FIGHTING FOODS (cont.)

Seafood

Fish

☐ Anchovy
☐ Black sea bass
☐ Black sea bream
☐ Chilean sea bass
☐ Cod
☐ Dover sole
☐ Gilt-head bream
☐ Hake
☐ Halibut
☐ Mackerel
☐ Mediterranean sea bass
☐ Salmon
☐ Sardines
☐ Striped bass
☐ Turbot

Claws and Shells

☐ Crab (blue, king, mitten, stone)
☐ Langoustine
☐ Lobster (Atlantic and European)
☐ Mantis shrimp
☐ Mussels
☐ Oysters
☐ Razor clams
☐ Sea scallops
☐ Shrimp
☐ Spiny lobster

Tubes and Tentacles

☐ Cuttlefish
☐ Octopus
☐ Sea cucumber
☐ Squid

Seaweed

☐ Dulse
☐ Kombu
☐ Nori
☐ Wakame

Roe

☐ Caviar
☐ Salmon roe
☐ Sea urchin roe
☐ Tarama

TABLE II.2. MEDITERASIAN FAT-FIGHTING FOODS (cont.)

Beverages

Tea
- ☐ Green tea
- ☐ Matcha
- ☐ Oolong tea
- ☐ Pu'er tea

Juice
- ☐ Concord grape juice
- ☐ Cranberry juice
- ☐ Orange juice
- ☐ Pomegranate juice
- ☐ Tomato juice
- ☐ Watermelon juice

Other
- ☐ Cocoa beverages
- ☐ Coffee
- ☐ Soy milk
- ☐ Water

Assess Your Baseline

Before you begin your two-week food journaling practice, take stock of where you are and record the some measurements that reflect the current state of your metabolism. Some of these are objective numbers (go ahead and use the measure most natural for you, such as inches, centimeters, pounds, or kilograms), while others are subjective and reflect how you feel.

Take Your Baseline Measurements

- Record your height:
  My height is: _____.
- Weigh yourself:
  My weight is: _____.
- Measure your waist size:
  My waist size is: _____.

- My general energy level is:

  1 2 3   4 5 6 7   8 9 10 (circle one)

  (very low)   (average)   (very good)

- I would rate my physical fitness level to be:

  1 2 3   4 5 6 7   8 9 10 (circle one)

  (very poor)   (average)   (very fit)

- After I eat, I usually feel:

  1 2 3   4 5 6 7   8 9 10 (circle one)

  (stuffed)   (full)   (satisfied)

- I know when I have eaten too much:

  ☐ Yes, but I don't realize it until it's too late

  ☐ Yes, and I always stop before I get to that point

  ☐ No, it's hard for me to know

- The meal I am most likely to overeat is (choose one, if any apply):

  ☐ Breakfast   ☐ Lunch   ☐ Dinner

- I can name the foods that make me feel uncomfortable (bloated, stomachache, crampy bowel, sluggish, etc.) after eating them:

  ☐ Yes   ☐ No   ☐ Unsure

- The foods that make me feel uncomfortable are (identify at least three):

  _____

  _____

  _____

  _____

Do Food Journaling for Two Full Weeks

Keeping a food journal in the first two weeks will help you notice and document the details of how you eat—details that you may not be aware of or have never recognized. Record information about which foods you eat using the template provided (you can download it from www.drwilliamli.com/foodjournal) and track how you are feeling by answering a series of questions every day.

Before you start journaling each meal, ask yourself the questions below to get a baseline for where you are right now.

More Baseline Questions to Ask and Record

What time do you wake up in the morning?

Are you hungry when you wake up?

At what times do you eat each meal: breakfast, lunch, dinner?

What exactly do you eat, and how much do you eat at each meal?

How hungry are you before each meal?

How do you feel after each meal?

What is your energy level throughout the day?

When and how many times a day do you snack?

What do you eat when you snack?

What time do you go to bed at night?

Now that you have some baseline data recorded, you can use journaling to become more aware of your behaviors and how you feel as you eat. Journaling is a great tool to help you identify feelings or the events that pull you off your plan. It will guide you to find strategies and tactics that can help you stay on your plan.

Documenting what and how much you eat also helps you to be conscious of your actual food intake. This is important, as most of us tend to grossly underestimate how much food we consume.

At the end of each day, you'll jot down how you felt about the day as a whole and document any insights gained. This can be a great place to add any strategies you tried that you found especially effective or inspiring so you can easily repeat them.

Use the following prompts to assist with your journaling.

Journaling Prompts

Day # ___ of 14: (fill in which Stage 1 day you're on)
Today's Date:

I woke up at _____ **(TIME)**
When I woke up, my energy level was _____
I felt _____
I noticed I _____ (use this prompt to add
   any other awareness you had)
I ate breakfast at _____ **(TIME)**

This is what I ate (list foods and quantities): _____
And I drank: _____
When I stopped eating, I felt _____
I noticed I _____ (use this prompt to add
   any other awareness you had)
An hour after eating, I felt (circle all that apply): sleepy, heavy,
   bloated, sluggish, foggy, headachy, focused, clear-headed,
   light, happy, energized (or write in your own).
I felt hungry again at _____ **(TIME)**
I did/did not (circle one) feel the urge to snack. So I
   _____ (write your response to the urge)
I ate lunch at _____ **(TIME)**

This is what I ate (list foods and quantities): _____
And I drank: _____
When I stopped eating, I felt _____
I noticed I _____ (use this prompt to add
   any other awareness you had)
An hour after eating, I felt (circle all that apply): sleepy, heavy,
   bloated, sluggish, foggy, headachy, focused, clear-headed,
   light, happy, energized.

I felt hungry again at _____(**TIME**)

I did/did not (circle one) feel the urge to snack. So I

_____ (write your response to the urge)

I ate dinner at _____(**TIME**)

This is what I ate (list foods and quantities): _____

And I drank: _____

When I stopped eating, I felt _____

I noticed I _____ (use this prompt to add any other awareness you had about your meal)

An hour after eating, I felt (circle all that apply): sleepy, heavy, bloated, sluggish, foggy, headachy, focused, clear-headed, happy, relaxed, comfortable

I felt hungry again at _____(**TIME**)

I did/did not (circle one) feel the urge to snack.

When the urge came on, I was _____

(What were you doing? What were you thinking about?)

So I _____ (write your response to the urge and be sure to note any strategies you find to be effective)

I went to bed at _____(**TIME**)

Reflecting on the day as a whole, I've become aware of

_____

What to Do

Food Swap

- For two weeks, avoid eating *all* foods in the Slow Down Foods column and add the Swap In Foods for each of your three daily meals.
- Choose as many of the Fat-Fighting Foods as you like from the 150 on the provided list to add to your diet. The more

Fat-Fighting Foods you eat, the less room you have for Slow Down Foods. Your metabolism will thank you.

- If you find yourself eating foods that are not on any of these lists, such as your favorite vegetables, legumes, and spices, carry on—those are fine.
- Use the Sample Meal Guide in Chapter 12 to help you plan and time your meals.

Journaling

(Optional: Download journal template pages to use as a guide from www.drwilliamli.com/foodjournal.)

- Keep your journal for at least two weeks, and answer the questions honestly.
- At the end of two weeks, sit down for thirty minutes to review all you've documented.
- Analyze what you recorded: Which foods and meals made you feel good? Which ones made you feel uncomfortable? Which food swaps did you enjoy the most? Were you mindful of your portion sizes, or did you get up from meals feeling overstuffed? When did you get hungry during the day? At what times were you eating? Were you eating when you were not hungry? Did you snack and, if so, when? What were the circumstances? What strategies did you discover and use that worked best to help you stay on track with the Swap In Foods and Fat-Fighting Foods?

The food journal reveals not just what you eat but also how you *connect* to food each day and how you *feel* about it. At the end of these two weeks, you (and your body) will be ready to commit to a program that elevates your metabolism and fights harmful body fat.

You will be able to use this information to support you as you enter Stage 2.

Stage 2: MediterAsian Intermittent Fasting (Four Weeks)

Now that you've raised your awareness and started using food swaps and eating more Fat-Fighting Foods, it's time to get to the real action by using the four weeks of MediterAsian Intermittent Fasting to reset your metabolism, burn down body fat, and activate your health defenses. By the end of this four-week period, you'll have established new healthy habits that will improve your metabolism and overall health—habits you can maintain for the rest of your life.

Here's a quick breakdown of the elements of Stage 2: set your eating window, plan your meals one week at a time, eat according to your meal plan, and do another self-assessment (Figure 11.2).

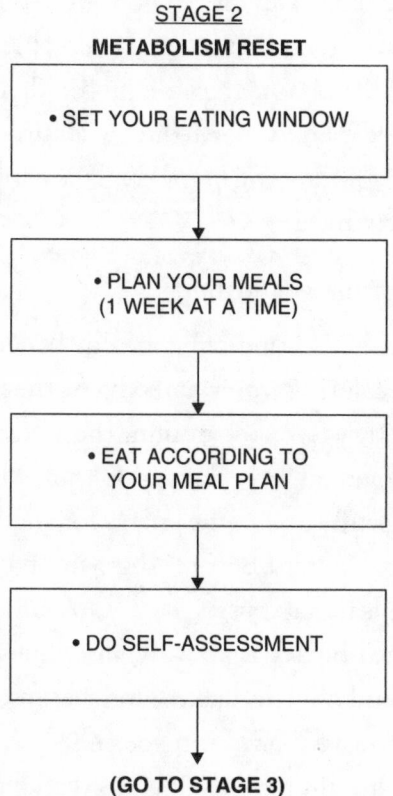

STAGE 2
METABOLISM RESET

• SET YOUR EATING WINDOW

• PLAN YOUR MEALS
(1 WEEK AT A TIME)

• EAT ACCORDING TO
YOUR MEAL PLAN

• DO SELF-ASSESSMENT

(GO TO STAGE 3)

Figure II.2 At-a-Glance: Metabolism reset.

MediterAsian Intermittent Fasting

Fasting is part of our natural behavior. When we sleep, we are fasting. And when we eat after waking up in the morning, we break that fast (that's why it's called "breakfast"). By definition, all humans practice *intermittent fasting*. So, although intermittent fasting has been popularized as a health trend, it is a routine part of how our body functions.

Intermittent fasting is a core part of the Eat to Beat Protocol and it fits inherently into the MediterAsian way of eating. The Mediterranean and Asian countries practice fasting as part of their religious traditions. Both cultures tend to eat lighter breakfasts and start the day with less of a calorie load. Most importantly, Mediterranean and Asian food culture is all about intentional eating: being aware of when and what you are eating, and not snacking mindlessly. Those who follow this way of eating are conscious of the food they eat and are highly selective about the quality of ingredients and how they are prepared. The absence of random snacking is logical and very MediterAsian in nature—why would you spoil your appetite when you know you'll be eating something really delicious for your next meal?

The Benefits of Intermittent Fasting

Here's why intermittent fasting offers health benefits. When you eat, you're loading fuel (calories) into your body. As the food breaks down in digestion, your pancreas secretes insulin, the hormone that tells your cells to absorb the ingested fuel (glucose) for immediate use. This keeps your organs running and supplies the energy for any physical and mental activities you may be doing. Beyond that, the fuel that's absorbed is stored in your fat cells for later use.

Your body is engineered so that, while insulin levels are high, it cannot tap that stored energy. This makes sense because while you are fueling up, you don't want to draw down your reserves; so the energy stays trapped in your fat. Insulin inhibits lipolysis (breaking down of fat), the process needed to access the energy stored in fat. Without lipolysis, you cannot access the fuel. In other words, when your insulin levels are up (while you are eating and for a period after eating while the fuel is being loaded into your cells), your fat cannot be tapped into and shrunk. It's like being at a gas station: when you pull up to the pump to fuel up, you have to turn off the engine. You are not permitted to burn away the fuel in the tank at the same time you are filling the tank.

On the other hand, you are fasting whenever you are not eating between meals, and this includes while you are sleeping. During this period, your blood levels of insulin run on the low side. Low insulin "unlocks" the fuel tank and allows lipolysis to occur. Your metabolism can access and break down your fat and use the energy as fuel. The longer you fast, the lower your blood insulin levels drop, and the more fat your body can burn. If you were shipwrecked on a desert island with no access to food, your fat stores would be quickly depleted. You'd burn your fat stores and lose a tremendous amount of weight in a short period of time. Fasting (and losing weight) and starvation (withering away) are on the same continuum; it's just a matter of intention and severity.

When we are not intermittently fasting, we are *intermittently eating* (this is the eating window of the Eat to Beat Protocol). This is the other half of a life plan that helps you to optimize your metabolism. An enormous body of scientific and clinical research has studied how switching between intermittent fasting and eating can support health, improve metabolism, aid in weight loss, fight body fat, suppress inflammation, increase longevity, fight cancer, and more.[1] It doesn't require you to starve. It merely reduces the time available to consume calories each day.[2]

The way the Eat to Beat Protocol works is simple: when you are not eating, insulin levels are lower, and your body can burn down fat and boost your metabolism. Eating foods that possess fat-fighting bioactives further activates your metabolism to burn down dangerous body fat. It takes metabolic advantage of the time when you are not eating, as well as the smart choices with foods you do consume while you are eating.

MediterAsian Intermittent Fasting also offers fringe benefits to the body's health defense systems: angiogenesis, regeneration, microbiome, DNA protection, and immunity. Your genetic machinery synchronizes itself during fasting to coordinate all the moving parts of your metabolism. Your DNA makes fewer inflammatory proteins during this time. When fasting, your body turns on the process of autophagy, which is a form of cellular housecleaning that sweeps up dead and dying cells.[3] At the same time, your stem cells swing into action to replace and regenerate any body tissues that need to be repaired or renewed, including your immune system.[4] Like a laptop rebooting, your microbiome resets itself during the fasted state.[5]

You'll get other important health benefits during the fasting/sleeping period when you are not eating. Burning fat by fasting helps your liver stay healthier. Cellular aging processes are slowed. Muscles are maintained and built up during fasting.[6] And your brain's neuroplasticity, its ability to form new connections from learning or to recover from injury, is optimized during intermittent fasting.[7]

The Eat to Beat Protocol is designed to help you benefit from all these metabolic healing advantages of fasting. In the morning, wait for a while before you eat anything. Use that time to brush your teeth, take a shower, get dressed, and prepare yourself for your day ahead *before* breakfast. If you need a reminder, set an alarm that goes off one hour (or more) after you wake up to alert you that your eating window is now open. The same principle applies to your evening routine. By not eating for three hours before bedtime, you gain more fasting time. Your body and your health will thank you.

Set Your Eating Window

This is the time period in each day within which you will do all your eating. You'll eat nothing before and nothing after. The time outside of this (when you are not eating) is when your body is fasting and performing critical functions for your metabolism that fight body fat. Adding calories to your system before or after your eating window interferes with these critical metabolic functions, so it's important not to snack during fasting hours.

To design your eating window, you must first decide at what time you will start and stop eating each day.

When to "open" your eating window: Wait at least one hour after you wake up before you take your first meal. If your alarm wakes you at 7:00 a.m., then open your eating window at 8:00 a.m. or any time afterward. Listen to your body. Most people discover that they are not hungry right after awakening. Still, this may cause you to break some long-standing habits. Many of us were taught as children that it is imperative to eat breakfast before school, so we learned to eat immediately after getting up. This is not optimal for your metabolism. Instead, you will extend your "noneating period" for as long as possible after you awaken. This lengthens the period of your overnight fast and improves your metabolism. Breakfast means you break your fast—plan on delaying this with a late breakfast, or even skip breakfast entirely. Discuss this with your doctor if you have diabetes or any health concerns; otherwise, it's fine.

When to "close" your eating window: The next step is to determine when your eating window *closes*. This is the time when you have your last bite of the day, which means when you finish your evening meal, not when you start it. Be aware that for optimal results, you should close your eating window no more than twelve hours after you opened it—or sooner. Let's say you get up at 7:00 a.m., and you decide to open your eating window at 8:00 a.m. This means you would need to close your eating window no later than 8:00 p.m., which is the twelve-hour time span. To meet this schedule, you could start dinner at 7:00 p.m., a reasonable time for most people. By 8:00 p.m., you are done. No late-night snacks.

If it suits your schedule, you should make the eating window even shorter than twelve hours. For example, if you eat dinner at 6:00 p.m., you could finish by 7:00 p.m. Your entire eating window would then be between 8:00 a.m. and 7:00 p.m. This is an eleven-hour window, well within the twelve-hour time span, and it is even better for your metabolism because it extends your fasting time. An eight-hour window is even better (you would eat a late breakfast at 10:00 a.m., say, then have an early dinner at 5:00 p.m. and be finished by 6:00 p.m.), though this is harder for most people to practice. You may need to experiment with different eating windows to find what works best with your schedule.

Whatever you do, make sure to stop eating at least two to three hours before bedtime. Not only will this improve the quality of your sleep, it also allows your body to finish its immediate work of digestion so it can start its fat-burning and other metabolic activities while you are asleep.

Let's review:

Example Twelve-Hour Eating Window:
7:00 a.m.:   Wake up (no eating for one hour)
8:00 a.m.:   Open eating window (eat breakfast)
8:00 p.m.:   Close eating period (finish dinner)
11:00 p.m.:   Bedtime

This eating window may be a close reflection of how you already eat, or you may need to tinker with the timing a bit to make it fit with your lifestyle. Experiment as needed—it's worth getting it right.

Just remember this: when you eat the MediterAsian Way, you are putting energy (calories) and bioactives (polyphenols, dietary fiber) into your body. When you are not eating, your body shifts into burning those calories that have been stored in fat, and the more time it has to do this, the more fat you will burn. To recap, to optimize your metabolism and turn your body's burners on high, wait at least one hour before you open your eating window in the morning. For best results, and a more restful night's sleep, have your last bite and close your eating window at least two to three hours before bedtime. For the entire four weeks of the Eat to Beat Protocol, eat all your meals within this time frame.

What to Do

- Fill out the worksheet below to determine the open and close times of your eating window.
- If it helps to remind you, set two alarms on your mobile device, fifteen minutes before the opening and closing times of your eating window.
- Use the Sample Meal Guide in Chapter 12 as a guide to set your mealtimes and know which meals you'll skip.

My Eating Window Worksheet

The time I wake up in the morning: _____ o'clock

The time my eating window starts (at least one hour after waking): _____ o'clock

The time my eating window closes (at least two hours before bedtime): _____ o'clock

The time I go to bed: _____ o'clock

Total hours of time I will eat (between start and close time): _____ hours

---

Plan (and Prep) Your Meals One Week at a Time

The best way to stay on track with the Eat to Beat Protocol is to plan ahead. Planning your meals in advance for the upcoming week is a smart way to prepare for grocery shopping and cooking and knowing what meals are coming up each day (and when you'll have leftovers to save time the next day!).

Here are four easy steps to help you plan and prep your meals a week at a time. I like to do these on the weekend when things are a little less hectic:

1. First, **select your recipes**. If you are looking for inspiration, you'll find thirty-seven delicious recipes in Chapter 12 that you can use as a starting point. I also recommend you add some healthy family favorites you already know how to prepare or go online to hunt for some new recipes. Look for ones that feature foods from the list of Fat-Fighting Foods. Avoid ingredients from the Slow Down Foods list and foods that are heavily processed or fried.

2. Once you have your recipes, **make a shopping list** of all the items you'll need to prepare all your meals for the week. (Pro tip: if you want to cut down on prep and cooking time, you can make more servings at a time and plan to make a few meals that will yield tasty leftovers.)

3. Take your shopping list to the market and **get all the ingredients**.

4. **Optional:** If you tend to have busy workweeks, take a little extra time and **do some of the prep work on the weekend to shorten your cooking time** during the workweek. For example, wash, peel, and cut carrots, onions, and other veggies for a soup and store them in the refrigerator in a glass container.

Eat According to Your Meal Plan

For a successful metabolism reset, it's important that you do your best to stick to your plan. While repeated efforts to lose weight do have benefits, as you've learned, starting and stopping will confuse your metabolism and make fighting body fat much harder to accomplish. Should you encounter an insurmountable obstacle that makes it impossible to eat the meal you planned, here are a few strategies you might try so that you don't veer too far off track.

- If you know ahead of time that making a meal will be difficult, pick out some fresh fruit or cut veggies you can eat instead.
- When presented with a meal that someone else prepared for you, look at all of the options being offered and choose only those that contain Fat-Fighting Foods and the foods on your Swap In Foods list.
- If you're at home and simply run out of time to cook a planned meal, swap it out for another meal you planned the same week but that is faster to prepare and access—or eat leftovers from a previous meal.
- If your only options are Slow Down Foods, you can just skip that meal and wait until you can access the food that you had planned to eat or that is more healthful. Drink a tall glass of water to subdue your hunger pangs. Do remember at your next meal not to overeat.

Do a Self-Assessment

At the end of these four weeks, you will have trained your body to take in fewer calories and to fuel itself with healthier Fat-Fighting Foods. Your body will also have had more time to burn down fat during your fasting periods. Your metabolism will soon be operating much more efficiently. Take note of how you feel and function. You should feel more energetic and alert and lighter on your feet.

Many people find it motivating to do quick evaluations along the way. You might remeasure your waist circumference or reweigh yourself, or, if you want to see how you're doing without obsessing over a number on the scale, try these helpful spot checks.

Pick a favorite clothing item that used to fit but has become too tight. Try it on once a week and see how it feels each time. If it's gradually getting easier to put on or zip up, or if it feels looser or is more comfortable, you're making progress!

Notice how your body moves. When you shed harmful body fat and get your metabolism going, you'll begin to notice it's easier to move. **Note any changes you experience in the following:**

- How much effort is required to stand up, sit, or get up off the floor?
- Does it feel easier to walk?
- Has your natural walking speed increased?
- Do you get less winded?
- Do you have more energy throughout the day?
- Can you bend over and breathe normally? (Without your stomach pressing into your diaphragm and forcing you to take short breaths?)

At the end of the four weeks, be sure to revisit the self-assessment and record your new data.

Self-Assessment After Four Weeks

- My current weight is: _____
- My waist size is: _____
- My current energy level is:

  1 2 3   4 5 6 7   8 9 10 (circle one)

  (very low)   (average)   (very good)
- I rate my physical fitness now to be:

  1 2 3   4 5 6 7   8 9 10 (circle one)

  (very poor)   (average)   (very fit)
- After I eat now, I feel:

  1 2 3   4 5 6 7   8 9 10 (circle one)

  (stuffed)   (full)   (satisfied)

Stage 3: Tailor Your Plan

Congratulations! You've completed the four-week program and now have the tools to fight extra body fat, improve your metabolism, and activate your health defenses. You've eliminated many foods that once harmed your metabolism and health defenses. You've figured out how to eat only within a designated time window so your body has time to conduct its important metabolic functions while you fast (and sleep). Importantly, you have been eating foods, prepared in ways that you enjoy, that science says help you burn away harmful fat.

Now your goal is to keep it going. And to do that, the protocol has to fit into your life circumstances, and you have to be able to adapt it when necessary (see Figure 11.3).

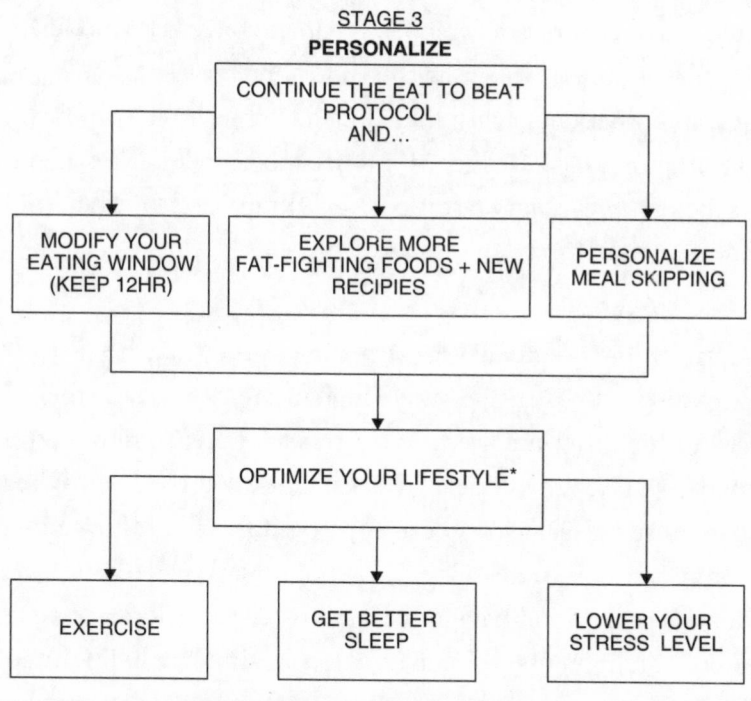

Figure 11.3 At-a-Glance: Personalize your plan.
*See chapter 13 for details.

Continue the Eat to Beat Protocol

Here are some tips to help you refine your protocol to better suit your preferences and keep the momentum going on your success.

Keep trying new foods and preparation methods. If you want to keep things interesting, try items on the Fat-Fighting Foods list that are less familiar and use new recipes to add variety to old standby foods. Keep delighting your palate with interesting tastes that will help you stay engaged with eating the foods that optimize your metabolism and boost your health.

Continue to avoid ultraprocessed foods. These are foods commonly found in a box, can, plastic wrapper, or jar and have been modified from their natural state and mixed with artificial preservatives, coloring, flavorings, and other chemicals, including added sugar, salt, and hydrogenated (saturated) fats. Most convenience foods, including frozen foods, snacks, boxed cereals, and fast foods, are ultraprocessed. They will slow down your metabolism.

Stay away from fried foods. As appealing as they may be (I really like crispy textures), deep-fried foods are high in calories because they absorb the fat in which they are fried. Avoid this food preparation method for any food, even healthy choices. For example, cod is a healthy seafood that contains omega-3 fatty acids. A piece of fried cod (fish-and-chips) can contain twelve times more fat—none of the added fats are the healthy omega-3s—and have more than twice the calories of a piece of baked cod. Frying any food makes it less healthy, including fried zucchini, fried tomatoes, fried calamari, fried shrimp, fried oysters, and so on. Oven crisping or air frying foods are much healthier ways to get the crunch without the fat.

Keep skipping a couple of meals each week. Try to skip a breakfast and, on a different day, a lunch each week. These already are commonly skipped meals. You may initially feel hungry as you get accustomed to this new eating pattern. One way to get around it is to drink a glass of water when you start to feel hungry. This will fool your brain and alter its release of the hunger hormone, ghrelin. You can also try going for a walk. You can power through it—just as millions of other people do when they skip a meal because they are too preoccupied to eat. Meal skipping is healthy because it helps lower your overall caloric intake, which tips your body's energy equation in favor of weight loss. Again, be aware that if you skip a meal, you may be tempted to overeat at the next meal, so watch your portions.

Each week's meal plan will look something like the one in Table 11.3.

Continue to avoid snacking. This means no mindless nibbling, no junk food bingeing in your car during a commute, no midnight snacks, and so on. Snacking triggers an insulin surge that blocks fat burning. Giving up snacks helps your body be more metabolically efficient.

Limit dining out. Eating at home will help you maintain the most control over your food choices, so dine in and prepare your own meals as much as possible. If you must dine out, refer to the Swap In Foods and Fat-Fighting Foods lists. Choose menu items wisely and eat moderate portions using the same principles as if you were at home.

TABLE 11.3. PERSONALIZED MEAL PLAN TEMPLATE

	Sunday	Monday	Tuesday	Wednesday	Thursday	Friday	Saturday
START eating 2 hours after wake-up	Breakfast	SKIP X	Breakfast	Breakfast	SKIP X	Breakfast	Breakfast
	Lunch	Lunch	Lunch	Lunch	Lunch	Lunch	SKIP X
STOP eating 3 hours before bedtime	Dinner	Dinner	Dinner	Dinner	Dinner	Dinner	Dinner

Continue to stop eating when you are satisfied but not full. The quality of the calories matters a lot when it comes to your metabolism, but so does the quantity. Overloading your body with calories damages your system. Portion control is vital to healthy eating and meeting your health goals.

Here are three additional ways to tailor the protocol to your liking:

1. **Modify the eating window as needed** to fit your wake-up and sleep times each day. Not everyone wakes up and goes to bed at the same time each day. For example, you may get up at 7 a.m. during the workweek, but on a weekend you may arise at 9 a.m. To adapt the plan, just make sure you delay eating for one hour after waking. So, during the workweek, you would not eat until 8 a.m., but on Saturday and Sunday, you would not eat until 10 a.m. (or you could skip breakfast and have an early lunch).

2. **Continue to explore new fat-fighting foods and find new recipes.** One of my greatest joys is to explore new foods. I have a saying: "Life is for the living," which to me means that we are meant to enjoy the plethora of delicious foods that are available to us. Make yourself a Fat-Fighting Food hunter (learn about new ones by signing up for my newsletter at www.drwilliamli.com) and continue to find new recipes to try. Who knows, some may become your new favorites.

3. **Personalize the meal-skipping schedule.** To adapt to real-life circumstances, you may need to change which meal you choose to skip on any given day of the week. That's fine, so long as you continue to skip a few meals per week. If you can only manage to skip one or two some weeks, that is fine. But aim to skip three the following week.

Return for a Reset

Even if you make a strong commitment to the Eat to Beat Protocol, you may wander off track from time to time. This can happen to anyone. Life throws unexpected curveballs all the time. Don't worry!

If you find yourself back to eating unhealthy foods and gaining weight, simply restart the protocol. Go back to Stage 1 and begin all over again. The Eat to Beat Protocol is designed to make it easy to start on the program and restart whenever needed. The good habits you learn from the protocol are like riding a bicycle—once you learn them, it's very easy to get back on track and do it again. The goal is to have a lifelong method to continuously improve your metabolism while fighting body fat.

Not All Calories Are Created Equal

There is one important added twist to the principle of moderation: not all calories are created equal. The *quality* of the food containing the calories makes a big difference.

You've heard of candy and soda referred to as "empty calories." They commonly contain high-fructose corn syrup, which is a simple sugar that, in excess, leads to metabolic syndrome. By the way, whole fruit also contains the same sugar and fructose but does not have this effect because, in addition to the calories from fructose, fruit has dietary fiber and bioactives that benefit your metabolism. The fat-fighting foods listed in this book will help guide you so that not only will you eat the right *quantity* of calories; you'll also be getting the *highest quality* of calories.

The concept of "nutrient density" is important when making food choices. Whole foods like fruits and vegetables contain fiber, bioactives, proteins, and other macro- and micronutrients, as well as natural sugars. The fiber makes you feel more satiated so you

(Continued)

---

won't feel as hungry over the course of a day. Eating less means putting fewer calories in your body. A hundred-calorie serving of a whole kiwifruit or red bell pepper is more nutrient-dense and has more health value than a hundred-calorie serving of candy. Aim for a high nutrient-to-calorie ratio when choosing what to eat. Protein is a macronutrient that takes more energy and time to digest, and this makes you feel fuller longer. All the Fat-Fighting Foods are nutrient-dense and contain bioactives that aid your metabolism.

In addition, "zero-calorie" on the food or beverage label does not mean it is healthier or that consuming it will prevent weight gain. Consuming sugar-free sodas and other foods that contain artificial sweeteners can have the opposite effect by harming your gut microbiome. This has been studied by researchers at the University of North Carolina at Chapel Hill, North Carolina State University, and the University of Georgia. Lab mice were given acesulfame potassium (Ace-K), an artificial sweetener used in sugar-free soda and foods. The chemical caused dysbiosis, a shift in makeup of gut bacteria in the mice. After four weeks of acesulfame, the mice gained weight.[8] When the researchers examined the genetic material of the gut bacteria after the mice consumed the artificial sweetener, they found that the bacteria's DNA responsible for metabolism had changed. Since these healthy bacteria normally help regulate insulin sensitivity, blood glucose levels, and blood lipids, throwing the microbiome off-balance disrupts your metabolism and can actually cause weight *gain*.

Other nonnutritive sweeteners, such as sucralose and saccharin, have also been shown to cause concerning changes in the gut microbiome and glucose intolerance.[9] Clinical studies of aspartame and acesulfame showed that individuals who consumed them had less of the important bacteria diversity in their gut that is linked to good health.[10]

The bottom line: if you want to lose weight and fight body fat, stay away from foods that harm your metabolism. Choose Fat-Fighting Foods, eat fewer calories, and burn more calories.[11] Eat smaller portions of high-quality, nutrient-dense foods. You don't have to count calories or obsess over the numbers. Look at the big picture, get into the habit of healthy eating, and enjoy your life!

Frequently Asked Questions

People often ask me how I adapt my approach to eating to fit real-life circumstances, when there are other considerations beyond simply planning, buying, and preparing food for myself. I've collected some of these questions and here are my answers to them:

What do I do if I'm also cooking for other people who do not eat like me?

The best way to approach this is to plan your own program—and ask if any of the Swap In Foods or Fat-Fighting Foods prepared with a healthy recipe would be appealing to your family members or friends. That way, everyone is bought into the program. There are enough tasty choices that you should be able to find something that will satisfy even picky eaters. The program will also improve the health of everyone you are feeding, so there is a benefit to sharing the plan.

In the event you have to prepare food for someone who is committed to an unhealthier way of eating or for someone who is very limited in what they are willing to eat—and you are willing to support that habit—you can always prepare a specific dish for that individual. Alternatively, invite them to bring or prepare their own meal.

When you are trying to get your metabolism elevated, you need to focus on yourself first. The good news is that I've found it's possible to get nearly everyone excited about delicious, healthy fat-fighting food.

What do I do if I'm on a tight budget?

Most of the foods in the Swap In Foods and Fat-Fighting Foods lists are found in almost every grocery store and are less expensive than heavily processed packaged foods—by eliminating snacks, sodas, and ultraprocessed foods and buying whole fresh foods and specific items from the grocery store middle aisles, you'll be saving money each time you go to the store. To that end, even if you're on a budget, you should still be able to buy the right foods for your metabolism. Certain healthy items, like dried and canned beans, are not only inexpensive, but also their recipes can make enough food for more than one meal. Also, when you are on a tight budget and want to eat as healthily as possible, you can save money by preparing your own meals and eating at home—you don't need to pay for someone else's labor using less-than-healthy ingredients, as is done in many restaurants.

What if I don't have time to prepare food for each meal?

The best way to tackle this challenge is to make enough at dinner for leftovers you can heat up and eat the next day. This can cut your meal preparation time in half over the course of a week. For example, if you make a dinner with leftovers on Monday, Wednesday, and Friday, you've cut out three days, or 40 percent, of cooking time from your entire week! Making easy lunches that can be eaten cold can eliminate cooking at lunchtime. And don't forget, when you skip a few meals, you are saving time as well. Also, remember the time-saving tip under "Plan (and Prep) Your Meals One Week at a Time." You can do all your meal prep work on, say, a Sunday so that all your ingredients are chopped, diced, washed, and measured. Then, on the day you cook the meal, all you have to do is put it all together. You can prepare some recipes ahead of time so they're ready to place in the oven or on the stovetop, and voilà! You've made delicious food more convenient!

What do I do if I'm dining out?

A simple way to stick with the Eat to Beat Protocol when dining out is to first take a photo of the Swap In Foods and Fat-Fighting Foods lists with your mobile device or keep the list stored as a note on your mobile device so you can quickly reference the menu when you are at a restaurant. Look for ingredients that match foods on these lists. Avoid fried foods, alcohol, and dairy products. If you have any questions about the way the menu item is prepared, or if the dish contains any of the ingredients to avoid, ask the server to check with the chef to see if modifications are possible.

One of the most important things to watch out for when you dine out is portion size. Many restaurants place way too much food on the plate. Don't feel like you need to eat it all. Remember, you've quit the clean plate club! You can take leftovers home for a time-saving meal the next day. And no matter how much or how little food is on the plate, eat slowly so your stomach can signal to your brain to stop the hunger hormone. Stop eating when you are satisfied but before you feel full. Sharing your food if you are dining with others is a great way to reduce how much you eat. Drink water with your meal to help you feel more satiated without devouring everything on the plate. Skip dessert. The Confucian concept *Hara hachi bun me* ("Stop eating when you are 80 percent full") is a great practice when dining at a restaurant.

What do I do if I'm invited to someone's home?

It's a treat to be invited to someone's home for a meal. Not only is the hospitality wonderful; it also saves you the time and effort of having to cook your own. Unfortunately, your host may not be as careful as you in choosing what to cook and serve, so it's up to you to safeguard your metabolism and take the right actions. Here are a few tips.

You could graciously thank your host for inviting you and let them know in advance that you are on an eating plan for your metabolism and need to be careful about what you eat. They will certainly ask you about your restrictions, and if you tell them honestly what you wish to avoid, your host may be able to prepare something suitable.

If snacks or appetizers are being served at someone's home, use your judgment. Avoid loading up on bite-sized offerings that may be made with unhealthy ingredients and go for the crudité, tree nuts, or fruit tray.

When sitting down at the table, if you serve yourself, go for the vegetables and healthiest foods first. They should be the dominant items on your plate. Take only two-thirds of what you might ordinarily take (no serving should fill more than one quarter of your plate). A good rule of thumb is that there should be plenty of "white space" on your plate. It should not be brimming with food. If you can avoid eating any of the foods on the Slow Down Foods list, that would be ideal, but I understand it is not always possible. In that case, take a very small portion, just enough for a gracious taste. Ask for water as your primary beverage. Skip dessert or take only a small portion and don't feel obliged to finish it. Don't add sugar to coffee or tea, but if you want to cut their strength and give them a creamy flavor, ask your host if they have a plant-based milk instead of dairy.

What do I do during the holidays?

During a holiday, it can be difficult to maintain a healthy eating pattern. Festive meals tend to be heavy on meats, processed meats, saturated fats, sugary foods, alcohol, and sweets in unrestrained quantities. Many traditions focus on homemade dishes, so at least the ultraprocessed element can be less dominant. Food is often part of the celebration, and each season in almost every culture recognizes at least one event in which abundant eating is a cherished tradition. For this reason, I do not recommend you start the four-week program around a major holiday.

Even so, you can use the principles of the plan to eat in a metabolically friendly way. Regardless of how everyone else is acting, keep to your eating window, don't snack, choose foods wisely to help and not harm your metabolism, eat slowly, and stop when you feel satisfied but before you are full.

What if I'm already on a diet?

The Eat to Beat Protocol is not a diet. It's a science-based, intuitive approach to elevate your health for a lifetime. But at some point, you might decide you want to try a diet. Tens of millions of people do it each year. You may already be on a diet that is working for you. That's great! The Eat to Beat Protocol can be used at the same time as almost any diet to improve your metabolism, fight body fat, and activate your health defenses. Simply adapt the protocol to fit the diet plan you've chosen. Whatever you are doing now, the Eat to Beat Protocol can make it work better.

Here are some practical tips for how to adapt:

1. **Compare the allowable foods.** Check to see which items on the Eat to Beat Protocol's Fat-Fighting Foods list are compatible with your chosen diet. Most will be fine, but there may be some that are contraindicated. The foods I've compiled all have scientific evidence for their benefits, but if there are any on my list that are not allowed on the diet you've chosen, just cross them off while you are on the diet. Choose from the ones that remain.

   Next, review the Slow Down Foods list. Continue to avoid them while you are on the diet. It is very unlikely that any diet plan aimed at true long-term health will force you to eat a Slow Down Food. Some trendy diets may emphasize certain ingredients that may be unhealthy, but you should limit or avoid them to protect your health.

2. **Check your eating times.** Review the diet you are choosing to see if it requires time-restricted feeding. If it does not, just keep to the eating window you created in Stage 2. If the diet increases

the amount of fasting time, that is fine. You will get even more metabolic benefits by extending the time you are not eating. Just remember not to overeat when you do.

I do not recommend diets that involve continuous eating throughout the day. This keeps your insulin levels elevated, which prevents your body from burning down body fat.

3. **Mind your caloric intake.** Many diets set a daily calorie limit. The Eat to Beat Protocol is more flexible and does not set limits, but it tells you to be mindful of them. Instead, it uses the elimination of Slow Down Foods, a time-restricted eating window, and skipping a few meals each week to lower caloric intake. If the diet you choose requires calorie counting or a specific form of calorie restriction, those can fit into the Eat to Beat Protocol. Just eat the Fat-Fighting Foods up to the diet-prescribed calorie limit.

Examples of Adaptations

Here are three examples of how to adapt the Eat to Beat Protocol if you are on a keto, Paleo, or vegan diet. I've chosen these because they are common and popular. Almost any diet can operate within the science-based protocol guidelines.

KETOGENIC DIET AND KETO LITE

To mimic fasting, the ketogenic diet is high in fat, moderate in protein, and very low in carbohydrates. As a result, it restricts your body's access to glucose from carbs and instead forces it to find alternative fuel through ketone bodies that are generated by burning fat. After a few days to a week, your body adjusts to use ketones as its main energy source. The ketogenic diet reduces insulin levels in your blood, burns fat, suppresses your appetite, and has been shown to be more effective for weight loss than eating a low-fat diet.[12]

Follow the guidelines for reducing carbohydrates (strict keto requires less than 20 grams of carbohydrates per day; keto lite is less restrictive and allows up to 50 grams per day) while eating allowable items from the Fat-Fighting Foods list.

Recommended foods include all vegetables, fresh herbs and spices, extra virgin olive oil, unsweetened dark chocolate, fresh and dried mushrooms, all seafood (prepared without using carbs), and tea and coffee (no sugar).

Some of the foods from the Fat-Fighting Foods list that you may need to eliminate with keto diets are fruits (small amounts of strawberries, raspberries, and blackberries are fine), beans and other legumes, pasta, rice, tomato paste with added sugar (without added sugar is okay), and all fruit juices.

Be mindful of the kind of fat and animal products you consume on the keto diet. In the long run and at high quantities, the fats used for keto—butter, ghee, lard, cream, cheese—will compromise your health.

Some tips to make keto healthier: choose leaner cuts of meat (top round beef, pork tenderloin, and skinless chicken or duck breast). Choose polyunsaturated fats like extra virgin olive oil instead of saturated fat like butter. For nonplant proteins, choose fish and seafood from the Fat-Fighting Foods list to benefit from their marine omega-3s. Skip the ultraprocessed and prepackaged keto foods, and avoid any products containing artificial sweeteners that can alter your microbiome.

The keto diets are very restrictive and not well balanced in terms of healthy nutrient-dense foods, since they prohibit whole grains and allow for only very small amounts of fruits. Be aware that keto can elevate your blood lipids, which increases your cardiovascular risk.[13] Because of the decreased intake of fiber, the keto diet can also alter the gut microbiome by decreasing levels of healthy bacteria.[14] A well-known keto side effect is the "keto flu," which can include nausea, headache, weakness, dizziness, irritability, and poor concentration. These symptoms occur as your body switches your metabolism from using glucose to using ketones as its main energy source.

PALEO

The Paleo diet is a low-carbohydrate pattern of eating that tries to mimic how humans were believed to have subsisted as hunter-gatherers 2.5 million years ago, long before the advent of agriculture ten thousand years ago. The idea for Paleo originally came from a 1985 article in the *New England Journal of Medicine* titled "Paleolithic Nutrition. A Consideration of Its Nature and Current Implications."[15]

The authors, Stanley Boyd Eaton, a radiologist, and Melvin Konner, an anthropologist, both from Emory University, argued that agriculture and food technology caused humans to radically deviate from the digestive traits of our Paleolithic ancestors who foraged as hunter-gatherers. They suggested that this derailment is the root cause of modern diet-related chronic diseases. Following their academic publication, they wrote a popular book, *The Paleolithic Prescription: A Program of Diet and Exercise and a Design for Living*, providing a diet plan for weight loss modeled after the way they imagined early humans ate.[16] The term "Paleo Diet" was trademarked by exercise physiologist Loren Cordain, who wrote the now-famous book by that title, and this set the stage for the popular diet called Paleo as it's known today.[17]

Many of the assumptions about what Paleolithic humans ate are inaccurate, but clinical studies do show that the Paleo diet is useful for losing weight.[18] A Swedish study of seventy middle-aged women who were obese and postmenopausal found that those who followed a Paleo diet for two years had a 59 percent greater reduction in body weight, compared to those who followed standard nutrition recommendations.[19]

The foods allowed in Paleo are minimally processed whole foods that are believed to be the ones available to early humans: fresh fruits and vegetables, fish and shellfish, nuts and oils (palm, coconut, olive), grass-fed meats and organ meats, free-range poultry and eggs.* Paleo is a very low-carb, low-fiber diet. Anything that was developed after the Paleolithic Age, such as processed foods and added sugar, is forbidden. Grains and legumes are domesticated foods, so they, too, are banned.

To adapt the Eat to Beat Protocol, simply identify the Fat-Fighting Foods permitted by Paleo. Cross off the foods that are disallowed. I want to point out that Paleo proponents instruct people not to eat foods that contain "antinutrients." These are identified as lectins (tomatoes), phytic acid (beans, nuts, seeds, root vegetables), and polyphenols (most vegetables and tea). The truth is, these all are useful bioactives that laboratory and clinical studies have proven to be beneficial for fighting body fat and improving overall health.[20] The term "antinutrient" carries no scientific weight, so I leave it up to you to determine whether or not to exclude the beneficial foods that contain them.

Because the original Paleo diet is so restrictive, a principle called 85/15 was developed to help people stay on the program. This means that 85 percent of your meals should be strict, hard-core Paleo foods, while the remaining 15 percent can be non-Paleo foods you can enjoy. This flexibility makes it possible to add back beneficial Fat-Fighting Foods that would otherwise be excluded. Stick to eating meals within your eating window—and don't snack.

Paleo embraces eating red meat, which is high in saturated fat, and over time this can contribute to adiposity and weight gain. The diet is also low in dietary fiber. Over the long term this is disadvantageous to your gut microbiome, which can weaken your metabolism. Strictly following the Paleo diet makes it challenging to dine at restaurants or eat

---

* Archaeological findings indicate that Paleolithic humans even practiced cannibalism and ate other now-extinct human species that lived at the same time, based on cutting marks on human bones discovered in Gough's Cave in the United Kingdom. (Source: R. Wallduck, et. al., "An Upper Paleolithic Engraved Human Bone Associated with Ritualistic Cannibalism," *PLOS One* 12, no. 8 [August 2017]: 1–180.)

as a guest in someone's home, since it can be hard to know which "modern age" ingredients have been used in a meal.

VEGAN

The term *vegan* was coined in 1944 by Donald Watson, a British animal rights activist, to define the beginning and the end of "veg-etari-an." It is a vegetarian diet that eliminates any use of animal products based on the moral belief that humans should not exploit animals. The diet is 100 percent plant based and forbids meat, fish, poultry, dairy, eggs, and even animal-produced products like honey.

While the vegan diet is a twentieth-century creation that has been popularized in books and films as well as studied in medical research, the principles of moralistic eating date back thousands of years across many cultures and religions. Greek philosopher and mathematician Pythagoras advocated eating plants and not animals two thousand years ago.[*] Ancient India gave birth to Jainism, a religion that espoused antiviolence toward all living things, including insects, birds, and all animals.[**]

Although veganism is based on preventing animal cruelty, its health benefits come from the consumption of plant-based whole foods.[21] These foods are loaded with fat-fighting bioactives that activate your body's health defense systems. Vegan diets (the ones that don't include ultraprocessed or fried foods) can be effective if you want to lose weight.[22] A study by researchers from the University of North Carolina

---

[*] A vegetarian diet was once known as the "Pythagorean diet" based on Pythagoras's ethical belief that animals are reasoning beings, so humans should avoid eating the meat of slaughtered animals. He also believed in metempsychosis, which is the migration of the soul upon death into another species. An animal could thus have the soul of a human being and therefore must not be harmed. Pythagoras himself lived on a diet of vegetables, bread, and honey. So, although he is best known for his mathematic theorem $a^2 + b^2 = c^2$, Pythagoras was one of the OGs of vegetarianism in the Western world.

[**] Followers of the religion known as Jainism are the strictest vegetarians in the world because they believe all living things possess a soul. They even avoid eating root vegetables because roots are viewed as containing "infinite lives" and should not be touched.

showed an almost threefold increase in weight loss from eating a vegan diet, compared to a low-fat diet.[23] Even non-strict vegan dieters lose more weight than people eating the typical Western diet.[24]

Adapting the Eat to Beat Protocol to the vegan diet is easy because many of the foods on the Fat-Fighting Foods list are plant based: fruits, vegetables, tree nuts, seeds, healthy oils, herbs, and spices. Eliminate the seafood items, and you are basically all set. If you follow strict vegan-ism, you'll need to check the ingredient labels for any middle-aisle foods to ensure no animal products were used in the processing, such as gela-tin, carmine, marine omega-3s, and shellac. Continue to eat within your eating window, continue to skip a few meals each week, and do not overeat.

A few health tips if you are considering a vegan diet. The quality of the plant-based food matters. Just because a food is plant based doesn't mean it's healthy. There are plenty of vegan junk foods (ice cream, can-dies, cookies, chips) with added sugar or high levels of sodium. Plant-based meats (burgers, nuggets, sausage, or meatballs) have the look and taste of meat and are suitable for vegans, but they are ultraprocessed foods. And all deep-fried vegetables are still fried in oil and laden with extra fat.

Being on a vegan diet requires you to do some extra planning to ensure you get adequate amounts of certain vitamins (B2, B3, B12, and D) and minerals (iron, calcium, iodine, selenium, and zinc) that are ordinarily consumed by eating animal products and seafood.[25] You can look up their levels in specific vegan-permitted foods and plan to include those in your diet—or take dietary supplements to make sure you get enough.

* * *

This is all to say that the Eat to Beat Protocol can be used on its own, or it can be combined with virtually any diet you choose to try. The way your metabolism and body fat respond to science-backed healthy foods and fasting does not change. It is hardwired in all of us. Remember, the diet that works is ultimately the one that you can stick to. Use the Eat to Beat Protocol as your guide.

In the next chapter, I will give you a Sample Meal Guide for the Eat to Beat Protocol and a schedule, and I'll share with you thirty-seven of my favorite recipes using Fat-Fighting Foods that I cook and enjoy myself.

To access more food lists that can benefit your metabolism and other resources, use your mobile device on this QR code:

CHAPTER 12

Sample Meal Guide and Recipes

To help you adopt the Eat to Beat Protocol and make it a natural part of your lifestyle, this chapter will provide you with Sample Meal Guides both for your two-week MediterAsian Swaps period and the four-week MediterAsian Intermittent Fasting program. This will help you learn and integrate the steps that were outlined in Chapter 11. The important part of my approach is that the structure and the habits will bring you *sustainable metabolic benefits*.

I've also included some delicious recipes that come from my own kitchen. These are built around fat-fighting foods and health-boosting bioactive compounds, but, equally important, they also include delicious ingredients. The recipes are easy to prepare. Be ready to delight yourself and your family and friends because the dishes taste great. And please note that these recipes are only a starting point—a way to inspire you to create your own MediterAsian repertoire.

Sample Eat to Beat Protocol Meal Guide

This Sample Meal Guide is not intended to be a rigid, set diet. You can follow it exactly if you wish, but the point is to understand the steps and then apply your own ideas to suit your preferences and life circumstances. Once you get the basics, you absolutely can personalize your own meal plan using the structure. Use this as a reference guide as you experiment and explore. Have fun with it!

The protocol is designed to provide a structure within which to build good habits you can stick to for a lifetime. It requires a little planning and awareness. To get started, just stick with the protocol structure. Once you have established Eat to Beat habits, they will become automatic.

Remember these few key components when you follow the sample plan and try the recipes:

1. Select foods that science has shown can activate your body's health defenses and ability to fight body fat.
2. Avoid foods that damage your metabolism.
3. Reduce portion sizes and be mindful at every meal not to overeat.
4. Give your body enough time during noneating (fasting) periods to draw on and burn down the energy from stored fat.
5. Try my recipes because they are easy to make and taste great. But above all, make sure the food you eat brings you joy.

How to Read the Sample Meal Guide

- Each column represents a day of the week.
- The rows are divided into the day's meals: breakfast, lunch, and dinner.
- On the left side, I recommend a start time and end time of your eating window, but you can adjust this to fit your schedule (just make sure to open your eating window one to two hours after you awaken and close the window two to three hours before bedtime).
- I have suggested which three meals to skip each week, but you can adjust to your schedule, so long as you make sure skipping meals is part of each week's program.

Sample MediterAsian Spot and Swap Plan

To complete Stage 1, follow this road map and repeat for two consecutive weeks (see Table 12.1). You can also download this road map on www .drwilliamli.com.

TABLE 12.1. SAMPLE MEDITERASIAN SPOT AND SWAP PLAN

☐ Identify Swap Out Foods ☐ Check desired Fat-Fighting Foods (FFF)	Sunday	Monday	Tuesday	Wednesday	Thursday	Friday	Saturday
Open Eating Window 2 hours after wake-up (Rise at 7 a.m. + 2 hours = start eating at 9 a.m.)	**Breakfast** ☐ EAT SWAPS + FFF (be careful of portion size)	**Breakfast** ☐ EAT SWAPS + FFF (be careful of portion size)	**Breakfast** ☐ EAT SWAPS + FFF (be careful of portion size)	**Breakfast** ☐ EAT SWAPS + FFF (be careful of portion size)	**Breakfast** ☐ EAT SWAPS + FFF (be careful of portion size)	**Breakfast** ☐ EAT SWAPS + FFF (be careful of portion size)	**Breakfast** ☐ EAT SWAPS + FFF (be careful of portion size)
No snacking	**Lunch** ☐ EAT SWAPS + FFF (be careful of portion size) ☐ Do Food Journaling	**Lunch** ☐ EAT SWAPS + FFF (be careful of portion size) ☐ Do Food Journaling	**Lunch** ☐ EAT SWAPS + FFF (be careful of portion size) ☐ Do Food Journaling	**Lunch** ☐ EAT SWAPS + FFF (be careful of portion size) ☐ Do Food Journaling	**Lunch** ☐ EAT SWAPS + FFF (be careful of portion size) ☐ Do Food Journaling	**Lunch** ☐ EAT SWAPS + FFF (be careful of portion size) ☐ Do Food Journaling	**Lunch** ☐ EAT SWAPS + FFF (be careful of portion size) ☐ Do Food Journaling
Close Eating Window 3 hours before bed (Bedtime at 11 p.m. – 3 hours = stop eating at 8 p.m.)	**Dinner** ☐ EAT SWAPS + FFF (be careful of portion size) ☐ Do Food Journaling	**Dinner** ☐ EAT SWAPS + FFF (be careful of portion size) ☐ Do Food Journaling	**Dinner** ☐ EAT SWAPS + FFF (be careful of portion size) ☐ Do Food Journaling	**Dinner** ☐ EAT SWAPS + FFF (be careful of portion size) ☐ Do Food Journaling	**Dinner** ☐ EAT SWAPS + FFF (be careful of portion size) ☐ Do Food Journaling	**Dinner** ☐ EAT SWAPS + FFF (be careful of portion size) ☐ Do Food Journaling	**Dinner** ☐ EAT SWAPS + FFF (be careful of portion size) ☐ Do Food Journaling

Sample MediterAsian Intermittent Fasting Meal Plan

Here is the week-by-week road map you will follow for Stage 2, Mediter-Asian Intermittant Fasting (see Table 12.2). I've given you specific guidance for each day. Take a look at the recipes listed for each meal and feel free to switch them around if you discover ones that you enjoy more.

In the rest of this chapter, you'll find thirty-seven of my favorite Eat to Beat recipes—organized by breakfast, lunch, and dinner and sorted alphabetically. These are inspired by my background, travels, passion for eating MediterAsian style, and knowledge of fat-fighting foods. I look forward to showing you examples of how you can combine simple and healthful ingredients in mouthwatering ways.

These dishes are easy to cook, look beautiful on the table, and are shareable—you do not have to be a trained chef to make a delicious meal. Even better, many of the recipes will create tasty leftovers for the next day. Making these meals will save you time and money. And all of the recipes feature ingredients from the fat-fighting foods list.

Here are just a few tips to help you use these recipes with the Eat to Beat Protocol. First, the recipes are designed to make enough for two to four servings. This allows you to share your creations with friends and family. If you are eating solo, eat one portion and save the rest for leftovers. This will help you save on time and food costs. Second, plan your meals one week at a time. This will allow you to buy what you need in advance, which also helps prevent impulse purchases while you shop at the last minute. The ingredients can be found in most grocery stores, or they are easily ordered online. Third, the recipes are very user-friendly and versatile to adapt to personal requirements, such as if you are dairy-free, lactose intolerant, vegetarian, or vegan. For easy identification, I've marked vegan-friendly recipes with (V). One last tip: these are not just for vegans—you can add chicken or seafood to any of the vegan-friendly dishes if you are an omnivore or pescatarian.

TABLE 12.2. SAMPLE PLANS: WEEKS ONE THROUGH FOUR

WEEK 1 OF 4

	Sunday	Monday	Tuesday	Wednesday	Thursday	Friday	Saturday
Use Swap Out Foods **Use desired Fat-Fighting Foods (FFF)** **Recipes should include them**							
Open Eating Window 2 hours after wake-up (Rise at 7 a.m. + 2 hours = start eating at 9 a.m.)	**Breakfast** Spiced quinoa porridge with blueberries and fig Coffee or tea	**Breakfast** ☐ SKIP X	**Breakfast** Strawberry lavender smoothie Coffee or tea	**Breakfast** Artichoke egg scramble Coffee or green tea	**Breakfast** ☐ SKIP X	**Breakfast** Berry walnut breakfast cookie Coffee or tea	**Breakfast** Jasmine wake-up Coffee or green tea
No snacking	**Lunch** Citrus trail mix	**Lunch** Mushroom pie	**Lunch** Mediterranean tuna caponata	**Lunch** Green papaya salad	**Lunch** Herb and avocado sandwich	**Lunch** Watermelon with chili lime	**Lunch** ☐ SKIP X
Close Eating Window 3 hours before bed (Bedtime at 11 p.m. − 3 hours = stop eating at 8 p.m.)	**Dinner** Vegetable chili	**Dinner** Chicken, white beans, and tomatoes with herbs	**Dinner** Pasta salad with sundried tomato and olives	**Dinner** Grilled spicy chicken with callaloo kale	**Dinner** Shakshuka with herbs and olives	**Dinner** Apricot coconut curry	**Dinner** Roasted fish, three ways

TABLE I2.2. SAMPLE PLANS: WEEKS ONE THROUGH FOUR (cont.)

WEEK 2 OF 4

	Sunday	Monday	Tuesday	Wednesday	Thursday	Friday	Saturday
Use Swap Out Foods **Use desired Fat-Fighting Foods** **Recipes should include them**							
Open Eating Window **2 hours after wake-up** (Rise at 7 a.m. + 2 hours = start eating at 9 a.m.)	**Breakfast** Dark chocolate coffee bark Coffee or tea	**Breakfast** ☐ **SKIP X**	**Breakfast** Berry walnut breakfast cookie Coffee or green tea	**Breakfast** Spiced quinoa porridge with blueberries and fig Coffee or green tea	**Breakfast** Strawberry lavender smoothie Coffee or green tea	**Breakfast** ☐ **SKIP X**	**Breakfast** Kiwi dragon fruit smoothie Coffee or green tea
No snacking	**Lunch** Mediterranean tuna caponata	**Lunch** Edamame hummus	**Lunch** Green papaya salad	**Lunch** Herb and avocado sandwich	**Lunch** Green salad, roasted shrimp, blood orange	**Lunch** Soba ramen	**Lunch** ☐ **SKIP X**
Close Eating Window **3 hours before bed** (Bedtime at 11 p.m. – 3 hours = stop eating at 8 p.m.)	**Dinner** Roasted mushrooms, beans, arugula	**Dinner** Tomato shrimp with apple cider vinegar	**Dinner** Ratatouille	**Dinner** Spiced chicken, rice, and kale	**Dinner** Wild mushroom barley stew	**Dinner** Chicken, white beans, tomatoes, and herbs	**Dinner** Tofu noodles with spicy sauce

	Sunday	Monday	Tuesday	Wednesday	Thursday	Friday	Saturday
Use Swap Out Foods **Use desired Fat-Fighting Foods** **Recipes should include them**							
Open Eating Window 2 hours after wake-up (Rise at 7 a.m. + 2 hours = start eating at 9 a.m.)	**Breakfast** Spiced quinoa porridge with blueberries and fig Coffee or tea	**Breakfast** ☐ **SKIP X**	**Breakfast** Strawberry lavender smoothie Coffee or tea	**Breakfast** Artichoke egg scramble Coffee or green tea	**Breakfast** ☐ **SKIP X**	**Breakfast** Kiwi dragon fruit smoothie Coffee or tea	**Breakfast** Berry walnut breakfast cookie Coffee or tea
No snacking	**Lunch** Chicha morada	**Lunch** Herb and avocado sandwich	**Lunch** Green papaya salad	**Lunch** Soba ramen	**Lunch** Mediterranean tuna caponata	**Lunch** Mushroom pie	**Lunch** ☐ **SKIP X**
Close Eating Window 3 hours before bed (Bedtime at 11 p.m. - 3 hours = stop eating at 8 p.m.)	**Dinner** Grilled spicy chicken with callaloo kale	**Dinner** Clams with black bean sauce	**Dinner** Wild mushroom barley stew	**Dinner** Roasted fish, three ways	**Dinner** Vegetable chili	**Dinner** Roasted mushrooms, beans, arugula	**Dinner** Edamame with tofu and snow cabbage

TABLE 12.2. SAMPLE PLANS: WEEKS ONE THROUGH FOUR (cont.)

WEEK 4 OF 4

Use Swap Out Foods Use desired Fat-Fighting Foods Recipes should include them	Sunday	Monday	Tuesday	Wednesday	Thursday	Friday	Saturday
Open Eating Window 2 hours after wake-up (Rise at 7 a.m. + 2 hours = start eating at 9 a.m.)	**Breakfast** Kiwi dragon fruit smoothie Coffee or tea	**Breakfast** ☐ **SKIP X**	**Breakfast** Artichoke egg scramble Coffee or tea	**Breakfast** Strawberry lavender smoothie Coffee or tea	**Breakfast** ☐ **SKIP X**	**Breakfast** Dark chocolate coffee bark Coffee or green tea	**Breakfast** Chicha morada Coffee or green tea
No snacking	**Lunch** Mediterranean tuna caponata	**Lunch** Soba ramen	**Lunch** Green papaya salad	**Lunch** Edamame hummus	**Lunch** Mushroom pie	**Lunch** Green salad, roasted shrimp, blood orange	**Lunch** ☐ **SKIP X**
Close Eating Window 3 hours before bed (Bedtime at 11 p.m. - 3 hours = stop eating at 8 p.m.)	**Dinner** Shakshuka with herbs and olives	**Dinner** Vegetarian chili	**Dinner** Grilled spicy chicken with callaloo kale	**Dinner** Clams with black bean sauce	**Dinner** Tomato shrimp with apple cider vinegar	**Dinner** Apricot coconut curry	**Dinner** Chicken, white beans, tomatoes, and herbs

Recipe List

BREAKFAST

LUNCH

DINNER

(V = *vegan*)

Breakfast

Artichoke Egg Scramble

This unexpected combination provides protein and fiber for breakfast. Parmesan is a low-lactose cheese and adds the perfect spicy edge to this easy egg dish. This recipe also works nicely with crumbled extra-firm tofu.

Serves: 2
Prep Time: 5 minutes
Cooking Time: 10 minutes

Ingredients:
1 tablespoon extra virgin olive oil
1 cup canned artichoke hearts, drained and roughly chopped
1 tablespoon chopped fresh oregano
¼ teaspoon kosher salt
½ teaspoon black pepper

4 large free-range chicken eggs, lightly beaten
¼ cup grated Parmesan cheese

Preparation:

Heat oil in a cast-iron skillet over medium heat. Add artichoke hearts and oregano, season with salt and pepper and sauté until edges of artichokes begin to turn crispy and golden, about 3–4 minutes. Add beaten eggs and 3 tablespoons of Parmesan to the skillet and gently scramble until eggs are fluffy, about 3 minutes more. Transfer to two plates and sprinkle with remaining Parmesan.

Berry Walnut Breakfast Cookies

A cookie sounds even better than a bar, and these are packed with delicious dried fruit and nuts. You can always swap out any of the dried fruits for dried figs, tart cherries, apples, or prunes and switch the walnuts to cashews, almonds, or pistachios. These cookies are the perfect grab-and-go breakfast with a cup of coffee or tea. (*Vegan-friendly*)

Serves: 12
Prep Time: 20 minutes
Cooking Time: 18 minutes

Ingredients:
1 ½ cups whole wheat flour
½ cup old-fashioned rolled oats
1 teaspoon ground cinnamon
1 teaspoon baking soda
½ teaspoon salt
1 cup almond butter
¼ cup 100% pure maple syrup
2 large eggs, beaten
1 teaspoon vanilla extract
¼ cup orange zest

¼ cup raw walnuts, coarsely chopped

½ cup dried cranberries

½ cup dried apricots, coarsely chopped

½ cup dried blueberries

½ cup cacao nibs

Preparation:

Preheat the oven to 350°F. Line a baking sheet with a silicone mat or parchment paper.

In a medium bowl, mix together the whole wheat flour, oats, cinnamon, baking soda, and salt. In a large bowl, whisk together the almond butter and maple syrup until well combined. Add the eggs, vanilla extract, and orange zest and whisk until smooth. Gently fold the dry ingredients into the wet ingredients and stir until just combined. Fold in the walnuts, cranberries, apricots, blueberries, and cacao nibs, evenly distributing throughout the dough.

Scoop out ⅓ cup of the batter and, using clean hands, roll into a ball. Place onto the prepared baking sheet and gently press down on the top to flatten slightly. Repeat with the rest of the batter, leaving about 2 inches between each cookie. Place baking sheets on separate shelves in the oven and bake until the cookies are soft and golden brown, and a tester inserted into the center of two cookies comes out clean, about 18 minutes. Remove the baking sheets from the oven and let cool on a wire rack for about 10 minutes before eating. Cut into servings the size of your palm.

Serve warm or store, covered, at room temperature for up to 5 days. Cookies also can be placed in a resealable bag and stored in the freezer for up to 2 months.

Chicha Morada

Chicha morada is a Peruvian beverage made by steeping a mixture of dried purple corn and aromatic spices. This version is sweetened with

100% fruit juice. Served over ice, this is a unique and healthy refresher. (*Vegan-friendly*)

Serves: Makes 12 cups
Prep Time: 10 minutes, plus 4 hours to chill
Cooking Time: 60 minutes

Ingredients:
1 pound dried purple maize
2 cinnamon sticks
1 vanilla bean, split
10 cups water
2 cups pomegranate juice
Juice of 2 limes
2 green apples, cored and diced

Preparation:

Place maize, cinnamon sticks, and vanilla bean in a large pot and cover with water. Bring mixture to a boil over high heat, then reduce heat and simmer for 60 minutes. Strain, transfer to a pitcher, stir in pomegranate juice and lime juice, and place in the refrigerator to chill. Add chunks of green apple and serve over ice.

Dark Chocolate Coffee Bark

A crave-able, crunchy breakfast treat with health benefits and a boost of caffeine. This recipe is the basic version, so feel free to add some chopped tree nuts or dried fruits for texture, extra flavor, and more metabolic kick. (*Vegan-friendly*)

Serves: 8
Prep Time: 30 minutes
Cooking Time: 15 minutes

Ingredients:

¼ cup roasted coffee beans

8 ounces dark chocolate, roughly chopped

½ teaspoon coarse sea salt

Preparation:

Line a baking sheet with parchment paper and set aside. Place coffee beans in a resealable bag and use a mallet or skillet to smash them into smaller pieces. Place chocolate in a double boiler and melt until smooth. Add coffee beans and stir to combine. Spread chocolate mixture onto the parchment-lined baking sheet. Sprinkle with sea salt. Allow to set until the chocolate is hardened. Place in the fridge or freezer for faster setting. Break into pieces and enjoy. Store in an airtight container in the refrigerator or freezer for up to 1 week.

Jasmine Wake-Up

A refreshing jasmine green tea beverage infused with fresh peaches and mint. You can swap the peaches for other stone fruit, such as plums, nectarines, apricots, or whatever is in season. (*Vegan-friendly*)

Serves: 4

Prep Time: 10 minutes, plus 20 minutes refrigeration

Cooking Time: 3 minutes

Ingredients:

4 bags jasmine tea

2 cups boiling water

3 cups ice

2 ripe peaches, sliced lengthwise, pits removed, and diced

2 cups cold water

2 tablespoons 100% maple syrup

4 mint leaves

Preparation:

In a heat-proof bowl, place the tea bags and carefully pour in the boiling water. Steep for exactly 3 minutes and discard tea bags. Set the tea aside and allow to cool for at least 10 minutes. In a medium pitcher, add the ice, jasmine tea, peaches, cold water, maple syrup, and mint and stir to combine.

Place the pitcher in the refrigerator for 20 minutes to allow flavors to combine. Serve cold.

Kiwi Dragon Fruit Smoothie

This exotic combo of kiwifruit and dragon fruit is a fiber-filled refresher. Look for packs of frozen dragon fruit in the freezer section of your favorite health food store. For an extra-thick smoothie, slice and freeze one of the kiwis ahead of time. (*Vegan-friendly*)

Serves: 1
Prep Time: 5 minutes
Cooking Time: 0 minutes

Ingredients:

1 (3.5-ounce) pack frozen dragon fruit puree
2 kiwifruit, peeled* and sliced
4 tablespoons orange juice, preferably freshly squeezed (1 large orange)
2 tablespoons coconut chips
1 tablespoon cacao nibs

Preparation:

Place dragon fruit, 1 kiwifruit, and orange juice in a blender and blend until smooth, stopping to scrape ingredients down with a spatula if needed. Add additional orange juice 1 tablespoon at a time if needed

---

* Note: Did you know the outer skin of kiwifruit is fiber-rich and edible? Peeling is optional.

to reach desired consistency. Scoop into a bowl and top with remaining kiwi, coconut chips, and cacao nibs.

Spiced Quinoa Porridge with Blueberries and Figs

This breakfast is packed with whole-grain nutrients and fiber. With gorgeous figs and blueberries, it is a delicious and warming meal to start the day. (*Vegan-friendly*)

Serves: 2
Prep Time: 5 minutes
Cooking Time: 20 minutes

Ingredients:

1/2 cup dried figs, thinly sliced
I bag green tea
1/2 cup hot water
I cup unsweetened almond milk
3/4 cup dried quinoa
I tablespoon honey
1/2 teaspoon ground turmeric
1/8 teaspoon ground ginger
1/8 teaspoon ground cardamom
1/8 teaspoon salt
1/2 cup fresh blueberries
2 tablespoons unsweetened coconut flakes

Preparation:

Slice dried figs, set aside.

Place the green tea bag in a mug or heat-proof bowl and add the hot water. Allow to steep for exactly 3 minutes. Remove the green tea bag and discard.

In a medium saucepan, add the prepared green tea, almond milk, quinoa, honey, turmeric, ginger, cardamom, and salt. Stir to combine.

Bring the mixture to a boil over high heat. Reduce the heat to medium-low and simmer, covered, until the quinoa is tender and liquid is absorbed, about 15 minutes.

Spoon half the quinoa into each of two bowls. Top each bowl with ¼ cup each of the fresh blueberries and figs and 1 tablespoon each of coconut flakes. Serve warm.

Strawberry Lavender Smoothie

The floral essence of lavender is the perfect complement to strawberries. Soy milk adds flavor as well as additional fat-fighting power. Be sure to purchase food-grade lavender, available in specialty food shops, spice markets, or online. (*Vegan-friendly*)

Serves: 1 (10 fluid ounce smoothie)
Prep Time: 5 minutes
Cooking Time: 0 minutes

Ingredients:
1 cup frozen strawberries
1 cup unsweetened soy milk
1 tablespoon honey
2 teaspoons dried lavender leaves

Preparation:
Place strawberries, soy milk, honey, and lavender in the blender and blend until smooth. Pour into a glass and serve.

Tomato Watermelon Juice

This is a delicious blend of two powerhouse sources of lycopene—a perfect way to jump-start your day. (*Vegan-friendly*)

Serves: 6
Prep Time: 15 minutes, plus 20–30 minutes refrigeration
Cooking Time: 0 minutes

Ingredients:

1 ½ pounds beefsteak tomatoes, seeded and chopped
6 cups cubed seedless watermelon
1 medium cucumber, sliced
1 cup ice cubes
2 teaspoons lemon juice
1 teaspoon honey
⅛ teaspoon kosher salt
Watermelon wedges, for garnish

Preparation:

Place the tomatoes, watermelon, cucumber, and ice cubes in a blender and blend until smooth, about 45 seconds. Add the lemon juice, honey, and salt and blend until combined, 30 seconds more. Using a mesh sieve, strain the juice and place in a pitcher in the refrigerator for 20–30 minutes to allow the flavors to combine.

To serve, pour 1 cup of the juice into each of four glasses. Garnish each glass with a watermelon wedge. Serve immediately.

Lunch

Citrus Trail Mix Lunch

Turn this snack into your lunch, since it is loaded with fat-fighting ingredients. Elevate the flavor with the zest of lemon, orange, or even grapefruit. (Remember: make a snack your lunch!) (*Vegan-friendly*)

Serves: 6
Prep Time: 15 minutes, plus 24 hours at room temperature
Cooking Time: 0 minutes

Ingredients:

¼ cup dry-roasted unsalted almonds

¼ cup dry-roasted unsalted shelled pistachios

2 tablespoons unsalted pumpkin seeds

¼ cup dried blueberries

¼ cup dried apples

Zest of 1 lemon

Preparation:

In a medium bowl, mix together the almonds, pistachios, pumpkin seeds, blueberries, and apples. Sprinkle the lemon zest over the top and allow the bowl to sit at room temperature, uncovered, for 24 hours. Toss to combine.

To serve, scoop ¼ cup of the trail mix into a small bowl and enjoy.

Edamame Hummus

Truly MediterAsian. Use fresh or frozen soybeans to make this twist on a classic dip. Serve with vegetables like zucchini, carrots, jicama, or bell peppers. (*Vegan-friendly*)

Serves: 6

Prep Time: 10 minutes

Cooking Time: 5 minutes

Ingredients:

1 ½ cups frozen shelled edamame

⅓ cup extra virgin olive oil

2 tablespoons tahini

1 clove garlic, crushed

2 tablespoons lemon juice

½ teaspoon lemon zest

¼ cup fresh parsley, roughly chopped

2 tablespoons fresh cilantro, roughly chopped

6 basil leaves
½ teaspoon honey
⅛ teaspoon cayenne pepper
½ teaspoon kosher salt

Preparation:

Fill a medium saucepan ¾ of the way with water and bring to a boil over high heat. Add the edamame and cook for 5 minutes. Drain and set aside to cool for 5 minutes.

Place the edamame into a food processor (fitted with a steel blade) or a blender and pulse until blended and smooth. Add the olive oil, tahini, garlic, lemon juice and zest, parsley, cilantro, basil, honey, cayenne, and kosher salt and pulse until smooth. Serve immediately or store, covered, up to 4 days in the refrigerator.

Green Papaya Salad

A fresh, tropical salad that will quickly become a favorite. The firm flesh of underripe papaya is the base for this simple dish. For an extra fat-fighting kick, add a finely chopped red chili to the dressing. (*Vegan-friendly*)

Serves: 4
Prep Time: 15 minutes
Cooking Time: 0 minutes

Ingredients:

Juice of 1 lime
2 teaspoons honey
1 tablespoon fish sauce
1 small green (unripe) papaya, julienned*
1 cup finely diced mango
1 cup cherry tomatoes, halved

---

* Note: Use a handheld julienne peeler for convenient peeling.

2 tablespoons chopped fresh mint

¼ cup shelled pistachios, chopped

Preparation:

In a large bowl, whisk lime juice, honey, and fish sauce until well combined. Add papaya, mango, tomatoes, mint, and pistachios. Toss well and serve. Store in the refrigerator for up to 3 days.

Green Salad with Roasted Shrimp and Blood Orange

Take your salad to the next level with some omega-3-rich seafood and citrus. All the elements of this dish can be prepared ahead of time; once assembled, refrigerate for up to 8 hours before serving.

Serves: 2

Prep Time: 10 minutes

Cooking Time: 10 minutes

Roasted Shrimp Ingredients:

½ pound large shrimp, peeled and deveined

2 teaspoons olive oil

¼ teaspoon kosher salt

¼ teaspoon black pepper

Dressing Ingredients:

3 tablespoons olive oil

Juice and zest of 1 blood orange

1 clove garlic, minced

¼ teaspoon kosher salt

¼ teaspoon black pepper

Salad Ingredients:

4 cups baby arugula

1 cup flatleaf parsley leaves

1 cup grapefruit segments

I bulb fennel, thinly sliced

½ cup shaved Parmesan cheese

Preparation:

Preheat oven to 400°F. Place the shrimp on a sheet pan, drizzle with olive oil, and season with salt and pepper. Roast for 10 minutes or until shrimp is pink, firm, and opaque. Remove from oven and set aside to cool slightly.

To make the dressing, combine olive oil, blood orange juice and zest, garlic, salt, and pepper in a small jar with a lid. Cover and shake well to combine.

To assemble the salad, place arugula, parsley, grapefruit, and fennel in a large bowl. Add Parmesan and cooked shrimp. Drizzle with dressing and toss gently.

Herb and Avocado Sandwich

These tasty finger sandwiches require virtually no time to prepare. The crunchy sunflower seeds complement the creamy texture of avocado. Add thinly sliced cucumbers for even more crunch or serve with sliced vegetables. (*Vegan-friendly*)

Serves: 2

Prep Time: 10 minutes

Cooking Time: 0 minutes

Ingredients:

I Haas avocado, sliced lengthwise and pit removed

I tablespoon fresh lime juice

I tablespoon chopped basil leaves

I tablespoon chopped fresh cilantro

I tablespoon chopped fresh parsley

⅛ teaspoon crushed pepper flakes
⅛ teaspoon salt
1 teaspoon unsalted sunflower seeds
4 slices 100% whole wheat bread

Preparation:

In a medium bowl, spoon the avocado flesh and drizzle with the lime juice. Add the basil, cilantro, parsley, crushed pepper flakes, and salt. Use a potato masher or back of a fork to mash the avocado until smooth. Add the sunflower seeds and stir to combine.

Place 1 slice of bread on each of two plates. Spread 2 tablespoons of the avocado mixture onto each slice of bread and top with the second slice of bread. Slice in half and serve immediately.

Mediterranean Tuna Caponata

An easy meal with the true flavors of the Mediterranean. Makes a tasty lunch that takes only minutes to create. Substitute olive oil–packed sardines or mackerel for variety.

Serves: 2
Prep Time: 15 minutes
Cooking Time: 0 minutes

Ingredients:

1 tablespoon extra virgin olive oil
Juice of ½ lemon
1 teaspoon mustard
⅛ teaspoon honey
⅛ teaspoon salt
5 ounces canned tuna in olive oil, drained
½ cup cherry tomatoes, quartered
2 ribs celery with the leaves, finely chopped

¼ cup kalamata olives, pitted and quartered

2 tablespoons finely chopped red onion

1 tablespoon chopped dill

1 tablespoon chopped parsley

2 slices of crusty sourdough bread

Preparation:

In a small bowl, whisk together the oil, lemon juice, mustard, honey, and salt. In a medium bowl, mix together the tuna, tomatoes, celery, olives, red onion, dill, and parsley until combined. Add the dressing and toss to evenly coat.

Divide the caponata on each of two plates, and serve with a slice of crusty sourdough bread.

Mushroom Pies

Pockets of vegan-friendly pastry stuffed with a fiery mushroom filling—these pies are scrumptious. Make the filling and dough up to 24 hours in advance, then simply assemble and bake. These pies can be frozen for up to 3 months. (*Vegan-friendly*)

Makes 8 pies

Cooking Time: 40 minutes

Prep Time: 60 minutes

Filling Ingredients:

1 pound sliced mushrooms (shiitake, maitake, portobello, cremini, use your favorite)

2 Scotch bonnet or habanero peppers, stems removed and cut in half*

½ small red onion, sliced

1 tablespoon olive oil

---

* Be careful when handling hot peppers; avoid touching face or eyes.

1/2 teaspoon kosher salt

3/4 teaspoon ground allspice

Dough Ingredients:

2 cups all-purpose flour

2 teaspoons kosher salt

1/2 teaspoon baking powder

2 teaspoons turmeric

1/4 cup olive oil

8–10 tablespoons ice water

Preparation:

Preheat oven to 400°F. Place mushrooms, chili peppers, and onion on a sheet pan. Drizzle with olive oil and season with salt. Bake for 20 minutes. Turn off the oven, remove, and set aside to cool. Once cool, transfer to a food processor, add allspice, and pulse until finely chopped.

While mushrooms are cooking, prepare the dough. In a large bowl, combine flour, salt, baking powder, and turmeric. Add olive oil and mix well until mixture appears crumbly. Then while mixing with clean hands, slowly add ice water 1–2 tablespoons at a time until a soft dough forms. Turn dough out onto a lightly floured surface and knead until smooth. Shape into a ball, wrap in plastic wrap, and place in the refrigerator to chill for 20 minutes. After 20 minutes, remove plastic wrap, divide evenly into eight pieces. Roll out each piece to a 4-inch circle. Add 2 tablespoons of the mushroom mixture onto each piece of dough. Fold in half and gently press the edges closed with a fork. Heat oven to 350°F. Place pies on a sheet pan and bake for 15–18 minutes, until golden brown and edges are crispy. Serve warm.

Soba Ramen

This health-elevated version of ramen gets a bomb of umami flavor from tomato paste, dried mushrooms, and kombu seaweed. Whole-grain soba noodles and vegetables complete the dish. Make a large batch of the flavorful broth and store in the freezer for up to 3 months. *(Vegan-friendly)*

Serves: 4
Prep Time: 15 minutes
Cooking Time: 15 minutes

Ingredients:

8 cups water
2 tablespoons white miso paste
2 tablespoons reduced-sodium soy sauce
2 tablespoons tomato paste
2 cloves garlic
1 sheet kombu
2 scallions, trimmed
1 ounce dried shiitake mushrooms (about 10 pieces)
2 slices ginger root
4 cups chopped bok choy
2 cups sliced or chopped carrots
4 cups cooked soba noodles*

Preparation:

In a large pot, combine water, miso, soy sauce, and tomato paste. Whisk well to combine. Add garlic, kombu, scallions, dried mushrooms, and ginger. Bring mixture to a boil over high heat and cook for 5 minutes. Reduce heat to low and cook for 10 minutes more. Use a slotted spoon to remove the mushrooms, set aside, and slice once cool enough to handle. Strain broth and discard remaining solids. To serve, place hot broth in four bowls with sliced mushrooms, bok choy, carrots, and cooked soba noodles. Finish with a light drizzle of olive oil, if desired. Add additional soy sauce or miso paste to taste.

---

* To prepare soba noodles, place in a large bowl and cover with boiling water. Allow to sit for 5 minutes or until noodles are tender.

Watermelon with Chili Lime Salt

An ultralight lunch that is a fiesta of flavors and colors! This is a mouth-watering and brown-fat-activating twist on one of my favorite summer fruits. (*Vegan-friendly*)

Serves: 8 pieces
Prep Time: 5 minutes plus 24 hours to dry lime zest
Cooking Time: 0 minutes

Ingredients:

Zest of 1 lime, grated and dried at room temperature for 24 hours*
2 teaspoons coarse sea salt
2 teaspoons red chili flakes
8 slices watermelon

Preparation:

To make the salt, place the air-dried lime zest, salt, and chili flakes in a mortar and pestle and grind until ingredients are well combined and at desired consistency. If you don't have a mortar and pestle, pulse ingredients in a spice grinder or food processor. Sprinkle ⅛ teaspoon of the mixture over 1 slice of watermelon and serve. Reserve leftover salt to flavor dips, salads, sauces, and marinades.

---

* Drying the zest makes the spice mixture easier to sprinkle and allows you to store it for later. If you plan to use it all at once, the drying step is optional.

Dinner

Apricot Coconut Curry

A spicy mix of aromatic veggies, warm spices, and creamy chickpeas, this dish could become your new comfort food. (*Vegan-friendly*)

Serves: 4
Prep Time: 15 minutes
Cooking Time: 25 minutes

Ingredients:

1 tablespoon olive oil
½ cup chopped onion
1 clove garlic, finely chopped
2 teaspoons curry powder
¼ teaspoon red pepper flakes
1 tablespoon reduced-sodium soy sauce
8 dried apricots, quartered
½ cup canned coconut milk
½ cup no-salt-added tomato sauce
1 head cauliflower, stemmed and florets halved lengthwise
1 cup diced carrots
1 (15-ounce) can chickpeas, drained and rinsed
½ cup chopped cilantro
½ cup chopped cashews
4 cups cooked brown rice
Lime wedges (optional)

Preparation:

Heat oil in a large skillet or Dutch oven over medium heat. Add onion, garlic, curry powder, and red pepper flakes. Cook for 5 minutes. Add soy sauce, apricots, coconut milk, tomato sauce, and ½ cup water; stir to combine. Add cauliflower, carrots, and chickpeas. Bring to a simmer and cook partially covered for 20 minutes. Top with cilantro and cashews and serve over rice with a squeeze of fresh lime juice, if desired.

Baby Bok Choy with Oyster Sauce

This is a family favorite, a simple green vegetable with an intensely flavorful sauce. It's really quick to make and is a great stand-alone meal with brown rice, or easy to pair with other MediterAsian dishes.

Serves: 4
Prep Time: 5 minutes
Cooking Time: 5 minutes

Bok Choy Ingredients:
6 bunches baby bok choy
1 tablespoon extra virgin olive oil
2 garlic cloves, thinly sliced
2 tablespoons Shaoxing rice wine*

Sauce Ingredients:
½ teaspoon cornstarch
¼ cup vegetable stock
1 tablespoon soy sauce
2 tablespoons oyster sauce*

Preparation:
Clean bok choy by rinsing well, dry, and slice off a ½ inch of the white ends. Cut the greens lengthwise to separate the leaves. Dissolve cornstarch in vegetable stock, add soy sauce and oyster sauce, mix well, and set sauce aside.

---

* Lee Kum Kee Premium Oyster Sauce and Shaoxing Rice Cooking Wine are available online.

Heat olive oil in a wok on high until shimmering. Add garlic. When garlic starts to turn golden brown, add the bok choy and stir-fry for 2 minutes until leaves turn an intense green color. Add the rice wine, stir-fry for 1 minute. Then add the sauce. Turn the bok choy leaves a few times in the sauce as it thickens, about 2 minutes. Take off heat and serve immediately. Add additional oyster sauce on top, if desired.

Chicken with White Beans, Tomatoes, and Herbs

This is an entire meal on a single baking sheet, one of the easiest recipes to prepare. The beans develop a crispy skin but have a soft center, the tomatoes burst with bright flavors, and the herbs give a distinct Mediterranean aroma. You'll love this dish, and, even better, it makes delicious leftovers for the next day.

Serves: 4
Prep Time: 10 minutes
Cooking Time: 40 minutes

Ingredients:
3 cans white beans, drained and rinsed
2 pints cherry tomatoes
1 tablespoon dried oregano
4 sprigs fresh thyme
3 cloves garlic, crushed
¼ teaspoon red pepper flakes
3 tablespoons extra virgin olive oil
½ cup dry white wine (optional)
½ teaspoon salt
½ teaspoon fresh cracked black pepper
8 chicken thighs, bone in, skin removed
(Reserve a pinch each of salt, fresh thyme, oregano, and black pepper to sprinkle to taste on top of the chicken.)

Preparation:

Preheat the oven to 425°F. In a large metal bowl, gently combine the beans, tomatoes, oregano, thyme, garlic, red pepper flakes, olive oil, white wine, salt, and black pepper. Spread the mixture thinly on the surface of a large baking pan that has a rim.

Place the chicken thighs on top of the beans and tomato mixture, taking care not to overlap them. Add a dash of olive oil on the top of the chicken. Sprinkle a pinch of salt, some black pepper, dried oregano, and fresh thyme on top of the chicken.

Place the pan in the oven and roast until the chicken is done, about 40 minutes. The internal temperature should read 165°F. Remove from oven and garnish with thyme sprigs. Serve immediately.

Clams with Black Bean Sauce

This is a classic dish served in dim sum houses of southern China. What a great way to serve up clams with a tasty sauce! The recipe requires fresh live clams, which can be hard to find, but they are worth the effort.

Serves: 4
Prep Time: 30 minutes
Cooking Time: 15 minutes

Ingredients:
20 fresh live clams (littleneck, Manila, cockles)
2 tablespoons extra virgin olive oil
2 slices fresh ginger
4 cloves garlic, sliced
2 tablespoons black bean and garlic sauce*

---

* Lee Kum Kee Black Bean Garlic Sauce, Lee Kum Kee Premium Oyster Sauce, and Shaoxing Rice Cooking Wine are available online.

1 cup clam juice

2 tablespoons premium oyster sauce

½ cup Shaoxing rice wine*

2 ½ tablespoons cornstarch dissolved in 5 tablespoons clam juice

2 scallions, chopped

Preparation:

Wash clams, then soak in water for 30 minutes. Heat olive oil in a wok and add ginger, garlic, and black bean and garlic sauce, and stir-fry over high heat for 1 minute. Drain clams and add to the wok along with clam juice. Place cover on wok and allow clams to steam cook for 10 minutes. Check periodically and shake wok or gently stir clams to allow them to open and release their fluid. Add oyster sauce, rice wine, and cornstarch dissolved in clam juice (make sure it is fully dissolved). Cook for 2 minutes. When all clams are open, sprinkle in chopped scallions, pour onto platter, and serve immediately.

Edamame and Arugula Pasta

This light MediterAsian pasta salad is an entire meal all on its own.

Serves: 4

Prep Time: 10 minutes

Cooking Time: 20 minutes

Ingredients:

2 ½ cups fresh or frozen shelled edamame (soybean)

12 ounces whole-grain short pasta (casarecce, fusilli, rotini, radiatore, penne, gemelli)*

6 tablespoons extra virgin olive oil, divided

5 ounces baby arugula, washed and dried

2 tablespoons sherry or white wine vinegar

---

* For added healthfulness, try a red lentil pasta.

1 teaspoon salt

½ teaspoon black pepper, freshly ground

¼ cup toasted walnuts, coarsely chopped

1 cup feta cheese, crumbled (eliminate for vegan version)

1 lemon

Preparation:

In a large pot, boil water over high heat and cook edamame for 3 minutes. Drain and let cool. Cook pasta to al dente per instructions on package (approximately 8–10 minutes) and drain. You can combine the pasta and edamame cooking process by timing pasta for 6 minutes, then adding edamame to water. Mix drained pasta and edamame in large mixing bowl with 2 tablespoons of olive oil. Add baby arugula and gently combine.

In a separate bowl, whisk remaining 4 tablespoons olive oil with vinegar, salt, and pepper. Add to bowl with pasta and edamame and gently mix together. Add toasted walnuts. Gently add crumbled feta and toss. Squeeze lemon juice to taste.

Edamame with Tofu and Snow Cabbage

This is a Shanghainese pasta-like dish that combines different vegetable flavors and textures to create a whole that is more delicious than its parts! The main thing is to find an Asian market where you can get the dried tofu skins and preserved snow cabbage. (*Vegan-friendly*)

Serves: 4

Prep Time: 45 minutes, mostly soaking

Cooking Time: 5 minutes

Ingredients:

9 ounces dried tofu skin (dried bean curd), soaked and sliced into strips*

1 teaspoon baking soda

---

* You can find tofu skins and jarred or canned preserved snow cabbage in most Asian markets. Shaoxing Rice Cooking Wine is available online.

2 tablespoons extra virgin olive oil

I cup preserved snow cabbage, coarsely chopped*

2 tablespoons Shaoxing rice wine

4 tablespoons vegetable stock

½ cup shelled edamame (fresh or frozen)

I teaspoon soy sauce

½ tablespoon cornstarch

2 tablespoons water

White pepper, to taste

Sesame oil, to taste

Preparation:

Soak the dried tofu skin in a bowl containing enough warm water to cover the skins and the baking soda for 30 minutes. The baking soda helps to soften and rehydrate the tofu. Replace with fresh warm water, continue soaking for another 15 minutes. Drain and cut the tofu skins into ½-inch-wide ribbons (about twice as wide as fettuccine).

Heat oil in wok on high until shimmering. Add snow cabbage and stir-fry for 1 minute. Add rice wine. After 30 seconds, add the tofu ribbons and vegetable stock and allow to boil. Then add edamame and soy sauce.

Thicken by dissolving cornstarch in 4 tablespoons of water and slowly stir into dish. The sauce will thicken after 1 minute. Add white pepper to taste and a few drops of sesame oil.

Remove from heat and serve.

Grilled Spicy Chicken with Callaloo Kale

A warm and earthy mix of spices, vegetables, and chicken thighs. Callaloo is a Caribbean-style vegetable dish, but I'm including it here in the spirit of embracing different culinary traditions.

Serves: 4

Prep Time: 30 minutes (plus 60 minutes to marinate)

Cooking Time: 30 minutes

Ingredients:

¼ teaspoon ground cinnamon

¼ teaspoon ground allspice

¼ teaspoon ground ginger

¼ teaspoon kosher salt

1 tablespoon low-sodium soy sauce or tamari

1 ½ pounds boneless, skinless chicken thighs

1 tablespoon extra virgin olive oil

2 cloves garlic, chopped

½ medium onion, sliced

1 Scotch bonnet or habanero pepper, stems removed and cut in half*

1 tablespoon fresh thyme leaves, chopped

1 cup chopped tomatoes

1 bunch kale, stemmed and roughly chopped (about 6 cups)

½ teaspoon kosher salt

2 teaspoons apple cider vinegar

Preparation:

In a small bowl, mix cinnamon, allspice, ginger, salt, and soy sauce. Place chicken thighs in a resealable bag and add spice mixture. Seal bag and store in the refrigerator to marinate for 1 hour or up to 24 hours. When ready to cook, preheat grill to 500°F. Grill for 6–7 minutes per side or until internal temperature reads 165°F on a meat thermometer. Remove from grill and allow to cool slightly before serving.

While the chicken is cooking, heat oil in a large skillet over medium heat. Add garlic, onion, chili pepper, and thyme; sauté 2–3 minutes. Add tomatoes and kale; season with salt and continue to sauté for another 5–8 minutes until onions soften and kale is wilted. Add a splash of vinegar and cook for 2–3 minutes more. Serve warm.

---

* Be careful when handling hot peppers; avoid touching face or eyes.

Olive Caper Tapenade

This is a Mediterranean topping that delivers great flavors and texture to any dish. Serve a generous dollop on a piece of chicken or fish and place the rest in a bowl on the table so people can add more if they like. You can even spread it like a relish on a tuna sandwich.

Serves: 4
Prep Time: 15 minutes
Cooking Time: 0 minutes

Ingredients:

½ cup green olives, chopped (Cerignola, Frescatrano, Castelvetrano, Picholine)
2 tablespoons capers, rinsed of salt and lightly chopped
½ lemon, juice and zest
1 tablespoon chives, chopped
1 tablespoon flat-leaf parsley, chopped
2 tablespoons extra virgin olive oil
Fresh cracked black pepper

Preparation:

Clean and chop all ingredients. Mix in a small metal bowl. Add fresh cracked pepper to taste. This can be prepared the day before and kept overnight in the refrigerator. Let it come up to room temperature before serving.

Pasta Salad with Sundried Tomatoes and Olives

A simple, beautiful pasta salad. Leftovers store well in the refrigerator overnight so you can enjoy them at lunch the next day. (*Vegan-friendly*)

Serves: 4
Prep Time: 15 minutes, plus 20 minutes refrigeration
Cooking Time: 10 minutes

Ingredients:

8 ounces whole wheat gemelli pasta

1 cup frozen shelled edamame

2 tablespoons red wine vinegar

2 tablespoons chopped basil

1 clove garlic, minced

1/8 teaspoon honey

1/2 teaspoon Dijon mustard

1/8 teaspoon salt

3 tablespoons extra virgin olive oil

1 medium orange or yellow bell pepper, chopped

1/3 cup pitted kalamata olives, halved

1/3 cup sundried tomatoes packed in oil, chopped

1/4 red onion, chopped

Preparation:

Bring 4 quarts of water to a boil in a large pot over high heat. Add the pasta and bring back to a boil. Reduce the heat to medium and cook, stirring occasionally, for 5 minutes. Add the edamame and bring back to a boil over high heat. Reduce the heat to medium-low and cook until al dente, about 5 minutes more. Drain completely and place in a large bowl to cool for about 10 minutes.

In a small bowl, whisk together the red wine vinegar, basil, garlic, honey, mustard, and salt. While whisking vigorously, slowly drizzle in the oil until combined.

Add the peppers, olives, tomatoes, and red onion to the cooled pasta and toss to combine. Drizzle the dressing over the pasta and toss to coat evenly. Cover the pasta salad and place in the refrigerator for at least 20 minutes to allow the flavors to marinate together. Serve cold.

Ratatouille

This classic vegetable-based Mediterranean dish can be eaten alone or served with roasted fish, chicken, or a side of white beans. Definitely leftover-friendly. (*Vegan-friendly*)

Serves: 4
Prep Time: 20 minutes
Cooking Time: 50 minutes

Ingredients:

3 tablespoons olive oil, divided
½ medium eggplant, cut into 1-inch dice
¼ teaspoon plus ⅛ teaspoon salt, divided
¼ teaspoon plus ⅛ teaspoon ground black pepper, divided
1 medium zucchini, cut into 1-inch dice
1 medium yellow squash, cut into 1-inch dice
1 red onion, chopped
2 cloves garlic, minced
2 cups shredded green cabbage
1 red bell pepper, chopped
¼ cup kalamata olives, pitted and halved lengthwise
1 (14.5-ounce) can no-added-salt fire-roasted diced
    tomatoes
2 tablespoons apple cider vinegar
2 thyme sprigs
3 bay leaves

Preparation:

In a medium sauté pan, heat 1 tablespoon of the olive oil over medium heat. When the oil is shimmering, add the eggplant and sprinkle with ⅛ teaspoon each of the salt and pepper. Cook the eggplant until browned on all sides, about 3 minutes. Use a slotted spoon to transfer the eggplant into a clean bowl.

Heat the second 1 tablespoon of the olive oil in the same sauté pan over medium heat. When the oil is shimmering, add the zucchini and yellow squash and sprinkle with ⅛ teaspoon each of the salt and pepper. Cook until browned on all sides, about 3 minutes. Use a slotted spoon to transfer the zucchini and yellow squash to the same bowl as the eggplant.

Heat the remaining 1 tablespoon of olive oil in the same sauté pan over medium heat. When the oil is shimmering, add the onion and garlic and cook until softened and translucent, about 3 minutes. Add the eggplant, zucchini, and yellow squash, cabbage, bell pepper, olives, diced tomatoes, apple cider vinegar, thyme sprigs, bay leaves, and remaining ⅛ teaspoon each of the salt and pepper and stir to combine. Raise the heat to high and bring the mixture to a boil. Lower to medium-low heat, covered, and allow the flavors to combine for 40 minutes. Remove bay leaves and thyme sprigs and discard. Serve warm.

Roasted Fish, Three Ways

Match your favorite fish with a tasty sauce. You can substitute salmon or sea bass fillets for the halibut. Cooking times will vary slightly depending on the thickness of the fillet. Use a thermometer to check when the internal cooking temperature reaches 145°F. To get the fillets the size you want, ask your fishmonger to slice them for you. If you are short on time, just make one of the sauces.

Serves: 4

Prep Time: 30 minutes

Cooking Time: 45 minutes (for all three sauces)

Roasted Fish Ingredients:

4 (5-ounce) halibut fillets

1 tablespoon olive oil

⅛ teaspoon salt

⅛ teaspoon ground black pepper

Arugula-Broccoli Sprout Pesto Ingredients:
1 cup fresh basil leaves
1/2 cup broccoli sprouts
1/4 cup grated Parmesan cheese
1/4 cup pine nuts
3 cloves garlic, crushed
1 teaspoon fresh lemon juice
1/4 teaspoon salt
1/3 cup extra virgin olive oil

Mango Chutney Ingredients:
1 mango, diced (about 1 1/2 cups)
2 pitted dates, chopped
1 1/2 tablespoons white wine vinegar
1 tablespoon lemon juice
1/2 teaspoon lemon zest
1 clove garlic, minced
2 teaspoons grated ginger
1/3 teaspoon crushed red pepper flakes

Quick Tzatziki Ingredients:
1/2 large English or hothouse cucumber, grated
1 cup nonfat plain Greek yogurt
1 clove garlic, minced
1 tablespoon chopped dill
1 teaspoon lemon juice
1/2 teaspoon kosher salt
1/8 teaspoon ground black pepper

Preparation:

To make the roasted fish, preheat the oven to 400°F.

Brush the halibut fillets with the olive oil and sprinkle both sides with the salt and black pepper. Place on a sheet pan skin-side down and bake in the preheated oven until the internal cooking temperature reaches 145°F, 12–15 minutes. Remove the sheet pan from the oven and allow the fish to slightly cool.

To make the pesto, place the basil, sprouts, Parmesan cheese, pine nuts, garlic, lemon juice, and salt in a blender and blend until smooth. While the machine is running, drizzle in the olive oil until it is incorporated.

Store the pesto in a resealable container in the refrigerator for up to 1 week. Makes ½ cup.

To make the chutney, in a medium saucepan, add the mango, dates, vinegar, lemon juice and zest, garlic, ginger, and red pepper flakes and stir to combine. Bring to a boil over high heat and then reduce the heat to low, cover, and simmer, stirring occasionally, for 30 minutes Remove the saucepan from the heat and allow to cool for 10–15 minutes.

Place the chutney in a blender and blend until mostly smooth, leaving some chunks. Makes 1 cup.

To make the tzatziki, place the grated cucumber in a colander. Using clean hands, press down to drain the excess liquid.

In a medium bowl, whisk together the cucumber, Greek yogurt, garlic, dill, lemon juice, salt, and pepper. Cover the bowl and refrigerate for at least 30 minutes to allow the flavors to blend.

Serve cold. Makes 1 ½ cups.

Roasted Mushrooms with Beans and Arugula

Roasted mushrooms add umami to this dish, complemented by the spicy arugula, tender beans, and salty anchovies in the dressing.

Serves: 4
Prep Time: 20 minutes
Cooking Time: 15 minutes

Mushroom and Bean Ingredients:
3 tablespoons extra virgin olive oil
2 cloves garlic, minced

1 tablespoon fresh parsley, chopped

1 teaspoon fresh thyme, leaves only

1/4 teaspoon salt

8 ounces cremini mushrooms, quartered

4 ounces shiitake mushrooms, quartered

4 cups arugula

1 (15.5-ounce) can low-sodium cannellini or white beans, drained and rinsed

Anchovy Dressing Ingredients:

2 tablespoons white wine vinegar

2 canned anchovy fillets

1 tablespoon fresh lemon juice

1 clove garlic, crushed

1/2 teaspoon Dijon mustard

2 tablespoons extra virgin olive oil

Note: to make this vegan-friendly, eliminate the anchovy and use a vegan
mustard.

Preparation:

To make the roasted mushrooms, preheat the oven to 375°F. Line a baking sheet with parchment paper.

In a medium bowl, add the oil, garlic, parsley, thyme, and salt and whisk to combine. Add the cremini and shiitake mushrooms and toss to evenly coat. Spoon the mushrooms onto the prepared baking sheet in a single layer and roast in the preheated oven until the mushrooms are slightly browned, 15 minutes. Remove the baking sheet from the oven and allow the mushrooms to cool for 10 minutes.

To make the dressing, in a food processor or blender, add the white wine vinegar, anchovy fillets, lemon juice, garlic, and Dijon mustard and pulse until smooth. With the motor running, slowly add the oil and pulse for at least 30 seconds to combine.

In a large serving bowl, mix together the arugula, beans, and roasted mushrooms. Drizzle the dressing over the salad and toss to evenly coat. Serve immediately.

Shakshuka with Herbs and Olives

This Mediterranean dish, originating from Tunisia, is made by poaching eggs in a tomato-based sauce flavored with vegetables and fresh herbs (*shakshuka* is an Arabic word meaning "mixture"). Serve with a crusty piece of whole-grain bread.

Serves: 6
Prep Time: 15 minutes
Cooking Time: 20 minutes

Ingredients:
1 tablespoon olive oil
1 medium red onion, cut into 1-inch-wide strips
2 green bell peppers, cut into 1-inch-wide strips
2 cloves garlic, minced
1 (28-ounce) can crushed tomatoes
¼ cup kalamata olives, pitted and halved
2 tablespoons chopped fresh cilantro
2 tablespoons chopped fresh basil leaves
¼ teaspoon salt
⅛ teaspoon freshly ground black pepper
⅛ teaspoon crushed red pepper flakes
6 large free-range chicken eggs

Preparation:

In a large sauté pan over medium heat, heat the olive oil until it shimmers. Add the onions and bell pepper and cook until softened, about 5 minutes. Add the garlic and cook until fragrant, about 30 seconds. Stir in the crushed tomatoes, olives, cilantro, basil, salt, black pepper, and red pepper flakes. Increase the heat to medium-high and bring the mixture to a boil, then reduce the heat to medium-low. Cover the pan and simmer for about 10 minutes to let the flavors blend together.

Use a wooden spoon to create six pockets in the sauce around the outer edge. Break 1 egg into a small glass bowl. Gently pour the egg into the pocket along the outer edge of the pan. Repeat with the remaining 5 eggs so that the eggs form a circle around the outer edge of the pan. Reduce the heat to low, cover the pan, and cook until the eggs are poached, about 6 minutes.

To serve, spoon 1 egg and an even amount of the sauce onto each of six plates.

Shellfish with Three Sauces

Cooking shellfish is very easy. Select the best fresh shellfish you can find from the seafood section, pick a sauce, and prepare a simple but elegant seafood dish in minutes. Each of these flavorful sauces is made with only five ingredients.

Serves: 2
Prep Time: 15 minutes
Cooking Time: 10 minutes

Caponata Ingredients:
1 tablespoon extra virgin olive oil
2 cloves garlic, finely chopped
1 small Japanese eggplant, finely diced
1 cup canned no-salt-added diced tomatoes
2 tablespoons capers

Chimichurri Ingredients:
1 tablespoon extra virgin olive oil
2 cloves garlic, finely chopped
1 Fresno chili, finely chopped
Juice of 1 lemon
¼ cup dry white wine (optional)
1 cup chopped fresh herbs (cilantro, parsley, dill, basil)

Coconut Lemongrass Ingredients:

1 tablespoon extra virgin olive oil

2 cloves garlic, finely chopped

1 tablespoon finely chopped fresh ginger

1 small stalk lemongrass, finely chopped

½ cup canned coconut milk

Shellfish Ingredients:

2 pounds shellfish (mussels, littleneck or other clams) scrubbed and rinsed

Preparation:

Heat oil in a large Dutch oven or soup pot with a lid over medium-high heat. Add remaining sauce ingredients for whichever sauce you choose, bring to a simmer, and cook for 2–3 minutes. Add mussels or clams and toss in the sauce. Cover and allow to steam for 5–6 minutes or until shells open.

Serve with fresh lemon or lime wedges and crusty bread.

Spiced Chicken, Rice, and Kale

This is a one-pot meal inspired by rice dishes from Central Asia that is aromatic and satisfying. If you wish to go meatless, swap the chicken with slices of firm tofu. There will be leftovers, which you can use for lunch or dinner the next day.

Serves: 4

Prep Time: 45 minutes

Cooking Time: 50 minutes

Ingredients:

1 ½ cups basmati rice

2 tablespoons extra virgin olive oil

2 garlic cloves, minced

2 shallots, finely chopped

1 pound skinless and boneless chicken thighs

1 teaspoon turmeric powder

½ teaspoon cayenne pepper

Salt, to taste

1 cup vegetable stock

2 cinnamon sticks

1 can (13.5-ounce) unsweetened coconut milk

1 can (15-ounce) chickpeas, drained

2 cups kale, coarsely chopped with ribs and stems removed

¼ cup Calabrian chili peppers, marinated in oil, sliced thinly*

½ lime, for juice

1 lime, cut into wedges

Preparation:

In a metal bowl, rinse rice in cold water until cloudiness disappears. Drain completely, then add water until it is 1 inch above the rice. Let soak for 45 minutes.

Using a 12-inch-wide cast-iron pan with 2-½-inch-tall sides (or a Dutch oven), heat olive oil over medium heat and add garlic and shallots. Cook for 3 minutes, until shallots become translucent and soft. Add chicken, turmeric, cayenne pepper, and a pinch of salt. Cook chicken for 2 minutes on each side. Add vegetable stock and cinnamon sticks. Turn up heat until liquid boils, then immediately reduce heat to low and simmer for 20 minutes.

Drain the rice and add to the pan with the chicken. Add coconut milk and stir with a wooden spoon to combine. Add chickpeas, kale, and chili peppers and stir to incorporate. Add the juice from ½ lime. Turn heat to high until liquid boils, then turn heat to low and place lid on pan. Simmer for 20 minutes, then turn off heat. Remove lid from pan and allow moisture to evaporate for 5 minutes.

Serve while hot, with lime wedges to squeeze on each serving.

---

* Sliced Calabrian chili peppers packed in oil can be ordered online.

Tofu Noodles with Spicy Sauce

If you've ever wondered how to use tofu in new ways, look no further than this mouthwatering dish that has complex flavors yet is simple to make.

This noodle dish is meatless, but the tofu provides the same protein and texture as meat. It's the OG of plant-based "meat" dishes. The topping is warm, but the noodles can be served hot or cold. *(Vegan-friendly)*

Serves: 2
Prep Time: 10 minutes
Cooking Time: 15 minutes

Ingredients:
3 tablespoons dark soy sauce*
3 tablespoons black vinegar*
1 ½ tablespoons honey
1 ½ tablespoons spicy chili crisp sauce*
Pinch ground Szechuan peppercorns
½ pound firm tofu
1 tablespoon extra virgin olive oil
3 garlic cloves, thinly sliced
8 ounces soba noodles
1 scallion, chopped, as garnish

Preparation:

Mix soy sauce, vinegar, honey, chili crisp sauce, and peppercorns in a small bowl and set aside.

Rinse tofu and pat dry. Press down to remove as much liquid as possible using paper towels. Cut the pressed tofu into ½-inch cubes.

Heat olive oil in a pan or wok until shimmering. Add garlic and sauté until it turns golden. Add cubed tofu and sear until slightly

---

* Lao Gan Ma Spicy Chili Crisp Sauce (chili oil sauce), Chinkiang Black Vinegar, and Lee Kum Kee Premium Dark Soy Sauce are available online.

browned, about 3 minutes, turning once or twice. Then pour in sauce and gently turn tofu and sauce with a wooden spoon to combine. Cook for 2 minutes, mixing gently.

Bring water to boil in a pot and cook the noodles until tender, then drain. If you are serving cold noodles, rinse under cold water until noodles are cold.

Place the noodles in a serving bowl, pour the sauce on top of noodles, toss lightly to mix. Sprinkle chopped scallions on top and serve.

Tomato and Shrimp with Sweet-and-Sour Cider Sauce

This classic Chinese dish is often made with ketchup, but I've switched it out for intensely flavored tomato paste and punched up the flavor with apple cider vinegar. Use shell-on shrimp to get the most out of this recipe—the tangy, sweet-and-sour sauce will coat the shells nicely— finger-licking good!

Serves: 2
Prep Time: 10 minutes
Cooking Time: 7 minutes

Ingredients:
8 jumbo shrimp, shells on*
4 tablespoons Shaoxing rice wine, divided**
3 tablespoons double-concentrated tomato paste**
1 tablespoon Chinkiang black vinegar**

---

* If you really can't deal with shell-on shrimp, you'll want to devein the shelled shrimp, slice halfway along the length of their bodies, and marinate them with double the amount of rice wine in the bowl before cooking.
** Double-concentrated tomato paste is sold in tubes, usually in supermarkets next to the jarred tomato sauces, or you can easily find it online, as with the Shaoxing Rice Cooking Wine and the Chinkiang black vinegar.

2 tablespoons apple cider vinegar

½ teaspoon soy sauce

White pepper, to taste

3 tablespoons extra virgin olive oil

2 garlic cloves, thickly sliced

2 slices fresh ginger

2 green scallions, cut into ½-inch pieces

½ teaspoon cornstarch

4 tablespoons water

Preparation:

Rinse shrimp under cold water. Remove legs with scissors and devein each shrimp. Rinse again, dry with a paper towel, and set aside in a small bowl. Add 2 tablespoons of the Shaoxing rice wine to marinate.

In another bowl, mix together the tomato paste, both vinegars, soy sauce, remaining 2 tablespoons Shaoxing rice wine, and a pinch of white pepper.

In a wok or pan, heat the oil on high until shimmering. Add the garlic and ginger and sauté for about 15 seconds. Add the shrimp and cook on one side for 2 minutes, then turn over and cook the other side for the same amount of time. Add the sauce and scallions. Place a cover on the wok and cook for 2 minutes.

Remove the cover. Dissolve the cornstarch in water, and slowly pour into wok, mixing with the sauce to thicken. Allow to boil, then turn off heat. Serve immediately, with a small bowl for shells after they have been licked clean.

Vegetable Chili

This warming meal of chili is made with black and white beans, plus anthocyanin-rich purple potatoes. Leftovers are perfect for the next day. (*Vegan-friendly*)

Serves: 4
Prep Time: 20 minutes
Cooking Time: 45 minutes

Ingredients:

2 tablespoons extra virgin olive oil

1 red onion, coarsely chopped

3 garlic cloves, minced

2 ribs celery, coarsely chopped

2 carrots, peeled and coarsely chopped

1 green bell pepper, coarsely chopped

6 small purple potatoes, cut into eighths

1 (28-ounce) can crushed tomatoes with the liquid

1 (15-ounce) can black beans, drained and rinsed

1 (15-ounce) can Great Northern beans, drained and rinsed

2 tablespoons chili powder

1 teaspoon ground cumin

1 teaspoon paprika

2 tablespoons fresh oregano leaves, chopped (dried can be substituted)

¼ cup basil, sliced into thin strips

¼ teaspoon salt

1 cup water

Preparation:

Heat the oil in a large pot over medium heat. When the oil is shimmering, add the onion and cook until soft and translucent, about 3 minutes. Add the garlic and cook until fragrant, 30 seconds. Add the celery, carrots, and pepper and cook until vegetables have softened, about 5 minutes. Add the purple potatoes, crushed tomatoes, black beans, Great Northern beans, chili powder, cumin, paprika, oregano, basil, and salt and stir to combine. Add water. Raise the heat to high and bring the mixture to a boil, then lower the heat to medium-low and simmer, covered, until the potatoes have softened and flavors combine, about 30–35 minutes.

Wild Mushroom Barley Stew

Wild mushrooms and barley make this a tasty comfort food. Dried mushrooms will give more umami flavor than fresh. Use whichever varieties are available at your local market or order your favorites online. (*Vegan-friendly*)

Serves: 4

Prep Time: 15 minutes, plus 30 minutes soaking time

Cooking Time: 1 hour

Ingredients:

1 ounce dried shiitake mushrooms

½ ounce dried porcini mushrooms

½ ounce dried morels

2 tablespoons extra virgin olive oil

1 medium red onion, chopped

1 clove garlic, minced

2 ribs celery, chopped

2 carrots, peeled and chopped

1 cup dried pearled barley

3 cups low-sodium vegetable broth

1 ½ cups tomato puree

½ teaspoon honey

1 teaspoon smoked paprika

1 teaspoon ground cumin

¼ teaspoon cayenne pepper

¼ teaspoon salt

¼ cup chopped fresh parsley

1 tablespoon chopped rosemary leaves

Preparation:

Place the dried mushrooms in a medium bowl. Pour hot water over the mushrooms until just fully covered. Allow to steep until soft, about

20–30 minutes. Drain the water using a mesh strainer and roughly chop the mushrooms.

In a large sauté pan, heat the olive oil over medium heat. When the oil is shimmering, add the onion and cook until soft and translucent, about 3 minutes. Add the garlic and continue cooking until fragrant, an additional 30 seconds. Add the celery and carrots and cook until softened, about 5 minutes. Add the mushrooms and cook until water is released, about 8 minutes. Add the barley, broth, tomato puree, honey, smoked paprika, cumin, cayenne, and salt and stir to combine. Raise the heat to high and bring mixture to a boil, then lower the heat to medium-low and simmer, covered, until the barley is tender, 40–45 minutes.

Add the fresh parsley and rosemary and stir to combine. Serve warm.

*   *   *

I hope reading (and eating) these recipes will prove to you that my MediterAsian Way of eating can make your health journey pleasurable. If you are a novice in the kitchen, keep in mind that everyone starts at the beginning.

And as you explore further and plan your own meals, you may find ingredients in this book or at the market that you want to try but are not sure how to cook them or what recipe to use the ingredients in. These days, it's easy to find guidance—just search online using "[ingredient name]" and "recipe" and "Mediterranean" or "Asian." You'll be rewarded with a long list of results, including cooking videos. Home-cooked dishes are passed down from one generation to the next. But I also love watching videos of people showing me how to cook a recipe. Once you make a new dish that you like, you'll want to tell other people about it, too. In medicine, we say, "See one, do one, teach one."

A final note about eating to beat your diet: you are not alone. Eating can be a powerful shared experience. I encourage you to adopt the Mediterranean and Asian cultural practice of eating with family or friends, especially those who appreciate good food. Along the way, you can share what you've learned about fat-fighting and health-boosting foods and bring more people along with you on your journey.

There's one last stop: eating to beat your diet involves fine-tuning your diet and lifestyle. In the last chapter, I'm going to tell you how to refine the techniques you've learned, so your metabolism can be optimized now and for years to come.

CHAPTER 13

Optimize Your Metabolism

Even if you believe you're in peak health, there is always room for improvement. Your body's ability to benefit from what you eat is affected by your lifestyle. That's why the terms "diet" and "lifestyle" are often used together. To optimize your metabolism and get to your next level of health, you'll need to attend to both. I call this a metabolism tune-up. Think of this chapter as an advanced protocol that can take you further than the basic Eat to Beat Protocol.

Your metabolism tune-up is divided into five categories: when you eat, how much you eat, how well you sleep, how you stay physically active, and how you manage stress. Let's go over how to optimize each of these areas to help you get the most benefit from the Eat to Beat Protocol.

When You Eat: Advanced Fasting

You can improve your metabolism by going beyond the twelve-hour fast that's built into the Eat to Beat Protocol and try even more ambitious forms of intermittent fasting. Don't be afraid to schedule your personal eating window so that it is even shorter in duration, as this will yield even better results. For example, if you wake up at 7 a.m. but start your daily eating window even later, at, say, 10 a.m. (instead of 9 a.m.), with a late breakfast, and you finish with an early dinner that concludes at 6 p.m., you'll have created a sixteen-hour window in which you are fasting and grooming your metabolism. Remember, shortening the duration of your eating window is important—your body needs time to fight fat and improve metabolism.[1] After a late breakfast, for example, you might choose to skip lunch, thus lowering your calorie intake that day even more. Or you could even skip breakfast and eat an early lunch and an early dinner. If you are aiming to hit your excess body fat hard, go for longer windows of fasting.

How Long Should You Fast?

When you research intermittent fasting, you'll come across the "16/8" rule.[2] Per this rule, you eat within an eight-hour window and then fast for sixteen hours. The 16/8 fasting period is longer than the Eat to Beat Protocol, which has a "12/12" schedule (twelve hours eating, twelve hours not eating). So which is better: 12/12 or 16/8?

Actually, there is no magic number for the hours you need to fast. The more, the better, but it has to fit into your life. While 16/8 does work for weight loss in mice and humans, it's not a rule set in stone. In fact, "sixteen hours" and "eight hours" were originally chosen for non-scientific reasons. The number came from a landmark experiment on intermittent fasting conducted on mice at the Salk Institute for Biological Studies in La Jolla, California.[3] According to a podcast episode on fasting by Stanford medical professor Andrew Huberman, the backstory behind 16/8 is that eight hours was the time "allowed" by the significant other of the graduate student who was running the experiment, in order for the student to have a reasonable work-life balance (lab experiments involving mice can be extremely time-intensive).[4] I can confirm from my own research experience that lab experiments are often influenced by the lifestyle of the person performing the study. Sometimes the science has to fit into a scientist's personal schedule.

Clinical studies have shown that a variety of time-restricted eating windows work to help your metabolism. A study of ninety individuals who were obese was conducted at the Weight Loss Medicine Clinic at the University of Alabama at Birmingham Hospital.[5] The study examined two fasting/eating windows: 12/12 and 16/8. After fourteen weeks, both groups lost weight—those who had fasted twelve hours lost 8.8 pounds, but those who fasted sixteen hours lost even more weight, 13.9 pounds. Another clinical study by a group at Maastricht University Medical Center in the Netherlands showed that a fourteen-hour fasting window was effective for improving fasting blood glucose levels.[6]

I recommend starting with the 12/12 time frame because it's an easier fit for the schedules and lifestyles of most people. But feel free to follow a 14/10 or 16/8 time frame, or an even longer fasting window, if that works for you. The most important thing is to make your eating window consistent and sustainable. The Eat to Beat Protocol helps build a program that can last a lifetime, and fasting is only one component.

The Metabolic Benefits of Not Snacking

One recommendation I give for the metabolic tune-up is to give up snacking. You've seen this in the Eat to Beat Protocol. Here's why: every time you have a snack, your insulin spikes. Repeated, continuous spikes of insulin throughout the day and at night wear down your metabolism and can eventually lead to insulin resistance. This is where your cells become less sensitive to insulin, so they are less able to absorb glucose from your bloodstream.

When your cells don't respond well to insulin, your body pumps out even more insulin to try to compensate. The presence of insulin hinders your body's ability to use fat for energy. The more insulin that's present, the harder it is for your metabolism to access and burn down fat.[7] With insulin resistance, your baseline blood sugar rises, and you're headed right toward the dangers of metabolic syndrome, type 2 diabetes, and obesity. The hormone insulin-like growth factor-1 also rises to abnormally high levels, which increases your risk for cardiovascular disease and cancer. When you quit snacking, your insulin levels decline during the day, and so does insulin-like growth factor. This unleashes your metabolism to burn fat, which further lowers your risk of developing insulin resistance—and other diseases as well. To bring it all together, here are five easy ways to optimize your fasting period:

1. Commit to your eating window.
2. Hold back on eating for two hours after you wake up in the morning.
3. Have your last bite of dinner at least three hours before bedtime.
4. Don't snack during your eating window.
5. Write a note to yourself and put it where you store your snacks!

Break the Cycle of Overeating

Controlling how much you eat is both the easiest and the most overlooked action you can take when it comes to metabolism. Almost all the clinical studies of fat-fighting foods showed benefits when the specific foods were combined *with* some form of controlled or reduced daily calorie intake. Yet we all have overindulged at some point in our lives, overloading our metabolism with excess calories (fuel), probably many times over.[8] We are all human, so it's important to pay even more attention during vulnerable times to how much food you load into your body at each meal. Personally, I'm most susceptible to this behavior during holiday gatherings when I am with family and friends and there are festive foods galore.

Perhaps you can relate to this situation. You sit down to a delicious meal and dig in without paying attention to the portions. What starts out as a delightful experience turns into an uncomfortable state of fullness because you ate too fast or just had a few too many bites of deliciousness before you could get yourself to stop. Your stomach is overstuffed, and you feel miserable just sitting in your chair. That discomfort happens because your stomach is pushing against the other organs in your abdomen. Your stomach is positioned directly beneath your diaphragm, a muscle whose action draws air into your lungs when you breathe. With your bulging stomach pushing up against your diaphragm, it's hard to inhale deeply. Until your stomach unloads its burden, you will feel uncomfortable in any position, except maybe lying down.

Your body is resilient, so it will recover from an *occasional* episode of overindulgence. But if overeating becomes a habit, as it is for many people, the extra calories will accumulate as stored fat, and you will surely gain weight, especially if the foods you overindulge in are heavy in carbohydrates and dietary fat.[9] Even if you follow the Eat to Beat Protocol, it doesn't take many rounds of overindulgence to undo your good work. Remember this the next time you feel tempted to finish that gigantic plate of pasta that's big enough for two people. Also remember that being on vacation does not give you a free pass to overeat. Researchers from Deakin University in Australia have discovered that even five days of gluttony can increase your harmful visceral fat by 15 percent.[10]

While on the Eat to Beat Protocol, on the days you skip a breakfast or a lunch, be extra careful not to overeat during the next meal. As I suggested in Chapter 9, drinking a glass of water before you eat is a good way to make your stomach feel full and make your brain signal you to be less hungry. Don't forget the benefit of drinking water in general: it triggers thermogenesis for fat burning all by itself.

Here are eight easy ways to avoid overeating without feeling deprived:

1. **Slow Down.** Wolfing your food makes it easy to overload your stomach before it has time to signal to your brain that you are full. Your stomach needs twenty minutes from the first bite for those critical satiety signals to be sent and received. Eat slowly. Take the time to savor your food. Your stomach and brain will tell you when to put down your fork.

2. **Focus on Your Food.** Don't be distracted when you eat. Reading, watching television, or scrolling on your phone takes your attention away from the act of eating. This is similar to distracted driving. It reduces your awareness of how fast and how much you are eating. When you pay attention to the road, you drive more safely. Being attentive to what you're eating helps to prevent overeating.[11]

3. **Watch Portion Sizes.** Whether you serve yourself or someone serves you, be aware of how much food is on your plate. A good rule of thumb is "You should eat no more than the size of your fist of anything except veggies or fruits." If you are dining out with others, sharing an entrée or ordering different small plates MediterAsian style allows you to eat a smaller portion of food.

4. **Quit the Clean Plate Club.** The value of finishing everything on your plate is an antiquated idea that originated in the United States after World War I and during the Great Depression when food was scarce.* The intent was definitely not to give people permission to gorge. Its goal (based on patriotism and shared sacrifice) was to encourage people to ration food and not let anything go to waste. The idea of piling food on your plate and eating every crumb is terribly misguided when it comes to health and is a surefire path to building fat and eroding your

---

* Here's the backstory on the Clean Plate Club: In 1917, the US government passed the Food and Fuel Control Act, also known as the Lever Act, which gave the president the power to regulate the distribution, purchase, and storage of food. From this act, the US Food Administration was created to ensure there was food conservation during World War I. Public campaigns were launched to decrease food consumption in the United States, and Americans signed pledges not to leave any scrap of food on their plate. The concept of the "clean plate" became synonymous with patriotism. Although the US Food Administration was dismantled after World War I ended, the clean plate idea was brought back to public attention after World War II during the rebuilding of Europe so that food could be directed to save starving Europeans. Clean Plate Clubs were formed in schools, and the idea that this is a virtuous and proper way of eating became entrenched in American society.

metabolism. When you are eating at home, portion size is easy to control, but you might still be tempted to take more than you should eat. At some restaurants, you may be served ridiculously large portion sizes. The solution is simple: don't eat it all—leave some on the plate, share some with whomever you're dining with, or take home the leftovers.

5. **Skip Second Helpings.** As a rule, I recommend that you never go for additional helpings of food. Even if you feel ecstatic about a dish, be mindful, and savor your first (and only!) serving by eating slowly.

6. **Eat Fiber-Rich Foods.** Plant-based foods like whole grains, legumes (beans, lentils, chickpeas), tree nuts and seeds, and whole fruits and leafy green vegetables can help you feel sated without overindulging. Studies have shown that eating dietary fiber earlier in the day, during lunch, has a satiating effect and makes you less likely to overeat during dinner.[12] High-protein foods also have a similar satiating effect.[13] These are abundant on the fat-fighting foods list.

7. **Use a Smaller Plate.** This is a simple way to retrain your habits on portion size. A study from Cornell University showed that the bigger the plate, the larger the serving people are tempted to take.[14] Counter that tendency by using a smaller plate, and you'll take a smaller portion of food. Tip: remind yourself to leave some "white space" showing on the plate.

8. **Continue Journaling.** In the Eat to Beat program, I have you do two weeks of food journaling at the beginning to develop awareness of what you eat and how you feel during and after eating. You can continue this or pick it up again anytime. Food journaling is a way to develop mindfulness. Making notes in a food journal after a meal can help you remember what you ate, how much, and how you felt after eating. Journaling makes you aware of the triggers and emotions you feel when you overeat, so you can

avoid doing it in the future. You can journal using pen and paper, make an electronic note, or use one of the many food journaling apps available.

Get the Right Amount (and Quality) of Sleep

What and how you eat are important for fine-tuning your metabolism, and so is sleeping. Sleep has a powerful impact on your metabolism, including how your body stores fat and how well your health defense systems operate. The bad news is that many of us do not get enough high-quality sleep, and we suffer as a result. Making sure that you are getting good-quality sleep is an important goal for your metabolism tune-up.

Research shows that teenagers and adults need between seven and nine hours of sleep each night, and younger children need even more.[15] In our modern world, however, a sleep crisis is sweeping across the globe, threatening the health of society.[16] Insufficient sleep not only increases the risk of heart disease, mental health issues, cancer, and premature death; it also disrupts your metabolism and increases your chances of becoming obese. Getting a good night's sleep not only helps us be more alert during the day; it also aids our metabolism in fighting excess body fat.

There are many reasons for our sleep-deprived state in the modern world, including social issues—stress about wars, pandemics, the economy—plus being online late at night or shift work, or medical causes like cancer, chronic pain, and sleep apnea.[17] Not getting enough sleep increases your risk for obesity, and having too much body fat also interferes with sleep. It's a vicious cycle.

Sleep deprivation compromises your metabolism and causes weight gain for many reasons.[18] For one, poor sleep interferes with your body's ability to burn fat during what is supposed to be your low insulin period.

Poor sleep causes your blood glucose to rise, and thus your insulin levels to rise with it, which then suppresses your body's ability to burn fat. This compromises the value of the intermittent fasting period during sleep in the Eat to Beat Protocol.

Researchers from Sapienza University in Rome, Italy, analyzed twenty clinical studies involving 307,128 people, and they found that those who slept fewer than seven hours per night had a 41 percent greater risk for obesity, compared to people who slept seven to nine hours per night.[19] In the lab, poor sleep quality has been shown to lead to an increase in visceral fat and abnormal changes in metabolism.[20]

When you don't get enough sleep, your body's circadian clock becomes derailed, and your hunger hormones fall out of sync with your body's energy needs. Remember pulling that all-nighter during college and the junk food you ate? Being tired makes you reach for sugary foods to gain energy. Sleep deprivation causes your stomach and brain to produce more ghrelin, the hunger hormone, making you want more food. It also decreases your levels of leptin, the hormone that makes you feel full.[21] When your circadian clock is confused, it throws your liver's ability to orchestrate metabolism out of whack.[22] Your blood lipids, ability to store energy with insulin, and secretion of adiponectin—the fat hormone responsible for health—all become uncoordinated, tipping your metabolism into chaos.[23]

Being sleep deprived also interferes with good judgment when it comes to food.[24] You become less choosy about what and how much you eat. Clarity of thinking results from having a good night's sleep. You may not know this, but while you are in deep sleep, a hidden drainage system in the brain called the glymphatic system opens up and flushes out the toxins that accumulated in the brain from the day before.[25] This happens *only* during deep sleep. If your brain's toxins are not drained, they sit there through the next day. The result is impaired cognition and brain fog. This interferes with good decision-making, including the ability to choose wisely and exercise restraint when it comes to food, as well as with other decisions related to your health that you might make during the day.

How do you know if you are not getting good-quality sleep? Here are a few questions you can ask yourself:

- Does it take you more than thirty minutes to fall asleep once you're in bed?
- Do you wake up repeatedly in the middle of the night?
- Do you feel tired and unusually sluggish during the day?
- Are you often irritable and stressed?

If you answered yes to any of the above, then make improving your sleep part of your metabolic tune-up. Here are seven easy ways to do it:

1. **Stick to a sleep schedule.** Go to bed at the same time every night. You may set an alarm to wake up in the morning, but try setting an alarm to remind you to go to bed at night. This will be especially helpful while following the Eat to Beat Protocol, so you know when to close your eating window.

2. **Avoid technology** (mobile device, laptop, gaming, television) for at least one hour before bedtime. I recommend that you do not bring your device to bed. The blue light coming from these devices disrupts your brain waves and sets off a neural chain reaction that interferes with your natural sleep pattern. If you are food journaling on a digital device, avoid doing it just before bedtime.

3. **Read a print book instead.** Studies show that reading a print book increases melatonin production in the brain naturally and helps you sleep better.[26]

4. **Avoid naps during the day.** Napping disturbs your body's circadian clocks, and this throws off your metabolism.

5. **Avoid food and drink (except for water)** for three hours before bedtime. This is an essential part of the Eat to Beat Protocol.

Food or drink just before bedtime raises blood glucose and, hence, insulin levels, which interferes with quality sleep as well as fat burning.[27]

6. **Take a relaxing walk.** Doing this after your evening meal helps you sleep.

7. **Sleep in a dark, cool room.** When you go to bed at night, turn off all the lights, shut your curtains, and close the bedroom door. Ambient light interferes with deep sleep. You might also sleep with a fan or open a window to keep the room cool, as this not only improves sleep but, if cool enough, it may even stimulate thermogenesis.

Get More Physically Active, in Big and Little Ways

Your metabolic tune-up should involve physical activity. Many of the clinical studies on fat-fighting foods have shown efficacy when combined with some form of exercise. Some people squirm a little when they hear this kind of advice. They hate going to the gym, find it inconvenient, or just don't know where they'll find the time. Here's the good news: going to work out in the gym is not the only way to do this. There are many ways to incorporate physical activity into your lifestyle. Any type of movement that requires your body to consume energy by its very nature will help you burn fat. And I mean *any* movement.

You may be surprised to learn that even *fidgeting*—moving "restlessly" in a way not necessary to perform a task (that's right: tapping your fingers, shaking your leg)—can spark thermogenesis and help you burn fat.[28] Researchers from the Mayo Clinic showed that fidgeting while sitting turns on thermogenesis and increases your resting calorie burn by 29 percent.[29] Remarkably, fidgeting while standing is more effective than doing it while sitting—it increases the burn rate by 38 percent.

To drill the point home, researchers from the United Kingdom studied 12,778 women over twelve years and discovered the negative health consequences of just sitting around. They found that people who sat more than seven hours a day (bus driver, airline pilot, computer programmer, gamer) had an increased mortality from *any cause* by 30 percent!

But they also discovered that people who fidgeted while they sat had a *decreased* mortality by 37 percent.[30] I am not telling you to fidget for health (people around you may find it annoying), but this is another example of how even small actions can have big effects when it comes to your metabolism.

Even better than fidgeting, regular, purposeful physical activity offers a windfall of benefits for your metabolism. Whether you like to go to the gym and lift weights, go for a run, swim, or ride your stationary bike, the idea of movement is more important than the concept of "working out." You can find lots of ways—like dancing, yoga, gardening, practicing tai chi, hiking—to remain agile and maintain strength by being in motion over a lifetime. The general wisdom is to exercise at least three times per week, each time for a minimum of twenty to thirty minutes. If you want to do more, do it! You'll feel better, and it will help your metabolism.

If you visit locations in the Mediterranean and Asia with exceptional longevity, the so-called Blue Zones—Sardinia, Ikaria, Okinawa—you'll notice that people who live there are constantly on the move: walking up and down hills, gardening, maintaining their homes, and strolling to meet up with friends and family. Burning more calories than you consume is key to fighting body fat and optimizing your metabolism.

Exercise also helps fight visceral fat. A review of 117 clinical studies showed that regular workouts reduced visceral fat by 6.1 percent, even without weight loss.[32] Lab studies also suggest that exercise promotes more useful brown fat to develop.[33] In the long run, regular exercise prevents weight gain and promotes many other health benefits by

Activities and Calories Burned

According to Harvard Medical School's consumer health division, here are some activities and the calories burned per hour for someone of average weight (155 pounds):[31]

- 200 cal/hr.: Playing golf, bowling, playing Frisbee
- 300 cal/hr.: Walking, practicing tai chi
- 400 cal/hr.: Hiking, swimming, ballroom dancing
- 500 cal/hr.: Ice skating, scuba diving, playing soccer
- 600 cal/hr.: Bicycling, running, practicing martial arts

activating your body's health defenses, including better circulation and regeneration. Physical activity also improves your gut microbiome and immunity.[34]

If you have any underlying health conditions, such as cardiovascular disease, bone and joint diseases, or a metabolic disease like diabetes, make sure you speak with your doctor before embarking on a new exercise program. Certain health conditions may require adjustments to your plan. But that should not discourage you from staying physically active. Exercise is vital to your metabolic tune-up.[35]

A word of caution: vigorous exercise can bring on a big appetite. This makes it doubly important to be mindful not to overeat and to control your portion sizes. You cannot exercise your way out of gluttony and its negative health consequences. If you need suggestions for where to start, here are seven practical tips for increasing physical activity within the Eat to Beat framework:

1. **Take a walk** every day after a meal. Enjoy the outdoors, and use the activity to clear your mind while burning some calories at the same time. It will also help you sleep.

2. **Go for a jog or a run.** If you don't enjoy running, a good alternative is to invest in a standing desk with a walking treadmill. You can be a metabolic multitasker.

3. **Ride your bicycle.** This is also great for commuting! In cold or bad weather, you can use an indoor stationary cycle instead.

4. **Swim.** If you can find a local pool and fit it into your schedule, swimming is a joint-friendly way to get a great workout that strengthens muscles all over your body. Swimming also trains your breathing, which is important for mental wellness.

5. **Take the stairs** instead of using the elevator or escalator.

6. **Do some gardening or make house cleaning** part of your physical activity plan.

7. **Fidget** if it comes naturally, preferably when you're alone.

Stress Less

Stress is a normal part of life, and we all experience it at some point. A little psychological stress is inevitable and may actually be beneficial, as it keeps you on your toes. Research from the University of California at Berkeley has shown that short-term stress can prime the brain by causing stem cells to create nerve connections, which will help improve mental agility and performance.[36] But excess stress can interfere with your metabolism, so stress must be addressed as part of your tune-up.

Chronic stress promotes inflammation that smolders everywhere in your body. It disrupts your hormones and interferes with your body's ability to combat obesity. Long-term stress actually leads to the loss of brain neurons, so not surprisingly the ability to make good decisions can be compromised.[37] Let's take a look at how this all happens.

Life's stressors cause your adrenal glands to release stress hormones—adrenaline and cortisol—as part of the "fight-or-flight" response that evolution hardwired in us. This helps us react quickly to potentially dangerous situations as part of our survival instinct. Adrenaline increases your heart rate, makes you breathe faster, and pumps up your blood pressure so you are ready to fight or run. The hormone cortisol stimulates your metabolism to release energy as part of this response. It inhibits insulin's effects, which makes your blood sugar level rise so the energy can be immediately used by your muscles if you need to go into combat.

While adrenaline blunts your appetite (your body is wired so you can't fight and eat at the same time), cortisol does the opposite. It stimulates hunger so you'll feel the urge to take in more energy, specifically sugary and fatty foods, to keep building up your body's fuel stores in case the threat persists. When the danger has subsided, adrenaline and cortisol hormones recede to their normal levels, and your metabolism winds back down to its normal function.

This process is advantageous when you're being chased by a tiger. But the kinds of tigers we face today don't go away (some might argue there is no escape). Today's stress tigers show up at work and at home, and they can be everywhere, all the time. This can result in a chronic stressed-out state, which keeps adrenaline and cortisol constantly elevated. Your body learns to ignore the adrenaline, but the cortisol makes you hungry all the time, increasing the risk that you will overeat and end up gaining weight.[38] Too much cortisol also sends a signal to your pituitary gland, a tiny organ located underneath your brain that turns down your thyroid gland. Because thyroid hormones help run your metabolism, your metabolism slows down.

Constant high levels of cortisol make your cells more resistant to insulin. When stressed, blood sugar levels tend to run higher, even when you are fasting. Stress also provokes inflammation in your body, which can be made worse when your stress spikes. Researchers from Concordia University in Montreal, Canada, studied 130 older adults over a period of ten years and found that those who had large fluctuations in cortisol on top of high baseline levels of cortisol had higher inflammatory markers in their blood.[39]

Chronic stress has so many causes, it's impossible to name them all: chronic illness, anxiety disorders, depression, and job burnout are just a few. Even worse, stress leads to poor decision-making, including making poor food choices, overeating, not getting enough sleep, and getting less exercise—which leads to more stress. All of this interferes with an efficient metabolism, not only making it harder for you to shed fat but also compromising your health defenses.

Anger is another cause of stress, and in extreme cases you may require professional help to manage it. Being overly stressed can trigger anger, leading to more stress. Acute anger causes adrenaline to flow in your blood and causes blood pressure to rise. The veins in your forehead may even bulge for short periods of time. Chronic anger, the kind that is held inside and smolders for years, is not only destructive to mental well-being; it disrupts your hormones and metabolism, making it harder to fight body fat. If you want to be metabolically healthier, it is time to let your anger go. Your health is more important than any grudge.

A study from the University of Pittsburgh examined 157 physically healthy postmenopausal women to determine the connection between anger and fat.[40] A CT scan was performed on each to determine the amount of visceral fat in their belly. Then a standardized test was given to assess their anger intensity and frequency and their style of anger (holding it in versus letting it out), and it measured the degree to which they possessed a hostile attitude. The results showed a striking correlation between higher levels of anger and increased amounts of visceral fat. In the lab, anger damages brain neurons while it triggers the growth of new blood vessels that can bring blood flow to support the growth of adipose tissue.[41] Repressed anger is associated with insulin resistance, a marker for metabolic stress, as well as self-destructive behaviors like overeating and making poor food choices.[42]

Everyone has different triggers for stress, so there is no universal solution to manage this complex emotional and physical response to the hardships of life. But here are ten broad strategies that can help:

1. **Get support.** Ask friends and family members you trust to help you find ways to lower your stress. Just sharing your situation can be a useful release valve. If you need more support, you may benefit from seeking out a trained therapist.
2. **Meditate.** Many of us stress ourselves out by putting too much attention on the past (what already happened) and the future (what we fear might happen). Meditation slows your mind and allows you, and your thoughts, to be present in the moment. Studies have shown mindfulness (being present with what you're doing, like when you eat) is itself an intervention that can aid in weight loss.[43]
3. **Do yoga.** The physical movement, breathing exercises, and mental training of yoga relieve stress, burn calories, and can even reduce waist size.[44]
4. **Have a cup of tea.** Clinical studies have shown drinking low-caffeine green tea and/or chamomile tea helps to reduce stress and anxiety.[45]
5. **Sleep well.** Poor sleep not only disrupts your metabolism; it also contributes to stress.
6. **Get regular exercise.** Physical activity helps reduce tension levels and lower stress. Exercise also helps you sleep better. Tai chi is a form of meditative exercise from China that can be very calming and keep you in shape. It has been used to lower stress from posttraumatic stress disorder as well as the stress from chronic pain.[46]
7. **Delegate.** Remember, you don't have to do it all, and if you feel like there is too much piled up on your shoulders, hand off some

of the tasks to someone else. It can feel more stressful to do this at first, but an important part of stress (and anger) management is learning to let certain things go. Not everything has to be under your control—and not everything has to be done by you.

8. **Take deep breaths** when you feel highly stressed. Deep breathing exercises can reduce cortisol levels.[47]

9. **Manage anger.** When you feel angry, take a step back from the situation and allow your anger to subside. Try to find humor in the situation. Avoid people and activities that trigger your anger. Go for a walk. Exercise can help you lower anger and stress. Don't be afraid to seek professional help or try anger management therapy.

10. **Practice self-care.** We all have little ways that only we know to help ourselves relax. Taking care of yourself in this way, so long as it is not dangerous or harmful, can lower your stress. Be assertive in caring for yourself. Take at least a few minutes each day to tend to your own needs.

Should Dietary Supplements Be Part of Your Tune-Up?

Many people incorporate dietary supplements into their lifestyle, and I am asked all the time, "What dietary supplements should I take for better health?"

Here's my simple and direct answer: eating whole food is your best approach. Supplements are for "topping off" what you can achieve using foods.[48] Getting the bioactives from food rather than supplements is preferable on multiple levels. Eating brings people together, creating the social bonds that are important for wellness and overall health. Food tastes good, and it smells good, so eating becomes a sensory experience that can bring joy and pleasure. Taking supplements does not achieve any of these results.

Food is also the *safest* way to get the macronutrients and bioactives our bodies need for health. Supplements are produced by many manufacturers, and the quality of ingredients used varies greatly. Investigations by Loyola University examined twenty-nine supplements and found that 60 percent of them contained contaminating fungi.[49] The presence of heavy metals, like cadmium, mercury, lead, barium, thallium, cesium, and arsenic is another concern with dietary supplements. One study of 121 dietary supplements found that 5 percent contained arsenic above the threshold of safe levels, with the highest level more than two hundred times the allowable limit set by the US Food and Drug Administration.[50]

Let me be very clear: I am not opposed at all to dietary supplements. Multivitamins, vitamin C, vitamin D_3, omega-3s, probiotics—these are all useful, and I've taken them all.[51] You may have your own list of supplements that you've used for years that you swear are helpful. That's perfectly fine! But if you are going to start taking a new supplement, or if you have any doubts about the ones you're already taking, I recommend that you do your homework on the quality of the product and the manufacturer's reputation.

Be aware that successful supplement brands often are acquired by other companies, so a supplement that was a great product when you first discovered it might be under new ownership that isn't as concerned with quality and safety as the original company. When it comes to dietary supplements for weight loss or burning body fat, I have yet to be convinced that *any* supplements are better for your overall health than food.

The one exception may be probiotics, which can help restore an ailing gut microbiome. Antibiotic use is so rampant in modern society, through excessive prescribing by physicians as well as being used throughout the livestock, dairy, and aquaculture industries, that we need to be on guard to protect our gut microbiome.[52] Choosing fiber-containing foods is a good prebiotic approach to care for and feed our healthy gut bacteria. Most of us, however, don't regularly eat enough probiotic foods (fermented foods, yogurt, pickles) to nurture our gut health. That said, it is not clear which of the thousands of probiotics available on the market are the best.

So perhaps a better question is: "What are the supplements I should *not* take?"

This would be a long list.

Here's the deal: dietary supplements are not regulated with the same degree of rigor and scrutiny as pharmaceuticals. Because of this, the quality control of supplements can be highly variable. Poor oversight can lead to problems like accidental contamination by bacteria and fungus.[53]

I witnessed this problem firsthand when I accepted an invitation to take a private tour of a dietary supplement factory. It seemed sanitary, and the owner and his workers spoke about their work in a highly professional manner. We wore shoe covers and hairnets in the facility. As we walked to a huge machine packing capsules into plastic bottles, I asked about their quality control. Just as the tour guide was describing how the company had "the most rigorous standards of the industry," I saw a few full yet unsealed bottles fall off the assembly line and clatter onto the floor—whereupon an ungloved, unmasked technician picked them up and dusted them off on his pant leg before placing the bottles back on the line to be capped, boxed, and shipped to customers!

Supplements can also contain hidden and illicit ingredients, including pharmaceuticals deemed unsafe for use without a prescription. Libido-enhancing supplements sold online have been discovered to contain unapproved synthetic chemicals similar to the prescription drugs sildenafil (Viagra) and tadalafil (Cialis), which can have dangerous interactions with other medications.[54] Because there is no government verification of supplement ingredients, dodgy products are being sold without restraint. Unless problems are discovered by chance, disclosed by an informant, or sometimes revealed through a medical tragedy, no one bothers to check.

The bottom line: if you decide you want to use supplements, go with reputable supplement manufacturers, be skeptical of grandiose too-good-to-be-true marketing claims, and do your due diligence by searching online for information about the manufacturer. Try typing in the keywords "[manufacturer's name]" with "complaint" and "warning." You will quickly find out whether they have had problems in the past or are under investigation.

You can also check to see if clinical trials have been conducted and published on the supplement or the main ingredient. A good resource is the PubMed search engine of the National Library of Medicine (https:// pubmed.ncbi.nlm.nih.gov). Type in the "[name of the supplement]" and "clinical trial." If studies have been published, read the abstract to see if the supplement was found to be effective and if there were any side effects of concern. You can also search for clinical trials using www.clinicaltrials.gov, which is a global database of human studies.

Be especially wary of dietary supplements making wondrous claims about weight loss. Some of these products are outright dangerous and contain ingredients that you should avoid without exception. The trade names of the supplements can change, but you should always check the ingredient label to know what's inside.

The following are three of the most dangerous ingredients to avoid at all costs in weight-loss products:

DNP, or 2,4-Dinitrophenol. This chemical is found in products sold online to weightlifters, bodybuilders, and extreme dieters. DNP is an industrial chemical used for making explosives, pesticides, fertilizers, and fabric dyes. It was discovered to cause weight loss in the 1930s but was swiftly banned because of its toxicity, which includes hyperthermia, cardiac arrest, coma, and organ failure.[55] It is true that DNP can cause the mitochondria in your cells to ignite and burn calories more rapidly, but it does so in an uncontrollable fashion, similar to a nuclear meltdown like Chernobyl or Fukushima. Reports of deaths have come from abuse of products containing DNP.[56] The International Criminal Police Organization (INTERPOL) in association with the World Anti-Doping Agency has issued a global alert warning of its dangers. Stay away from DNP. It's a lethal chemical.

DMAA, or 1,3-dimethylamylamine. This synthetic amphetamine is used in some weight loss and sports nutrition cocktails and as an illegal doping agent for high-performance athletes. Another name for DMAA is methylhexanamine. It is prohibited to sell DMAA as a dietary supplement, but it can still be found in online products marketed for slimming and weight loss.[57] Sometimes, however, sneaky manufacturers disguise it by identifying DMAA as a natural stimulant from geranium extracts. In fact, the chemical is synthesized in a factory. The pharmaceutical company Eli Lilly originally created DMAA as a nasal decongestant drug in 1944 but then voluntarily withdrew it from the market in the 1980s due to its potentially lethal side effects.* DMAA is a stimulant and does have thermogenic properties, but its amphetamine-like effects can cause increased heart rate, palpitations, hypertension, seizures, and cardiac arrest.[58] The US Food and Drug Administration has issued a warning, and numerous countries have banned its use in consumer products. Be very careful about online weight-loss products that contain designer amphetamines. Read the ingredient label and be on the lookout for DMAA by any name.

Ephedra/ephedrine. This is a central nervous system stimulant derived from an herb (ma huang) that is used in traditional Chinese medicine. Ephedra has appeared in weight-loss products in combination with caffeine and other natural substances. The chemical does promote short-term weight loss, but due to its side effects—nausea, vomiting, and anxiety are the most common, but stroke, heart attack, arrhythmia,

---

* The original Eli Lilly drug was called Forthane.

brain hemorrhage, seizures, and death have also been reported—it is a banned ingredient in dietary supplements sold in the United States.[59]

If you do decide to take a dietary supplement, here are some tips:

1. **Do your research.** Make sure the manufacturer is legitimate and has no history of fraud, consumer complaints, or regulatory violations.
2. **Read the ingredient label.** You may think you are only getting one specific micronutrient, but dietary supplements are often formulated with many other substances you don't want or need, including some that could be outright harmful to your health.
3. **Don't take too many.** You do not want to risk overdosing on a dietary supplement any more than you want to risk overdosing on a prescription medicine. More is not necessarily better. Check the label for recommended daily dosing or look up the information online through a reputable source such as a government agency or academic medical center.
4. **Be skeptical of claims** that seem too good to be true. Supplements can support one or more health functions in your body, but they are far from miracle cures. Any marketing that suggests a supplement can achieve an unrealistic result is probably fraudulent.
5. **Don't mix supplements** together with prescription medicines in the same container because the tablets or capsules can look similar. To avoid the risk of a medication overdose, keep supplements and medicines in separate easily identifiable containers.

* * *

You have learned about the Eat to Beat Protocol and ways to conduct a metabolic tune-up, so you now have all the essential *knowledge* to fight fat and boost your health. You know what to eat, how to eat, when to eat, and not to eat too much. You've learned about the importance of quality sleep; staying physically active; managing stress; and putting foods first, before dietary supplements. Now it's time to make it a regular part of your life!

Put your newfound knowledge to work and eat to beat your diet. By taking action to improve your metabolism, you'll fight that excess body fat and elevate your health to the next level.

The best part?

You can love your food and love your metabolism!

S cience empowers us by revealing how we can live better lives. Making the best food choices we can allows us to harness our body's hardwired systems to strengthen our health, become more resistant to disease, and recover faster and better from illness. In my first book, *Eat to Beat Disease*, I shared how eating certain foods to activate your body's health defenses can keep at bay the dangers of cancer, heart disease, stroke, blindness, and arthritis—fates that you want to avoid. In this book, you've learned that you can use the latest scientific insights about food and your body to take charge of your metabolism.

The present state of your metabolism is not your fate. You can optimize your metabolism by controlling body fat as the means to get to your next level of health. Foods that feed and heal your metabolism can help you beat obesity, metabolic syndrome, diabetes, and a host of other chronic illnesses while simultaneously strengthening your health defenses. It's a winning situation across the board.

The scientific progress being made in the field of food as medicine is stunning because it keeps expanding our ability to direct our own health destiny. As the gate to these new scientific frontiers opens, we will continue to discover new paths that take us toward a brighter and healthier future. What's next? Beyond fighting disease and strengthening metabolism, the next great goal in human health is to overcome the aging process itself. We are now learning how using food as medicine can not only extend our life span but also keep us vibrant and youthful well into what was once considered old age.

Science tells us the best is yet to come. Stay tuned.

Acknowledgments

In the same way that your metabolism has many critical parts, many individuals have made vital contributions to this book. I could not have written *Eat to Beat Your Diet* without them. I'd like to express my appreciation and gratitude to my research team: Emily Yeo, Michelle Hutnik, Shruti Shertukde, and Delaney King Schurr. They were indefatigable in analyzing the hundreds of complex food and metabolism studies that I've described throughout *Eat to Beat Your Diet*. Emily was truly a standout contributor—she helped develop the different methodologies used to calculate the effective doses of foods from human metabolism studies so that I could present them as practical amounts that any reader can easily grasp. Others who contributed their expertise were Tiffany Chag and Dasha Agoulnik, who gave me key insights on nutrition, metabolism, and fitness; Robert N. Spengler III of the Max Planck Institute for the Science of Human History, who shared his knowledge on the foods that were exchanged on the ancient Silk Road; and Dr. Aaron Cypess of the US National Institutes of Health and Dr. Silvia Corvera of the UMass Chan Medical School, who gave me permission to use their research images and supplied me with additional scientific references on the biology and physiology of human adipose tissue—to these individuals, I am deeply grateful.

Because my work on food and health celebrates the joy of eating, I must thank my chef friends who shared their wisdom on how to approach and prepare ingredients that are important in the MediterAsian Way of cooking and eating: Regis Bourdon, Amanda Cohen, Nonie Favero, Sally Ling, Natalie Liu Spellman, Michael Pagliarini, and Michael Schlow. Special thanks go to Dana White and Tobi Amidor for their help with the recipes that I've included to inspire my readers.

I would like to thank Robin Colucci, Corey Powell, and John Maas. They were my editorial team—and instrumental in helping me refine my narrative and polish my prose. I'd like to acknowledge Diana Saville for her assistance with graphics and maps, and Courtney Martel and Sydney Mittiga for their hard work and attention to detail in curating the hundreds of scientific references that are cited.

Few authors are as fortunate as me to have a literary agent as phenomenal as Celeste Fine. She and her team at Park Fine Literary and Media gave me their incisive wisdom whenever I needed it throughout the book-writing process. I'd like to thank them for their support and invaluable guidance. I'd like to express my appreciation to Nana Twumasi, my editor at Hachette Book Group, and to Ike John Williams and Paul Sennott for their legal assistance. I'd also like to give special thanks to Costis Psychas and the staff at Perivolas in Oia, Santorini. They provided me with an actual writing cave in which I could finish writing this book in a truly inspirational and tranquil Mediterranean setting.

Finally, writing a book is a privilege with a cost. The privilege is being given the chance to share my knowledge and ideas with the world. The cost is that doing so takes precious time away from my family. To them, I'd like to express my heartfelt thanks for allowing me to spend not only the countless hours over invaluable years doing the research but also the many months of time away spent writing. Without their love and support, this book would not have been possible.

Notes

Chapter 1: The Surprising Science of Fat, Health, and Disease

1. M. A. Rupnick, D. Panigrahy, et al., "Adipose Tissue Mass Can Be Regulated Through the Vasculature," *Proceedings of the National Academy of Sciences USA* 99, no. 16 (2002): 10730–10735.
2. E. Bråkenhielm, R. Cao, et al., "Angiogenesis Inhibitor, TNP-470, Prevents Diet-Induced and Genetic Obesity in Mice," *Circulation Research* 94, no. 12 (2004): 1579–1588; K. F. Barnhart, D. R. Christianson, et al., "A Peptidomimetic Targeting White Fat Causes Weight Loss and Improved Insulin Resistance in Obese Monkeys," *Science Translational Medicine* 3, no. 108 (2011): 108–112.
3. Y. Cao and R. Cao, "Angiogenesis Inhibited by Drinking Tea," *Nature* 398 (1999): 381.
4. K. C. Maki, M. S. Reeves, et al., "Green Tea Catechin Consumption Enhances Exercise-Induced Abdominal Fat Loss in Overweight and Obese Adults," *Journal of Nutrition* 139, no. 2 (2009): 264–270; H. Wang, Y. Wen, et al., "Effects of Catechin Enriched Green Tea on Body Composition," *Obesity* 18, no. 4 (2010): 773–779.
5. J. Kwak and D. Shin, "Association Between Green Tea Consumption and Abdominal Obesity Risk in Middle-Aged Korean Population: Findings from the Korean Genome and Epidemiology Study," *International Journal of Environmental Research and Public Health* 19, no. 5 (2022): 2735.
6. A. Y. Lemoine, S. Ledoux, et al., "Link Between Adipose Tissue Angiogenesis and Fat Accumulation in Severely Obese Subjects," *Journal of Clinical Endocrinology and Metabolism* 97, no. 5 (2012): E775–E780.
7. M. E. T. Williams, M. A. Sahin, et al., "Matcha Green Tea Drinks Enhance Fat Oxidation During Brisk Walking in Females," *International Journal of Sport Nutrition and Exercise Metabolism* 28, no. 5 (2018): 536–541; F. Di Pierro, A. Bressan, et al., "Potential Role of Bioavailable Curcumin in Weight Loss and Omental Adipose Tissue Decrease: Preliminary Data of a Randomized, Controlled Trial in Overweight People with Metabolic Syndrome. Preliminary Study," *European Review for Medical and Pharmacological Sciences* 19, no. 21 (2015): 4195–4202; J. Tan, C. Huang, et al., "Soy Isoflavones Ameliorate Fatty Acid Metabolism of Visceral Adipose Tissue by Increasing the AMPK Activity in Male Rats with Diet-Induced Obesity (DIO)," *Molecules* 24, no. 15 (2019): 2809; H. Lee, M. Kim, et al., "Ginseng Treatment Reverses Obesity and Related Disorders by Inhibiting Angiogenesis in Female DB/DB Mice," *Journal of Ethnopharmacology* 155, no. 2 (2014): 1342–1352; Q. Li, J. Xia, et al., "Sulforaphane Inhibits Mammary Adipogenesis by Targeting Adipose Mesenchymal Stem Cells," *Breast Cancer Research and Treatment* 141, no. 2 (2013): 317–324; W. Cheng, H. Huang, et al., "Genistein Inhibits Angiogenesis Developed During Rheumatoid Arthritis Through the IL-6/JAK2/STAT3/VEGF Signalling Pathway," *Journal of Orthopaedic Translation* 22 (2019):

92–100; Y. Cao and R. Cao, "Angiogenesis Inhibited by Drinking Tea," *Nature* 398, no. 6726 (1999): 381; S. T. J. Jackson, K. W. Singletary, et al., "Sulforaphane Suppresses Angiogenesis and Disrupts Endothelial Mitotic Progression and Microtubule Polymerization," *Vascular Pharmacology* 46, no. 2 (2007): 77–84.

8. A. W. Lee, T. L. Cheng, et al., "Ursolic Acid Induces Allograft Inflammatory Factor-1 Expression via a Nitric Oxide-Related Mechanism and Increases Neovascularization," *Journal of Agricultural and Food Chemistry* 58, no. 24 (2010): 12941–12949; V. Casieri, M. Matteucci, et al., "Long-Term Intake of Pasta Containing Barley (1-3) Beta-D-Glucan Increases Neovascularization-Mediated Cardioprotection Through Endothelial Upregulation of Vascular Endothelial Growth Factor and Parkin," *Scientific Reports* 7, no. 1 (2017): 13424; J. Chen, M. Jayachandran, et al., "Sea Bass (*Lateolabrax maculatus*) Accelerates Wound Healing: A Transition from Inflammation to Proliferation," *Journal of Ethnopharmacology* 236 (2019): 263–276.

9. C. Hepler, L. Vishvanath, et al., "Sorting Out Adipocyte Precursors and Their Role in Physiology and Disease," *Genes and Development* 31, no. 2 (2017): 127–140.

10. S. S. Moghe, S. Juma, et al., "Effect of Blueberry Polyphenols on 3T3-F442A Preadipocyte Differentiation," *Journal of Medicinal Food* 15, no. 5 (2012): 448–452; X. Xu, W. Chen, et al., "Inhibition of Preadipocyte Differentiation by *Lycium barbarum* Polysaccharide Treatment in 3T3-L1 Cultures," *Electronic Journal of Biotechnology* 50 (2021): 53–58; L. Y. Wu, C. W. Chen, et al., "Curcumin Attenuates Adipogenesis by Inducing Preadipocyte Apoptosis and Inhibiting Adipocyte Differentiation," *Nutrients* 11, no. 10 (2019): 2307.

11. A. A. Qayyum, A. B. Mathiasen, et al., "Autologous Adipose-Derived Stromal Cell Treatment for Patients with Refractory Angina (MyStromalCell Trial): 3-Years Follow-up Results," *Journal of Translational Medicine* 17, no. 360 (2019); K. Shigematsu, N. Komori, et al., "Repeated Infusion of Autologous Adipose Tissue-Derived Stem Cells for Parkinson's Disease," *Acta Neurologica Scandinavica* 145 (2022): 119–122.

12. M. Bydon, A. B. Dietz, et al., "CELLTOP Clinical Trial: First Report from a Phase 1 Trial of Autologous Adipose Tissue-Derived Mesenchymal Stem Cells in the Treatment of Paralysis Due to Traumatic Spinal Cord Injury," *Mayo Clinic Proceedings* 95, no. 2 (2020): 406–414.

13. H. Lin, E. D. Stanchina, et al., "Maitake Beta-Glucan Enhances Umbilical Cord Blood Stem Cell Transplantation in the NOD/SCID Mouse," *Experimental Biology and Medicine* 234, no. 3 (2009): 342–353; N. P. Fusté, M. Guasch, et al., "Barley β-Glucan Accelerates Wound Healing by Favoring Migration versus Proliferation of Human Dermal Fibroblasts," *Carbohydrate Polymers* 210 (2019): 389–398; V. Spigoni, C. Lombardi, et al., "N-3 PUFA Increase Bioavailability and Function of Endothelial Progenitor Cells," *Food and Function* 5, no. 8 (2014): 1881–1890; C. Heiss, S. Jahn, et al., "Improvement of Endothelial Function with Dietary Flavanols Is Associated with Mobilization of Circulating Angiogenic Cells in Patients with Coronary Artery Disease," *Journal of the American College of Cardiology* 56, no. 3 (2010): 218–224; I. Spyridopoulos, S. Fichtlscherer, et al., "Caffeine Enhances Endothelial Repair by an AMPK-Dependent Mechanism," *Arteriosclerosis, Thrombosis, and Vascular Biology* 28, no. 11 (2008): 1967–1974; W. Kim, M. H. Jeong, et al., "Effect of Green Tea Consumption on Endothelial Function and Circulating Endothelial Progenitor Cells in Chronic Smokers," *Circulation* 70, no. 8 (2006): 1052–1057; D. Grassi, R. Draijer, et al., "Black Tea Increases Circulating Endothelial Progenitor Cells and Improves Flow Mediated

Dilatation Counteracting Deleterious Effects from a Fat Load in Hypertensive Patients: A Randomized Controlled Study," *Nutrients* 8, no. 11 (2016): 727.

14. J. Mao, D. Wang, et al., "Gut Microbiome Is Associated with the Clinical Response to Anti-PD-1 Based Immunotherapy in Hepatobiliary Cancers," *Journal of Immunotherapy Cancer* 9 (2021): e003334.

15. P. J. Turnbaugh, M. Hamady, et al., "A Core Gut Microbiome in Obese and Lean Twins," *Nature* 457, no. 7228 (2009): 480–484.

16. H. Wein, "Gut Microbiomes Differ Between Obese and Lean People," NIH Research Matter, *National Institutes of Health*, December 8, 2008, https://www.nih.gov/news -events/nih-research-matters/gut-microbiomes-differ-between-obese-lean-people.

17. Y. Xu, N. Wang, et al., "Function of *Akkermansia muciniphila* in Obesity: Interactions with Lipid Metabolism, Immune Response and Gut Systems," *Frontiers in Microbiology* 11, no. 219 (2020).

18. M. C. Dao, A. Everard, et al., "Akkermansia Muciniphila and Improved Metabolic Health During a Dietary Intervention in Obesity: Relationship with Gut Microbiome Richness and Ecology," *Gut* 65 (2016): 426–436.

19. B. Routy, E. L. Chatelier, et al., "Gut Microbiome Influences Efficacy of PD-1-Based Immunotherapy Against Epithelial Tumors," *Science* 359, no. 6371 (2018): 91–97.

20. A. Fernández-Sánchez, E. Madrigal-Santillán, et al., "Inflammation, Oxidative Stress, and Obesity," *International Journal of Molecular Sciences* 12, no. 5 (2011): 3117–3132; C. Cerdá, C. Sánchez, et al., "Oxidative Stress and DNA Damage in Obesity-Related Tumorigenesis," *Advances in Experimental Medicine and Biology* 824 (2014): 5–17.

21. K. J. Royston and T. O. Tollefsbol, "The Epigenetic Impact of Cruciferous Vegetables on Cancer Prevention," *Current Pharmacology Reports* 1, no. 1 (2015): 46–51; S. Karsli-Ceppioglu, M. Ngollo, et al., "The Role of Soy Phytoestrogens on Genetic and Epigenetic Mechanisms of Prostate Cancer," *Enzymes* 37 (2015): 193–221.

22. K. Kvaløy, C. M. Page, et al., "Epigenome-wide Methylation Differences in a Group of Lean and Obese Women—A HUNT Study," *Scientific Reports* 8, no. 16330 (2018): 1–9.

23. C. Gallardo-Escribano, V. Buonaiuto, et al., "Epigenetic Approach in Obesity: DNA Methylation in a Prepubertal Population Which Underwent a Lifestyle Modification," *Clinical Epigenetics* 12, no. 144 (2020): 1–14.

24. M. C. Azcona-Sanjulian, "Telomere Length and Pediatric Obesity: A Review," *Genes* 12, no. 6 (2021): 946; D. B. P. Clemente, L. Maitre, et al., "Obesity Is Associated with Shorter Telomeres in 8-Year-Old Children," *Scientific Reports* 9, no. 18739 (2019): 1–8.

25. O. T. Njajou, R. M. Cawthon, et al., "Shorter Telomeres Are Associated with Obesity and Weight Gain in the Elderly," *International Journal of Obesity* 36, no. 9 (2012): 1176–1179.

26. J. Folkman and R. Kalluri, "Cancer Without Disease," *Nature* 427, no. 6977 (2004): 787.

27. P.-A. Dugué, M. Rebolj, et al., "Immunosuppression and Risk of Cervical Cancer," *Expert Review of Anticancer Therapy* 13, no. 1 (2013): 29–42; R. J. Biggar, A. K. Chaturvedi, et al., "AIDS-Related Cancer and Severity of Immunosuppression in Persons with AIDS," *Journal of the National Cancer Institute* 99, no. 12 (2007): 962–972; M. Taborelli, P. Piselli, et al., "Risk of Virus and Non-Virus-Related Malignancies Following Immunosuppression in a Cohort of Liver Transplant Recipients. Italy, 1985–2014," *International Journal of Cancer* 143, no. 7 (2018): 1588–1594.

28. R. Liu and B. S. Nikolajczyk, "Tissue Immune Cells Fuel Obesity-Associated Inflammation in Adipose Tissue and Beyond," *Frontiers in Immunology* 10, no. 1587 (2019): 1–16.

29. A. D. Ruggiero, C.-C. Chuang Key, et al., "Adipose Tissue Macrophage Polarization in Healthy and Unhealthy Obesity," *Frontiers in Immunology* 8, no. 625331 (2021): 1–14.

30. S. P. Weisberg, D. McCann, et al., "Obesity Is Associated with Macrophage Accumulation in Adipose Tissue," *Journal of Clinical Investigation* 112, no. 12 (2003): 1796–1808.

31. T. Worth, "Why Are Obese People More Vulnerable to COVID?" *Nature Portfolio*, June 24, 2021, doi:https://doi.org/10.1038/d42859-021-00051-w.

32. R. Cancello, C. Henegar, et al., "Reduction of Macrophage Infiltration and Chemoattractant Gene Expression Changes in White Adipose Tissue of Morbidly Obese Subjects After Surgery-Induced Weight Loss," *Diabetes* 54, no. 8 (2005): 2277–2286.

33. J. J. Milner and M. A. Beck, "The Impact of Obesity on the Immune Response to Infection," *Proceedings of the Nutrition Society* 71, no. 2 (2012): 298–306.

34. S. Kwok, S. Adam, et al., "Obesity: A Critical Risk Factor in the COVID-19 Pandemic," *Clinical Obesity* 10, no. 6 (2020): e12403.

35. R. Yu, J. W. Park, et al., "Modulation of Select Immune Responses by Dietary Capsaicin," *International Journal for Vitamin and Nutrition Research* 68, no. 2 (1998): 114–119.

36. T. Ohishi, S. Goto, et al., "Anti-inflammatory Action of Green Tea," *Anti-Inflammatory and Anti-Allergy Agents in Medicinal Chemistry* 15, no. 2 (2016): 74–90; B. O. Rennard, R. F. Ertl, et al., "Chicken Soup Inhibits Neutrophil Chemotaxis in Vitro," *Chest* 118, no. 4 (2000): 1150–1157.

37. N. M. Iyengar, K. A. Brown, et al., "Metabolic Obesity, Adipose Inflammation and Elevated Breast Aromatase in Women with Normal Body Mass Index," *Cancer Prevention Research* 10, no. 4 (2017): 235–243.

38. M. J. Gunter, D. R. Hoover, et al., "Insulin, Insulin-Like Growth Factor-I, and Risk of Breast Cancer in Postmenopausal Women," *Journal of the National Cancer Institute* 101, no. 1 (2009): 48–60.

39. T. Tsujimoto, H. Kajio, et al., "Association Between Hyperinsulinemia and Increased Risk of Cancer Death in Nonobese and Obese People: A Population-Based Observational Study," *International Journal of Cancer* 141, no. 1 (2017): 102–111.

40. E. J. Gallagher and D. LeRoith, "The Proliferating Role of Insulin and Insulin-Like Growth Factors in Cancer," *Trends in Endocrinology and Metabolism* 21, no. 10 (2010): 610–618.

41. Y. Wu, S. Yakar, et al., "Circulating Insulin-Like Growth Factor-I Levels Regulate Colon Cancer Growth and Metastasis," *Cancer Research* 62, no. 4 (2002): 1030–1035.

42. A. Szczeklik and Z. Podolec, "Central Regulation of Blood Eosinophilia by the Beta-Adrenergic System in Rats," *International Archives of Allergy and Applied Immunology* 50, no. 3 (1976): 328–340.

43. A. Gucalp, N. M. Iyengar, et al., "Periprostatic Adipose Inflammation Is Associated with High-Grade Prostate Cancer," *Prostate Cancer and Prostatic Diseases* 20, no. 4 (2017): 418–423.

44. GBD 2019 Cancer Risk Factor Collaborators, "The Global Risk of Cancer Attributable to Risk Factors, 2010–2019: A Systematic Analysis for the Global Burden of Disease Study 2019," *Lancet* 400 (2022): 563–591.

45. M. Esler, N. Straznicky, et al., "Mechanisms of Sympathetic Activation in Obesity-Related Hypertension," *Hypertension* 48, no. 5 (2006): 787–796.

46. M. C. Foster, S. J. Hwang, et al., "Fatty Kidney, Hypertension, and Chronic Kidney Disease: The Framingham Heart Study," *Hypertension* 58 (2011): 784–790.

47. J. B. Meigs, P. W. F. Wilson, et al., "Body Mass Index, Metabolic Syndrome, and Risk of Type 2 Diabetes or Cardiovascular Disease," *Journal of Clinical Endocrinology and Metabolism* 91, no. 8 (2006): 2906–2912.

48. A. Romero-Corral, F. H. Sert-Kuniyoshi, et al., "Modest Visceral Fat Gain Causes Endothelial Dysfunction in Healthy Humans," *Journal of the American College of Cardiology* 56, no. 8 (2010): 662–666.

49. G. Giannotti, C. Doerries, et al., "Impaired Endothelial Repair Capacity of Early Endothelial Progenitor Cells in Prehypertension: Relation to Endothelial Dysfunction," *Hypertension* 55, no. 6 (2010): 1389–1397.

50. M. Pirro, F. Bagaglia, et al., "Hypercholesterolemia-Associated Endothelial Progenitor Cell Dysfunction," *Therapeutic Advances in Cardiovascular Disease* 2, no. 5 (2008): 329–339.

51. U. Ozcan, Q. Cao, et al., "Endoplasmic Reticulum Stress Links Obesity, Insulin Action, and Type 2 Diabetes," *Science* 306, no. 5695 (2004): 457–461.

52. J. Yong, J. D. Johnson, et al., "Therapeutic Opportunities for Pancreatic β-cell ER Stress in Diabetes Mellitus," *Nature Reviews Endocrinology* 17 (2021): 455–467.

53. A. M. George, A. G. Jacob, et al., "Lean Diabetes Mellitus: An Emerging Entity in the Era of Obesity," *World Journal of Diabetes* 6, no. 4 (2015): 613–620.

54. C. Ding, Z. Chan, et al., "Visceral Adipose Tissue Tracks More Closely with Metabolic Dysfunction Than Intrahepatic Triglyceride in Lean Asians Without Diabetes," *Journal of Applied Physiology* 125, no. 3 (2018): 909–915.

55. V. Mohan and R. Vijayaprabha, "Clinical Profile of Lean NIDDM in South India," *Diabetes Research and Clinical Practice* 38, no. 2 (1997): 101–108.

56. B. Hartmann, S. Lanzinger, et al., "Lean Diabetes in Middle-Aged Adults: A Joint Analysis of the German DIVE and DPV Registries," *PloS One* 12, no. 8 (2017): 1–14.

57. M. Hamer and G. D. Batty, "Association of Body Mass Index and Waist-to-Hip Ratio with Brain Structure: UK Biobank Study," *Neurology* 92, no. 6 (2019): e594–e600.

58. M. I. Tolea, S. Chrisphonte, et al., "Sarcopenic Obesity and Cognitive Performance," *Clinical Interventions in Aging* 13 (2018): 1111–1119.

59. O. Ntlholang, K. McCarroll, et al., "The Relationship Between Adiposity and Cognitive Function in a Large Community-Dwelling Population: Data from the Trinity Ulster Department of Agriculture (TUDA) Ageing Cohort Study," *British Journal of Nutrition* 120, no. 5 (2018): 517–527.

60. S. S. Anand, M. G. Friedrich, et al., "Evaluation of Adiposity and Cognitive Function in Adults," *JAMA Network Open* 5, no. 2 (2022): 1–16.

61. S. S. Anand, M. G. Friedrich, et al., "Reduced Cognitive Assessment Scores Among Individuals with Magnetic Resonance Imaging-Detected Vascular Brain Injury," *Stroke* 51, no. 4 (2020): 1158–1165.

62. A. A. Miller and S. J. Spencer, "Obesity and Neuroinflammation: A Pathway to Cognitive Impairment," *Brain, Behavior, and Immunity* 42 (2014): 10–21.

63. A. E. Dixon and U. Peters, "The Effect of Obesity on Lung Function," *Expert Review of Respiratory Medicine* 12, no. 9 (2018): 755–767.

64. R. L. Jones and M.-M. U. Nzekwu, "The Effects of Body Mass Index on Lung Volumes," *Chest* 130, no. 3 (2006): 827–833.

65. J. G. Elliot, G. M. Donovan, et al., "Fatty Airways: Implications for Obstructive Disease," *European Respiratory Journal* 54, no. 6 (2019): 1–10.

66. Y. Yeghiazarians, H. Jneid, et al., "Obstructive Sleep Apnea and Cardiovascular Disease: A Scientific Statement from the American Heart Association," *Circulation* 144, no. 3 (2021): e56–e67.

67. N. Nashi, S. Kang, et al., "Lingual Fat at Autopsy," *Laryngoscope* 117, no. 8 (2007): 1467–1473.

68. A. M. Kim, B. T. Keenan, et al., "Tongue Fat and Its Relationship to Obstructive Sleep Apnea," *Sleep* 37, no. 10 (2014): 1639–1648.

69. T. D. Bradley and J. S. Floras, "Sleep Apnea and Heart Failure: Part I: Obstructive Sleep Apnea," *Circulation* 107, no. 12 (2003): 1671–1678.

70. T. Young, L. Finn, et al., "Sleep Disordered Breathing and Mortality: Eighteen-Year Follow-up of the Wisconsin Sleep Cohort," *Sleep* 31, no. 8 (2008): 1071–1078.

71. S. Pamidi, K. Wroblewski, et al., "Obstructive Sleep Apnea in Young Lean Men: Impact on Insulin Sensitivity and Secretion," *Diabetes Care* 35, no. 11 (2012): 2384–2389.

72. K. A. Franklin, C. Sahlin, et al., "Sleep Apnoea Is a Common Occurrence in Females," *European Respiratory Journal* 41, no. 3 (2013): 610–615.

73. S. Ryan, C. Arnaud, et al., "Adipose Tissue as a Key Player in Obstructive Sleep Apnoea," *European Respiratory Review: An Official Journal of the European Respiratory Society* 28, no. 152 (2019): 1–11.

74. S. H. Wang, B. T. Keenan, et al., "Effect of Weight Loss on Upper Airway Anatomy and the Apnea-Hypopnea Index. The Importance of Tongue Fat," *American Journal of Respiratory and Critical Care Medicine* 201, no. 6 (2020): 718–727.

75. W. Sawadogo, M. Tsegaye, et al., "Overweight and Obesity as Risk Factors for COVID-19-Associated Hospitalisations and Death: Systematic Review and Meta-Analysis," *BMJ Nutrition, Prevention and Health* 5, no. 1 (2022): 1–9.

76. G. J. Martínez-Colón, K. Ratnasiri, et al., "SARS-CoV-2 Infects Human Adipose Tissue and Elicits an Inflammatory Response Consistent with Severe COVID-19," *BioRxiv* 2021.10.24.465626; M. Reiterer, M. Rajan, et al., "Hyperglycemia in Acute COVID-19 Is Characterized by Insulin Resistance and Adipose Tissue Infectivity by SARS-CoV-2," *Cell Metabolism* 33, no. 11 (2021): 2174–2188.

77. D. Frasca and B. B. Blomberg, "Obesity Accelerates Age Defects in Mouse and Human B Cells," *Frontiers in Immunology* 11, no. 2060 (2020): 1–7; D. Frasca, F. Ferracci, et al., "Obesity Decreases B Cell Responses in Young and Elderly Individuals," *Obesity* 24, no. 3 (2016): 615–625; D. Frasca, L. Reidy, et al., "Influence of Obesity on Serum Levels of SARS-Cov-2-Specific Antibodies in COVID-19 Patients," *PloS One* 16, no. 3 (2021): 1–16.

78. M. Ackermann, S. E. Verleden, et al., "Pulmonary Vascular Endothelialitis, Thrombosis, and Angiogenesis in Covid-19," *New England Journal of Medicine* 383, no. 2 (2020): 120–128.

79. A. Virdis, "Endothelial Dysfunction in Obesity: Role of Inflammation," *High Blood Pressure and Cardiovascular Prevention* 23, no. 2 (2016): 83–85.

80. American Friends of Tel Aviv University, "Obesity Plays Major Role in Triggering Autoimmune Diseases," *ScienceDaily*, November 10, 2014, www.sciencedaily.com /releases/2014/11/141110110722.htm.

81. L. Vimercati, L. De Maria, et al., "Association Between Long COVID and Overweight/ Obesity," *Journal of Clinical Medicine* 10, no. 4143 (2021): 1–8.

82. S. G. Wannamethee, A. G. Shaper, et al., "Reasons for Intentional Weight Loss, Unintentional Weight Loss, and Mortality in Older Men," *Archives of Internal Medicine* 165, no. 9 (2005): 1035–1040.

83. J. E. Neter, B. E. Stam, et al., "Influence of Weight Reduction on Blood Pressure: A Meta-Analysis of Randomized Controlled Trials," *Hypertension* 42, no. 5 (2003): 878–884.

84. D. Ettehad, C. A. Emdin, et al., "Blood Pressure Lowering for Prevention of Cardiovascular Disease and Death: A Systematic Review and Meta-Analysis," *Lancet* 387, no. 10022:957–967.

85. L. R. Teras, A. V. Patel, et al., "Sustained Weight Loss and Risk of Breast Cancer in Women 50 Years and Older: A Pooled Analysis of Prospective Data," *Journal of the National Cancer Institute* 112, no. 9 (2020): 929–937.

86. "Obesity, Weight Gain, and Cancer Risk," *World Cancer Research Fund International*, www.wcrf.org/diet-activity-and-cancer/risk-factors/obesity-weight-gain-and-cancer/.

87. J. Luo, R. T. Chlebowski, et al., "Intentional Weight Loss and Endometrial Cancer Risk," *Journal of Clinical Oncology* 35, no. 11 (2017): 1189–1193.

88. J. D. Wright, "Preventing Endometrial Cancer: Weighing the Evidence," *Journal of Clinical Oncology* 35, no. 11 (2017): 1149–1150.

89. N. R. Cook, L. J. Appel, et al., "Weight Change and Mortality: Long-Term Results from the Trials of Hypertension Prevention," *Journal of Clinical Hypertension* 20, no. 12 (2018): 1666–1673.

90. S. B. Kritchevsky, K. M. Beavers, et al., "Intentional Weight Loss and All-Cause Mortality: A Meta-Analysis of Randomized Clinical Trials," *PloS One* 10, no. 3 (2015): 1–25.

91. A. Sasaki, N. Horiuchi, et al., "Mortality and Causes of Death in Type 2 Diabetic Patients. A Long-Term Follow-up Study in Osaka District, Japan," *Diabetes Research and Clinical Practice* 7, no. 1 (1989): 33–40; M. Zhu, J. Li, et al., "Mortality Rates and the Causes of Death Related to Diabetes Mellitus in Shanghai Songjiang District: An 11-Year Retrospective Analysis of Death Certificates," *BMC Endocrine Disorders* 15, no. 45 (2015): 1–8.

Chapter 2: Rethinking Body Fat

1. Gene Kim and Benji Jones, "Sumo Wrestlers Eat Up to 7,000 Calories a Day, Yet They Aren't Unhealthy," *Business Insider*, December 12, 2020, www.businessinsider.com /sumo-wrestlers-obesity-diet-calories-exercise-symptoms-2019-3.

2. "Underweight Associated with Highest Mortality and Costs After Cardiac Catheterisation," *European Society of Cardiology*, August 26, 2017, www.escardio.org/The-ESC /Press-Office/Press-releases/Underweight-associated-with-highest-mortality-and -costs-after-cardiac-catheterisation.

3. L. M. Rossow, D. H. Fukuda, et al., "Natural Bodybuilding Competition Preparation and Recovery: A 12-Month Case Study," *International Journal of Sports Physiology and Performance* 8, no. 5 (2013): 582–592.

4. K. E. Friedl, R. J. Moore, et al., "Lower Limit of Body Fat in Healthy Active Men," *Journal of Applied Physiology* 77, no. 2 (1994): 933–940.

5. S. Cao, R. Moineddin, et al., "J-shapedness: An Often Missed, Often Miscalculated Relation: The Example of Weight and Mortality," *Journal of Epidemiology and Community Health* 68, no. 7 (2014): 683–690.

6. A. Caliebe, A. Nebel, et al., "Insights into Early Pig Domestication Provided by Ancient DNA Analysis," *Scientific Reports* 7 (2017): 44550.

7. V. Di Nicola, "Omentum a Powerful Biological Source in Regenerative Surgery," *Regenerative Therapy* 11 (2019): 182–191.

8. C. Naylor and W. A. Petri Jr., "Leptin Regulation of Immune Responses," *Trends in Molecular Medicine* 22, no. 2 (2016): 88–98.

9. P. Fernández-Riejos, S. Najob, et al., "Role of Leptin in the Activation of Immune Cells," *Mediators of Inflammation* (2010): 568343.

10. Z. Tahergorabi and M. Khazaei, "Leptin and Its Cardiovascular Effects: Focus on Angiogenesis," *Advances in Biomedical Research* 4 (2015): 79.

11. W. Lieb, L. M. Sullivan, et al., "Relation of Serum Leptin with Cardiac Mass and Left Atrial Dimension in Individuals >70 Years of Age," *American Journal of Cardiology* 104, no. 4 (2009): 602–605.

12. D. H. Kim, C. Kim, et al., "Adiponectin Levels and the Risk of Hypertension: A Systematic Review and Meta-Analysis," *Hypertension* 62, no. 1 (2013): 27–32.

13. N. Ouchi and Kenneth Walsh, "Adiponectin as an Anti-Inflammatory Factor," *Clinica Chimica Acta* 380 (2007): 24–30.

14. K. Ohashi, N. Ouchi, et al., "Anti-Inflammatory and Anti-Atherogenic Properties of Adiponectin," *Biochimie* 94, no. 10 (2012): 2137–2142.

15. N. Ouchi, H. Kobayashi, et al., "Adiponectin Stimulates Angiogenesis by Promoting Cross-Talk Between AMP-Activated Protein Kinase and Akt Signaling in Endothelial Cells," *Journal of Biological Chemistry* 279, no. 2 (2004): 1304–1309.

16. K. Shimada, T. Miyazaki, et al., "Adiponectin and Atherosclerotic Disease," *Clinica Chimica Acta* 344 (2004): 1–12.

17. S. A. Robertson, C. J. Rae, et al., "Induction of Angiogenesis by Murine Resistin: Putative Role of PI3-Kinase and NO-Dependent Pathways," *Regulatory Peptides* 152 (2009): 41–47.

18. Y. He, Y. Guo, et al., "Resistin Promotes Cardiac Homing of Mesenchymal Stem Cells and Functional Recovery After Myocardial Ischemia-Reperfusion via the ERK1/2-MMP-9 Pathway," *American Journal of Physiology–Heart and Circulatory Physiology* 316, no. 1 (2019): H233–H244.

19. K. Gessner, Conradi Gesneri medici tigurine historiae animalium lib, *I de Quadrupedibus viviparis* (1551), 842, 1.6–9.

20. W. Arnold, "Social Thermoregulation During Hibernation in Alpine Marmots (Marmota marmota)," *Journal of Comparative Physiology. B, Biochemical, Systemic, and Environmental Physiology* 158, no. 2 (1988): 151–156.

21. A. T. Rasmussen, "The So-Called Hibernating Gland," *Journal of Morphology* 38 (1923): 147–205.

22. R. E. Smith, "Thermogenic Activity of the Hibernating Gland in the Cold-Acclimated Rat," *Physiologist* 4, no. 113 (1961): 187–196.

23. W. Aherne and D. Hull, "Brown Adipose Tissue and Heat Production in the Newborn Infant," *Journal of Pathology and Bacteriology* 91, no. 1 (1966): 223–234.

24. C. M. Poissonnet, A. R. Burdi, et al., "Growth and Development of Human Adipose Tissue During Early Gestation," *Early Human Development* 8, no. 1 (1983): 1–11.

25. X.-L. Cao, W. Zhao, et al., "Di-(2-ethylhexyl) Adipate and 20 Phthalates in Composite Food Samples from the 2013 Canadian Total Diet Study," *Food Additives and Contaminants. Part A, Chemistry, Analysis, Control, Exposure and Risk Assessment* 32, no. 11 (2015): 1893–1901.

26. L. Edwards and N. L. McCray, "Phthalate and Novel Plasticizer Concentrations in Food Items from U.S. Fast Food Chains: A Preliminary Analysis," *Journal of Exposure Science and Environmental Epidemiology* 32 (2022): 366–373.

27. R. da Silva Costa, T. S. M. Fernandes, et al., "Potential Risk of BPA and Phthalates in Commercial Water Bottles: A Minireview," *Journal of Water and Health* 19, no. 3 (2021): 411–435.

28. H. Gao, Y-F. Yang, et al., "Prenatal Phthalate Exposure Associated with Age-Specific Alterations in Markers of Adiposity in Offspring: A Systematic Review," *Ecotoxicology and Environmental Safety* 232 (2022): 1–11.

29. C. G. Brook, "Fat in the Newborn," *Archives of Disease in Childhood* 54, no. 11 (1979): 845–848.

30. S. J. Fomon, F. Haschke, et al., "Body Composition of Reference Children from Birth to Age 10 Years," *American Journal of Clinical Nutrition* 35 (1982): 1169–1175.

31. W. Shen, M. Punyanitya, et al., "Sexual Dimorphism of Adipose Tissue Distribution Across the Lifespan: A Cross-Sectional Whole-Body Magnetic Resonance Imaging Study," *Nutrition and Metabolism* 6, no. 17 (2009): 1–9.

32. B. P. Leitner, S. Huang, et al., "Mapping of Human Brown Adipose Tissue in Lean and Obese Young Men," *Proceedings of the National Academy of Sciences U.S.A.* 114, no. 32 (2017): 8649–8654.

33. R. J. F. Loos and G. S. H. Yeo, "The Bigger Picture of FTO: The First GWAS-Identified Obesity Gene," *Nature Reviews Endocrinology* 10, no. 1 (2014): 51–61.

34. N. Lan, Y. Lu, et al., "FTO—A Common Genetic Basis for Obesity and Cancer," *Frontiers in Genetics* 11, no. 559138 (2020): 1–12.

35. S. J. Melhorn, M. K. Askren, et al., "FTO Genotype Impacts Food Intake and Corticolimbic Activation," *American Journal of Clinical Nutrition* 107, no. 2 (2018): 145–154.

36. T. M. Frayling, N. J. Timpson, et al., "A Common Variant in the FTO Gene Is Associated with Body Mass Index and Predisposes to Childhood and Adult Obesity," *Science* 316, no. 5826 (2007): 889–894.

37. T. O. Kilpeläinen, L. Qi, et al., "Physical Activity Attenuates the Influence of FTO Variants on Obesity Risk: A Meta-Analysis of 218,166 Adults and 19,268 Children," *PLoS Medicine* 8, no. 11 (2011): e1001116.

38. K. M. Livingstone, C. Celis-Morales, et al., "FTO Genotype and Weight Loss: Systematic Review and Meta-Analysis of 9563 Individual Participant Data from Eight Randomised Controlled Trials," *British Medical Journal* 354, no. i4707 (2016).

39. A. C. P. da Fonseca, C. Mastronardi, et al., "Genetics of Non-Syndromic Childhood Obesity and the Use of High-Throughput DNA Sequencing Technologies," *Journal of Diabetes and Its Complications* 31, no. 10 (2017): 1549–1561; I. S. Farooqi and S. O'Rahilly, "Recent Advances in the Genetics of Severe Childhood Obesity," *Archives of Disease in Childhood* 83, no. 1 (2000): 31–34.

40. K. A. Irizarry and A. M. Haqq, "Syndromic Obesity," in *Pediatric Obesity*, ed. M. Freemark (New York: Humana, 2018), 153–182.

41. A. V. Khera, M. Chaffin, et al., "Polygenic Prediction of Weight and Obesity Trajectories from Birth to Adulthood," *Cell* 177, no. 3 (2019): 587–596.

42. D. Mozaffarian, T. Hao, et al,. "Changes in Diet and Lifestyle and Long-Term Weight Gain in Women and Men," *New England Journal of Medicine* 364, no. 25 (2011): 2392–2404; E. M. Taveras, C. S. Berkey, et al., "Association of Consumption of Fried Food

Away from Home with Body Mass Index and Diet Quality in Older Children and Adolescents," *Pediatrics* 116, no. 4 (2005): e518–e24; P. Guallar-Castillón, F. Rodríguez-Artalejo, et al., "Intake of Fried Foods Is Associated with Obesity in the Cohort of Spanish Adults from the European Prospective Investigation into Cancer and Nutrition," *American Journal of Clinical Nutrition* 86, no. 1 (2007): 198–205.

43. Q. Qi, A. Y. Chu, et al., "Fried Food Consumption, Genetic Risk, and Body Mass Index: Gene-Diet Interaction Analysis in Three US Cohort Studies," *British Medical Journal* 248 (2014): 1–12.

44. Q. Qi, A. Y. Chu, et al., "Sugar-Sweetened Beverages and Genetic Risk of Obesity," *New England Journal of Medicine* 367, no. 15 (2012): 1387–1396.

45. M. R. Lowe, M. L. Butryn, et al., "The Power of Food Scale. A New Measure of the Psychological Influence of the Food Environment," *Appetite* 53 (2009): 114–118.

46. L. Sominsky and S. J. Spencer, "Eating Behavior and Stress: A Pathway to Obesity," *Frontiers in Psychology* 5, no. 434 (2014): 1–8; E. Robinson, P. Aveyard, et al., "Eating Attentively: A Systematic Review and Meta-Analysis of the Effect of Food Intake Memory and Awareness on Eating," *American Journal of Clinical Nutrition* 97, no. 4 (2013): 728–742; D. Ferriday, M. L. Bosworth, et al., "Effects of Eating Rate on Satiety: A Role for Episodic Memory?" *Physiology and Behavior* 152 (2015): 389–396.

47. B. S. Samuel, A. Shaito, et al., "Effects of the Gut Microbiota on Host Adiposity Are Modulated by the Short-Chain Fatty-Acid Binding G Protein-Coupled Receptor, Gpr41," *Proceedings of the National Academy of Sciences of the United States of America* 105, no. 43 (2008): 16767–16772.

48. X.-L. Cao, W. Zhao, et al., "Di-(2-ethylhexyl) Adipate and 20 Phthalates in Composite Food Samples from the 2013 Canadian Total Diet Study," *Food Additives and Contaminants. Part A, Chemistry, Analysis, Control, Exposure and Risk Assessment* 32, no. 11 (2015): 1893–1901.

49. R. Kursawe, V. D. Dixit, et al., "A Role of the Inflammasome in the Low Storage Capacity of the Abdominal Subcutaneous Adipose Tissue in Obese Adolescents," *Diabetes* 65, no. 3 (2016): 610–618.

50. D. Q. Huang, H. B. El-Serag, et al., "Global Epidemiology of NAFLD-Related HCC: Trends, Predictions, Risk Factors and Prevention," *Nature Reviews Gastroenterology and Hepatology* 18, no. 4 (2021): 223–238.

51. B. Vandanmagsar, Y.-H. Youm, et al., "The NLRP3 Inflammasome Instigates Obesity-Induced Inflammation and Insulin Resistance," *Nature Medicine* 17, no. 2 (2011): 179–188.

52. H. Cui, M. López, et al., "The Cellular and Molecular Basis of Leptin and Ghrelin Resistance in Obesity," *Nature Reviews Endocrinology* 13, no. 6 (2017): 338–351.

53. D. Frasca, A. Diaz, et al., "Leptin Induces Immunosenescence in Human B Cells," *Cellular Immunology* 348 (2020): 1–17.

54. J. R. Vasselli, P. J. Scarpace, et al., "Dietary Components in the Development of Leptin Resistance," *Advances in Nutrition* 4, no. 2 (2013): 164–175.

55. G. M. Mackie, D. Samocha-Bonet, et al., "Does Weight Cycling Promote Obesity and Metabolic Risk Factors?" *Obesity Research and Clinical Practice* 11, no. 2 (2017): 131–139.

56. T. Pallister, M. A. Jackson, et al., "Untangling the Relationship Between Diet and Visceral Fat Mass Through Blood Metabolomics and Gut Microbiome Profiling," *International Journal of Obesity* 41, no. 7 (2017): 1106–1113.

57. E. A. Willis, W.-Y. Huang, et al., "Increased Frequency of Intentional Weight Loss Associated with Reduced Mortality: A Prospective Cohort Analysis," *BMC Medicine* 18, no. 248 (2020): 1–13.

Chapter 3: Heal Your Metabolism

1. R. Johnston and M. E. Valentinuzzi, "Metabolism: The Physiological Power-Generating Process: A History of Methods to Test Human Beings' 'Vital Capacity' [Retrospectroscope]," *IEEE Pulse* 7, no. 3 (2016): 50–57.
2. G. Eknoyan, "Santorio Sanctorius (1561–1636)—Founding Father of Metabolic Balance Studies," *American Journal of Nephrology* 19, no. 2 (1999): 226–233.
3. F. C. Bing, "The History of the Word 'Metabolism,'" *Journal of the History of Medicine and Allied Sciences* 26, no. 2 (1971): 158–180.
4. "What Is the Doubly-Labelled Water Method?" IAEA, https://doubly-labelled-water-database.iaea.org/about.
5. "Introduction to IAEA DLW Database," IAEA, https://doubly-labelled-water-database.iaea.org/home.
6. Graphic by Diana Saville, adapted from T. W. Rhoads and R. M. Anderson, "Taking the Long View on Metabolism," *Science* 373, no. 6556 (2021): 739.
7. S. Swarup, A. Goyal, et al., "Metabolic Syndrome," *StatPearls* (2022): 1–10.
8. M. G. Saklayen, "The Global Epidemic of the Metabolic Syndrome," *Current Hypertension Reports* 20, no. 2 (2018): 1–8.
9. L. B. Yates, L. Djoussé, et al., "Exceptional Longevity in Men: Modifiable Factors Associated with Survival and Function to Age 90 Years," *Archives of Internal Medicine* 168, no. 3 (2008): 284–290.
10. J. P. Cooke, "Endotheliopathy of Obesity," *Circulation* 142, no. 4 (2020): 380–383.
11. D. Konukoglu and H. Uzun, "Endothelial Dysfunction and Hypertension," *Advances in Experimental Medicine and Biology* 956 (2017): 511–540.
12. H. Kanai, K. Tokunaga, et al., "Decrease in Intra-Abdominal Visceral Fat May Reduce Blood Pressure in Obese Hypertensive Women," *Hypertension* 27, no. 1 (1996): 125–129.
13. J. M. Heaton, "The Distribution of Brown Adipose Tissue in the Human," *Journal of Anatomy* 112 (1972): 35–39.
14. A. M. Cypess, S. Lehman, et al., "Identification and Importance of Brown Adipose Tissue in Adult Humans," *New England Journal of Medicine* 360, no. 15 (2009): 1509–1517.
15. P. Huttunen, J. Hirvonen, et al., "The Occurrence of Brown Adipose Tissue in Outdoor Workers," *European Journal of Applied Physiology and Occupational Physiology* 46, no. 4 (1981): 339–345.
16. K. A. Virtanen, M. E. Lidell, et al., "Functional Brown Adipose Tissue in Healthy Adults," *New England Journal of Medicine* 360, no. 15 (2009): 1518–1525.
17. A. M. Cypess, L. S. Weiner, et al., "Activation of Human Brown Adipose Tissue by a β3-adrenergic Receptor Agonist," *Cell Metabolism* 21, no. 1 (2015): 33–38.
18. C. Torgan, "Drug Activates Brown Fat and Increases Metabolism," *National Institutes of Health*, January 26, 2015, www.nih.gov/news-events/news-releases/drug-activates-brown-fat-increases-metabolism.
19. S. Snitker, Y. Fujishima, et al., "Effects of Novel Capsinoid Treatment on Fatness and Energy Metabolism in Humans: Possible Pharmacogenetic Implications," *American Journal of Clinical Nutrition* 89, no. 1 (2009): 45–50.

20. Graphic by Diana Saville, adapted from S. Snitker, Y. Fujishima, et al., "Effects of Novel Capsinoid Treatment on Fatness and Energy Metabolism in Humans: Possible Pharmacogenetic Implications," *American Journal of Clinical Nutrition* 89, no. 1 (2009): 48.

21. M. Blaszkiewicz, J. W. Willows, et al., "The Importance of Peripheral Nerves in Adipose Tissue for the Regulation of Energy Balance," *Biology* 8, no. 1 (2019): 1–23.

22. Y. M Shuba, "Beyond Neuronal Heat Sensing: Diversity of TRPV1 Heat-Capsaicin Receptor-Channel Functions," *Frontiers in Cellular Neuroscience* 14, no. 612480 (2021): 1–17.

23. D. Ricquier, "Uncoupling Protein 1 of Brown Adipocytes, the Only Uncoupler: A Historical Perspective," *Frontiers in Endocrinology* 2, no. 85 (2011): 1–7.

24. J. M. O. Andrade, A. C. M. Frade, et al., "Resveratrol Increases Brown Adipose Tissue Thermogenesis Markers by Increasing SIRT1 and Energy Expenditure and Decreasing Fat Accumulation in Adipose Tissue of Mice Fed a Standard Diet," *European Journal of Nutrition* 53, no. 7 (2014): 1503–1510.

25. C. R. Cederroth, M. Vinciguerra, et al., "A Phytoestrogen-Rich Diet Increases Energy Expenditure and Decreases Adiposity in Mice," *Environmental Health Perspectives* 115, no. 10 (2007): 1467–1473.

26. Q. Shixian, B. VanCrey, et al., "Green Tea Extract Thermogenesis-Induced Weight Loss by Epigallocatechin Gallate Inhibition of Catechol-O-Methyltransferase," *Journal of Medicinal Food* 9, no. 4 (2006): 451–458.

27. S. Ma, H. Yu, et al., "Activation of the Cold-Sensing TRPM8 Channel Triggers UCP1-Dependent Thermogenesis and Prevents Obesity," *Journal of Molecular Cell Biology* 4, no. 2 (2012): 88–96.

28. J. Lone, J. H. Choi, et al., "Curcumin Induces Brown Fat-Like Phenotype in 3T3-L1 and Primary White Adipocytes," *Journal of Nutritional Biochemistry* 27 (2016): 193–202.

Chapter 4: You Can Eat to Beat Fat

1. S. Spalletta, V. Flati, et al., "Carvacrol Reduces Adipogenic Differentiation by Modulating Autophagy and Chrebp Expression," *PloS One* 13, no. 11 (2018): 1–21.

2. Y. Ting, W.-T. Chang, et al., "Antiobesity Efficacy of Quercetin-Rich Supplement on Diet-Induced Obese Rats: Effects on Body Composition, Serum Lipid Profile, and Gene Expression," *Journal of Agricultural and Food Chemistry* 66, no. 1 (2018): 70–80.

3. N. Xu, L. Zhang, et al., "Low-Dose Diet Supplement of a Natural Flavonoid, Luteolin, Ameliorates Diet-Induced Obesity and Insulin Resistance in Mice," *Molecular Nutrition and Food Research* 58, no. 6 (2014): 1258–1268.

4. M. Sudhakar, S. J. Sasikumar, et al., "Chlorogenic Acid Promotes Development of Brown Adipocyte-Like Phenotype in 3T3-L1 Adipocytes," *Journal of Functional Foods* 74 (2020): 1–8; X. He, S. Zheng, et al., "Chlorogenic Acid Ameliorates Obesity by Preventing Energy Balance Shift in High-Fat Diet-Induced Obese Mice," *Journal of the Science of Food and Agriculture* 101, no. 2 (2021): 631–637.

5. S. D. Kunkel, C. J. Elmore, et al., "Ursolic Acid Increases Skeletal Muscle and Brown Fat and Decreases Diet-Induced Obesity, Glucose Intolerance and Fatty Liver Disease," *PloS One* 7, no. 6 (2012): 1–8.

6. A. S. González-Garibay, A. López-Vázquez, et al., "Effect of Ursolic Acid on Insulin Resistance and Hyperinsulinemia in Rats with Diet-Induced Obesity: Role of Adipokines Expression," *Journal of Medicinal Food* 23, no. 3 (2020): 297–304.

7. A. J. Ahn, L. Wang, et al., "Dietary 23-Hydroxy Ursolic Acid Protects Against Diet-Induced Weight Gain and Hyperglycemia by Protecting Monocytes and Macrophages Against Nutrient Stress-Triggered Reprogramming and Dysfunction and Preventing Adipose Tissue Inflammation," *Journal of Nutritional Biochemistry* 86 (2020): 1–10.

8. H. Xiong, J. Wang, et al., "Hesperidin: A Therapeutic Agent for Obesity," *Drug Design, Development and Therapy* 13 (2019): 3855–3866.

9. Y.-C. Chou, C.-T. Ho, et al., "Immature Citrus Reticulata Extract Promotes Browning of Beige Adipocytes in High-Fat Diet-Induced C57BL/6 Mice," *Journal of Agricultural and Food Chemistry* 66, no. 37 (2018): 9697–9703.

10. J. F. Lu, M. Q. Zhu, et al., "Neohesperidin Attenuates Obesity by Altering the Composition of the Gut Microbiota in High-Fat Diet-Fed Mice," *FASEB Journal* 34, no. 9 (2020): 12053–12071.

11. M. Strączkowski, A. Nikołajuk, et al., "The Effect of Moderate Weight Loss, With or Without (1, 3)(1, 6)-B-Glucan Addition, on Subcutaneous Adipose Tissue Inflammatory Gene Expression in Young Subjects with Uncomplicated Obesity," *Endocrine* 61, no. 2 (2018): 275–284.

12. R. Mathews, V. Shete, et al., "The Effect of Cereal B-Glucan on Body Weight and Adiposity: A Review of Efficacy and Mechanism of Action," *Critical Reviews in Food Science and Nutrition* (2021): 1–13.

13. E. Gouranton, C. Thabuis, et al., "Lycopene Inhibits Proinflammatory Cytokine and Chemokine Expression in Adipose Tissue," *Journal of Nutritional Biochemistry* 22, no. 7 (2011): 642–648; R. Zhu, J. Wei, et al., "Lycopene Attenuates Body Weight Gain Through Induction of Browning via Regulation of Peroxisome Proliferator-Activated Receptor γ in High-Fat Diet-Induced Obese Mice," *Journal of Nutritional Biochemistry* 78 (2020): 1–13; R. Zhu, J. Wei, et al., "Lycopene Attenuates Body Weight Gain Through Induction of Browning via Regulation of Peroxisome Proliferator-Activated Receptor γ in High-Fat Diet-Induced Obese Mice," *Journal of Nutritional Biochemistry* 78 (2020): 1–13.

14. G. Chen, Y. Ni, et al., "Lycopene Alleviates Obesity-Induced Inflammation and Insulin Resistance by Regulating M1/M2 Status of Macrophages," *Molecular Nutrition and Food Research* 63, no. 21 (2019): e1900602; J. Wang, Y. Suo, et al., "Lycopene Supplementation Attenuates Western Diet-Induced Body Weight Gain Through Increasing the Expressions of Thermogenic/Mitochondrial Functional Genes and Improving Insulin Resistance in the Adipose Tissue of Obese Mice," *Journal of Nutritional Biochemistry* 69 (2019): 63–72.

15. E. I. Ugwor, A. S. James, et al., "Lycopene Alleviates Western Diet-Induced Elevations in Anthropometrical Indices of Obesity, Adipose Lipids, and Other Nutritional Parameters," *International Journal for Vitamin and Nutrition Research* (2021): 1–9.

16. A. Jahagirdar, D. Usharani, et al., "Sesaminol Diglucoside, a Water-Soluble Lignan from Sesame Seeds Induces Brown Fat Thermogenesis in Mice," *Biochemical and Biophysical Research Communications* 507 (2018): 155–160.

17. J. W. Kang, J. Park, et al., "Secoisolariciresinol Diglucoside Inhibits Adipogenesis Through the AMPK Pathway," *European Journal of Pharmacology* 820 (2018): 235–244.

18. S. Fukumitsu, K. Aida, et al., "Flaxseed Lignan Attenuates High-Fat Diet-Induced Fat Accumulation and Induces Adiponectin Expression in Mice," *British Journal of Nutrition* 100, no. 3 (2008): 669–676.

19. W. Y. Park, S.-K. Choe, et al., "Black Raspberry (*Rubuscoreanus* Miquel) Promotes Browning of Preadipocytes and Inguinal White Adipose Tissue in Cold-Induced Mice,"

Nutrients 11, no. 2154 (2019): 1–15; L. Wang, Y. Wei, et al., "Ellagic Acid Promotes Browning of White Adipose Tissues in High-Fat Diet-Induced Obesity in Rats Through Suppressing White Adipocyte Maintaining Genes," *Endocrine Journal* 66, no. 10 (2019): 923–936.

20. M. Okla, I. Kang, et al., "Ellagic Acid Modulates Lipid Accumulation in Primary Human Adipocytes and Human Hepatoma Huh7 Cells via Discrete Mechanisms," *Journal of Nutritional Biochemistry* 26, no. 1 (2015): 82–90; Y. Makino-Wakagi, Y. Yoshimura, et al., "Ellagic Acid in Pomegranate Suppresses Resistin Secretion by a Novel Regulatory Mechanism Involving the Degradation of Intracellular Resistin Protein in Adipocytes," *Biochemical and Biophysical Research Communications* 417, no. 2 (2012): 880–885; M. M. Michicotl-Meneses, M. D. R. Thompson-Bonilla, et al., "Inflammation Markers in Adipose Tissue and Cardiovascular Risk Reduction by Pomegranate Juice in Obesity Induced by a Hypercaloric Diet in Wistar Rats," *Nutrients* 13, no. 2577 (2021): 1–17.

21. X. Wu, G. R. Beecher, et al., "Concentrations of Anthocyanins in Common Foods in the United States and Estimation of Normal Consumption," *Journal of Agricultural and Food Chemistry* 54, no. 11 (2006): 4069–4075.

22. J. Liu, W. Hao, et al., "Blueberry and Cranberry Anthocyanin Extracts Reduce Bodyweight and Modulate Gut Microbiota in C57BL/6 J Mice Fed with a High-Fat Diet," *European Journal of Nutrition* 60, no. 5 (2021): 2735–2746.

23. R. A. van der Heijden, M. C. Morrison, et al., "Effects of Anthocyanin and Flavanol Compounds on Lipid Metabolism and Adipose Tissue Associated Systemic Inflammation in Diet-Induced Obesity," *Mediators of Inflammation* (2016): 1–10; Y. Liu, D. Li, et al., "Anthocyanin Increases Adiponectin Secretion and Protects Against Diabetes-Related Endothelial Dysfunction," *American Journal of Physiology–Endocrinology and Metabolism* 306, no. 8 (2014): E975–E988.

24. M. Lee and M. Lee, "The Effects of C3G and D3G Anthocyanin-Rich Black Soybean on Energy Metabolism in Beige-like Adipocytes," *Journal of Agricultural and Food Chemistry* 68, no. 43 (2020): 12011–12018.

25. N. Wang, Y. Ma, et al., "Hydroxytyrosol Prevents PM2.5-Induced Adiposity and Insulin Resistance by Restraining Oxidative Stress Related NF-κB Pathway and Modulation of Gut Microbiota in a Murine Model," *Free Radical Biology and Medicine* 141 (2019): 393–407; Z. Liu, N. Wang, et al., "Hydroxytyrosol Improves Obesity and Insulin Resistance by Modulating Gut Microbiota in High-Fat Diet-Induced Obese Mice," *Frontiers in Microbiology* 10, no. 390 (2019): 1–12.

26. B. Stefanon and M. Colitti, "Original Research: Hydroxytyrosol, an Ingredient of Olive Oil, Reduces Triglyceride Accumulation and Promotes Lipolysis in Human Primary Visceral Adipocytes During Differentiation," *Experimental Biology and Medicine* 241, no. 16 (2016): 1796–1802; E. Scoditti, S. Capri, et al., "Hydroxytyrosol Modulates Adipocyte Gene and Mirna Expression Under Inflammatory Condition," *Nutrients* 11, no. 10 (2019): 1–29.

27. Y. Liu, X. Fu, et al., "The Protective Effects of Sulforaphane on High-Fat Diet-Induced Obesity in Mice Through Browning of White Fat," *Frontiers in Pharmacology* 12, no. 665894 (2021): 1–13; L. Xu, N. Nagata, et al., "Glucoraphanin: A Broccoli Sprout Extract That Ameliorates Obesity-Induced Inflammation and Insulin Resistance," *Adipocyte* 7, no. 3 (2018): 218–225; H. Q. Zhang, S. Y. Chen, et al., "Sulforaphane

Induces Adipocyte Browning and Promotes Glucose and Lipid Utilization," *Molecular Nutrition and Food Research* 60, no. 10 (2016): 2185–2197.

28. I. Çakır, P. L. Pan, et al., "Sulforaphane Reduces Obesity by Reversing Leptin Resistance," *eLife* 11 (2022): 1–28.

29. J.-K. Min, K.-Y. Han, et al., "Capsaicin Inhibits in Vitro and in Vivo Angiogenesis," *Cancer Research* 64, no. 2 (2004): 644–651.

30. A. Aoun, F. Darwish, et al., "The Influence of the Gut Microbiome on Obesity in Adults and the Role of Probiotics, Prebiotics, and Synbiotics for Weight Loss," *Preventative Medicine and Food Science* 25, no. 2 (2020): 113–123.

31. H. C. Wastyk, G. K. Fragiadakis, et al., "Gut-Microbiota-Targeted Diets Modulate Human Immune Status," *Cell* 184, no. 16 (2021): 4137–4153.e14.

32. Y. Xu, N. Wang, et al., "Function of *Akkermansia muciniphila* in Obesity: Interactions with Lipid Metabolism, Immune Response and Gut Systems," *Frontiers in Microbiology* 11, no. 219 (2020): 1–12.

33. Q. Zhou, Y. Zhang, et al., "Gut Bacteria *Akkermansia* Is Associated with Reduced Risk of Obesity: Evidence from the American Gut Project," *Nutrition and Metabolism* 17, no. 90 (2020): 1–9.

34. M. C. Collado, M. Derrien, et al., "Intestinal Integrity and Akkermansia Muciniphila, a Mucin-Degrading Member of the Intestinal Microbiota Present in Infants, Adults, and the Elderly," *Applied and Environmental Microbiology* 73, no. 23 (2007): 7767–7770.

35. L.-H. Chen, Y.-H. Chen, et al., "Antiobesity Effect of Lactobacillus Reuteri 263 Associated with Energy Metabolism Remodeling of White Adipose Tissue in High-Energy-Diet-Fed Rats," *Journal of Nutritional Biochemistry* 54 (2018): 87–94.

36. X.-J. Kong, K. Liu, et al., "The Effects of Limosilactobacillus Reuteri LR-99 Supplementation on Body Mass Index, Social Communication, Fine Motor Function, and Gut Microbiome Composition in Individuals with Prader-Willi Syndrome: A Randomized Double-Blinded Placebo-Controlled Trial," *Probiotics and Antimicrobial Proteins* 13, no. 6 (2021): 1508–1520.

37. M. Calasso and M. Gobbetti, "Lactic Acid Bacteria | Lactobacillus spp.: Other Species," in *Encyclopedia of Dairy Sciences*, 2nd ed., ed. John W. Fuquay (Amsterdam: Elsevier, 2011), 1507–1511; R. Lu, M. Shang, et al., "Lactic Acid Bacteria Isolated from Korean Kimchi Activate the Vitamin D Receptor-Autophagy Signaling Pathways," *Inflammatory Bowel Diseases* 26, no. 8 (2020): 1199–1211; J. Zheng, X. Zhao, et al., "Comparative Genomics Lactobacillus Reuteri from Sourdough Reveals Adaptation of an Intestinal Symbiont to Food Fermentations," *Scientific Reports* 5, no. 18234 (2015): 1–11; S. R. Herbel, B. Lauzat, et al., "Species-Specific Quantification of Probiotic Lactobacilli in Yoghurt by Quantitative Real-Time PCR," *Journal of Applied Microbiology* 115, no. 6 (2013): 1402–1410.

38. D. A. Jones, S. L. Prior, et al., "Changes in Markers of Oxidative Stress and DNA Damage in Human Visceral Adipose Tissue from Subjects with Obesity and Type 2 Diabetes," *Diabetes Research and Clinical Practice* 106, no. 3 (2014): 627–633.

39. C. Gallardo-Escribano, V. Buonaiuto, et al., "Epigenetic Approach in Obesity: DNA Methylation in Prepubertal Population Which Underwent a Lifestyle Modification," *Clinical Epigenetics* 12, no. 144 (2020): 1–14.

40. L. P. Kozak, "The Genetics of Brown Adipocyte Induction in White Fat Depots," *Frontiers in Endocrinology* 2, no. 64 (2011): 1–13.

41. A.-C. Pilkington, H. A. Paz, et al., "Beige Adipose Tissue Identification and Marker Specificity-Overview," *Frontiers in Endocrinology* 12, no. 599134 (2021): 1–9.
42. M. A. Exley, L. Hand, et al., "Interplay Between the Immune System and Adipose Tissue in Obesity," *Journal of Endocrinology* 223, no. 2 (2014): R41–R48.
43. T. Kawai, M. V. Autieri, et al., "Adipose Tissue Inflammation and Metabolic Dysfunction in Obesity," *American Journal of Physiology. Cell Physiology* 320, no. 3 (2021): C375–C391.
44. Z. Shamekhi, R. Amani, et al., "A Randomized, Double-Blind, Placebo-Controlled Clinical Trial Examining the Effects of Green Tea Extract on Systemic Lupus Erythematosus Disease Activity and Quality of Life," *Phytotherapy Research: PTR* 31, no. 7 (2017): 1063–1071; Y. Minami, T. Sasaki, et al., "Diet and Systemic Lupus Erythematosus: A 4-Year Prospective Study of Japanese Patients," *Journal of Rheumatology* 30, no. 4 (2003): 747–754; R. Otton, A. P. Bolin, et al., "Polyphenol-Rich Green Tea Extract Improves Adipose Tissue Metabolism by Down-Regulating Mir-335 Expression and Mitigating Insulin Resistance and Inflammation," *Journal of Nutritional Biochemistry* 57 (2018): 170–179; M. S. Ellulu, A. Rahmat, et al., "Effect of Vitamin C on Inflammation and Metabolic Markers in Hypertensive and/or Diabetic Obese Adults: A Randomized Controlled Trial," *Drug Design, Development and Therapy* 9 (2015): 3405–3412.

Chapter 5: Eating the MediterAsian Way

1. R. Legrand, P. Manckoundia, et al., "Assessment of the Health Status of the Oldest Olds Living on the Greek Island of Ikaria: A Population-Based Study in a Blue Zone," *Current Gerontology and Geriatrics Research* 2019 (2019): 8194310.
2. R. N. Spengler, F. Maksudov, et al., "Arboreal Crops on the Medieval Silk Road: Archaeobotanical Studies at Tashbulak," *PLoS One* 13, no. 8 (2018): e0201409.
3. A. Keys and M. Keys, *How to Eat Well and Stay Well the Mediterranean Way* (Garden City, NY: Doubleday, 1975).
4. W. C. Willett, F. Sacks, et al., "Mediterranean Diet Pyramid: A Cultural Model for Healthy Eating," *American Journal of Clinical Nutrition* 61, no. 6 (1995): 1402S–1496S.
5. A. Ligouori, F. Petti, et al., "Effect of a Basic Chinese Traditional Diet in Overweight Patients," *Journal of Traditional Chinese Medicine* 33, no. 3 (2013): 322–324.
6. F. Leonetti, A. Liguori, et al., "Effects of Basic Traditional Chinese Diet on Body Mass Index, Lean Body Mass, and Eating and Hunger Behaviours in Overweight or Obese Individuals," *Journal of Traditional Chinese Medicine* 36, no. 4 (2016): 456–463.
7. S. Zhen, Y. Ma, et al., "Dietary Pattern Is Associated with Obesity in Chinese Children and Adolescents: Data from China Health and Nutrition Survey (CHNS)," *Nutrition Journal* 17, no. 68 (2018), https://doi.org/10.1186/s12937-018-0372-8.
8. K. Murakami, M. B. E. Livingstone, et al. "Thirteen-Year Trends in Dietary Patterns Among Japanese Adults in the National Health and Nutrition Survey 2003–2015: Continuous Westernization of the Japanese Diet." *Nutrients* 10, no. 8 (2018): 994.
9. S. Sugawara, M. Kushida, et al., "The 1975 Type Japanese Diet Improves Lipid Metabolic Parameters in Younger Adults: A Randomized Controlled Trial," *Journal of Oleo Science* 67, no. 5 (2018): 599–607.
10. M. Asano, M. Kushida, et al., "Abdominal Fat in Individuals with Overweight Reduced by Consumption of a 1975 Japanese Diet: A Randomized Controlled Trial," *Obesity* 27, no. 6 (2019): 899–907.

11. D. Romaguera, T. Norat, et al., "Adherence to the Mediterranean Diet Is Associated with Lower Abdominal Adiposity in European Men and Women," *Journal of Nutrition* 139, no. 9 (2009): 1728–1737.

12. D. B. Panagiotakos, C. Chrysohoou, et al., "Association Between the Prevalence of Obesity and Adherence to the Mediterranean Diet: The ATTICA Study," *Nutrition* 22, no. 5 (2006): 449–456.

13. K. Esposito, C.-M. Kastorini, et al., "Mediterranean Diet and Weight Loss: Meta-Analysis of Randomized Controlled Trials," *Metabolic Syndrome and Related Disorders* 9, no. 1 (2011): 1–12.

14. D. Poulimeneas, C. A. Anastasiou, et al., "Exploring the Relationship Between the Mediterranean Diet and Weight Loss Maintenance: The MedWeight Study," *British Journal of Nutrition* 124, no. 8 (2020): 874–880.

15. A. Crimarco, M. J. Lamdry, et al., "Ultra-Processed Foods, Weight Gain, and Co-Morbidity Risk," *Current Obesity Reports* 11, no. 3 (2022): 80–92.

16. D. L. Santos Ferreira, C. Hübel, et al., "Associations Between Blood Metabolic Profile at 7 Years Old and Eating Disorders in Adolescence: Findings from the Avon Longitudinal Study of Parents and Children," *Metabolites* 9, no. 9 (2019): 191.

17. G. S. Duaerte and A. Farah, "Effect of Simultaneous Consumption of Milk and Coffee on Chlorogenic Acids' Bioavailability in Humans," *Journal of Agricultural and Food Chemistry* 59, no. 14 (2011): 7925–7931.

18. K. R. Schell, K. E. Fernandes, et al., "The Potential of Honey as a Prebiotic Food to Re-Engineer the Gut Microbiome Toward a Healthy State," *Frontiers in Nutrition* 9 (2022): 957932.

19. V. Y. Njike, R. G. Ayettey, et al., "Egg Ingestion in Adults with Type 2 Diabetes: Effects on Glycemic Control, Anthropometry, and Diet Quality—A Randomized, Controlled, Crossover Trial," *BMJ Open Diabetes Research and Care* 4 (2016): e000281.

20. Age-Related Eye Diseases Study 2 Research Group, "Lutein + Zeaxanthin and Omega-3 Fatty Acids for Age-Related Macular Degeneration: The Age-Related Eye Disease Study 2 (AREDS2) Randomized Clinical Trial," *Journal of the American Medical Association* 309, no. 19 (2013): 2005–2015; B. Eisenhauer, S. Natoli, et al., "Lutein and Zeaxanthin-Food Sources, Bioavailability and Dietary Variety in Age-Related Macular Degeneration Protection," *Nutrients* 9, no. 2 (2017): 120.

21. M. Sugiyama, A. C. Tang, et al., "Glycemic Index of Single and Mixed Meal Foods Among Common Japanese Foods with White Rice as a Reference Food," *European Journal of Clinical Nutrition* 57, no. 6 (2003): 743–752.

22. J. A. Giménez-Bastida, H. Zielinski, et al., "Buckwheat Bioactive Compounds, Their Derived Phenolic Metabolites and Their Health Benefits," *Molecular Nutrition and Food Research* 61, no. 7 (2017). doi:10.1002/mnfr.201600475.

23. A. Bédard, P.-O. Lamarche, et al., "Can Eating Pleasure Be a Lever for Healthy Eating? A Systematic Scoping Review of Eating Pleasure and Its Links with Dietary Behaviors and Health," *PLoS One* 15, no. 12 (2020): e0244292.

24. F. Islami, H. Poustchi, et al., "A Prospective Study of Tea Drinking Temperature and Risk of Esophageal Squamous Cell Carcinoma," *International Journal of Cancer* 146, no. 1 (2020): 18–25.

25. Y. Yi, H. Liang, et al., "Green Tea Consumption and Esophageal Cancer Risk: A Meta-Analysis," *Nutrition and Cancer* 72, no. 3 (2020): 513–521.

Chapter 6: The Fresh Market

1. M. Vadiveloo, L. B. Dixon, et al., "Dietary Variety Is Inversely Associated with Body Adiposity Among US Adults Using a Novel Food Diversity Index," *Journal of Nutrition* 145, no. 3 (2015): 555–563.

2. S. Alinia, O. Hels, et al., "The Potential Association Between Fruit Intake and Body Weight—A Review," *Obesity Reviews* 10, no. 6 (2009): 639–647; L. Hebden, F. O'Leary, et al., "Fruit Consumption and Adiposity Status in Adults: A Systematic Review of Current Evidence," *Critical Reviews in Food Science and Nutrition* 57, no. 12 (2017): 2526–2540.

3. Z. Chen, D. Radjabzadeh, et al., "Association of Insulin Resistance and Type 2 Diabetes with Gut Microbial Diversity: A Microbiome-Wide Analysis from Population Studies," *JAMA Network Open* 4, no. 7 (2021): 1–13.

4. M. Conceição de Oliveira, R. Sichieri, et al., "Weight Loss Associated with a Daily Intake of Three Apples or Three Pears Among Overweight Women," *Nutrition* 19, no. 3 (2003): 253–256.

5. M. L. Bertoia, K. J. Mukamal, et al., "Changes in Intake of Fruits and Vegetables and Weight Change in United States Men and Women Followed for Up to 24 Years: Analysis from Three Prospective Cohort Studies," *PLoS Medicine* 12, no. 9 (2015).

6. S. C. Chai, S. Hooshmand, et al., "Daily Apple versus Dried Plum: Impact on Cardiovascular Disease Risk Factors in Postmenopausal Women," *Journal of the Academy of Nutrition and Dietetics* 112, no. 8 (2012): 1158–1168.

7. Z. Bian, H. Liu, et al., "Ursolic Acid Protects Against Anoxic Injury in Cardiac Microvascular Endothelial Cells by Regulating Intercellular Adhesion Molecule-1 and Toll-Like Receptor 4/MyD88/NF-κB Pathway," *Human and Experimental Toxicology* 41 (2022): 1–10; B. Liu, Y. Liu, et al., "Ursolic Acid Induces Neural Regeneration After Sciatic Nerve Injury," *Neural Regeneration Research* 8, no. 27 (2013): 2510–2519; M. S. Kiran, R. I. Viji, et al., "Modulation of Angiogenic Factors by Ursolic Acid," *Biochemical and Biophysical Research Communications* 371, no. 3 (2008): 556–560; Q. Sheng, F. Li, et al., "Ursolic Acid Regulates Intestinal Microbiota and Inflammatory Cell Infiltration to Prevent Ulcerative Colitis," *Journal of Immunology Research* 2021 (2021): 1–16.

8. T. Yang, J. Doherty, et al., "Effectiveness of Commercial and Homemade Washing Agents in Removing Pesticide Residues on and in Apples," *Journal of Agricultural and Food Chemistry* 65 (2017): 9744–9752.

9. B. A. Stracke, C. E. Rüfer, et al., "Three-Year Comparison of the Polyphenol Contents and Antioxidant Capacities in Organically and Conventionally Produced Apples (Malus domestica Bork. Cultivar 'Golden Delicious')," *Journal of Agricultural and Food Chemistry* 57, no. 11 (2009): 4598–4605.

10. J. Boyer and R. H. Liu., "Apple Phytochemicals and Their Health Benefits," *Nutrition Journal* 3, no. 5 (2004): 1–15.

11. D. Feskanich, R. G. Ziegler, et al., "Prospective Study of Fruit and Vegetable Consumption and Risk of Lung Cancer Among Men and Women," *Journal of the National Cancer Institute* 92, no. 22 (2000): 1812–1823.

12. A. Escarpa and M. C. González, "High-Performance Liquid Chromatography with Diode-Array Detection for the Determination of Phenolic Compounds in Peel and Pulp from Different Apple Varieties," *Journal of Chromatography* A 823 (1998): 331–337.

13. N. Navaei, S. Pourafshar, et al., "Influence of Daily Fresh Pear Consumption on Biomarkers of Cardiometabolic Health in Middle-Aged/Older Adults with Metabolic

Syndrome: A Randomized Controlled Trial," *Food and Function* 10, no. 2 (2019): 1062–1072.

14. S. Nishikawa, T. Hyodo, et al., "α-Monoglucosyl Hesperidin but Not Hesperidin Induces Brown-Like Adipocyte Formation and Suppresses White Adipose Tissue Accumulation in Mice," *Journal of Agricultural and Food Chemistry* 67, no. 7 (2019): 1948–1954; C. J. Rebello, F. L. Greenway, et al., "Naringenin Promotes Thermogenic Gene Expression in Human White Adipose Tissue," *Obesity* 27, no. 1 (2019): 103–111; M. S. Ellulu, A. Rahmat, et al., "Effect of Vitamin C on Inflammation and Metabolic Markers in Hypertensive and/or Diabetic Obese Adults: A Randomized Controlled Trial," *Drug Design, Development and Therapy* 9 (2015): 3405–3412; R. J. Sram, B. Binkova, et al., "Vitamin C for DNA Damage Prevention," *Mutation Research* 733 (2012): 39–49.

15. R. Zhu, B. Chen, et al., "Lycopene in Protection Against Obesity and Diabetes: A Mechanistic Review," *Pharmacological Research* 159 (2020): 1–15.

16. M. Afarideh, R. Thaler, et al., "Global Epigenetic Alterations of Mesenchymal Stem Cells in Obesity: The Role of Vitamin C Reprogramming," *Epigenetics* 16, no. 7 (2021): 705–717; C. J. Rebello, F. L. Greenway, et al., "Naringenin Promotes Thermogenic Gene Expression in Human White Adipose Tissue," *Obesity* 27, no. 1 (2019): 103–111; H. Xiong, J. Wang, et al., "Hesperidin: A Therapeutic Agent for Obesity," *Drug Design, Development and Therapy* 13 (2019): 3855–3866.

17. K. Fujioka, F. Greenway, et al., "The Effects of Grapefruit on Weight and Insulin Resistance: Relationship to the Metabolic Syndrome," *Journal of Medicinal Food* 9, no. 1 (2006): 49–54.

18. L. S. McAnulty, D. C. Nieman, et al., "Effect of Blueberry Ingestion on Natural Killer Cell Counts, Oxidative Stress, and Inflammation Prior to and After 2.5 h of Running," *Applied Physiology, Nutrition, and Metabolism = Physiologie Appliquee, Nutrition et Metabolisme* 36, no. 6 (2011): 976–984.

19. N. Istek and O. Gurbuz, "Investigation of the Impact of Blueberries on Metabolic Factors Influencing Health," *Journal of Functional Foods* 38 (2017): 298–307.

20. A. Jennings, A. MacGregor, et al., "Higher Dietary Flavonoid Intakes Are Associated with Lower Objectively Measured Body Composition in Women: Evidence from Discordant Monozygotic Twins," *American Journal of Clinical Nutrition* 105, no. 3 (2017): 626–634.

21. M. T. Ariza, P. Reboredo-Rodríguez, et al., "Strawberry Achenes Are an Important Source of Bioactive Compounds for Human Health," *International Journal of Molecular Sciences* 17, no. 1103 (2016): 1–14.

22. H. Jiang, W. Zhang, et al., "The Anti-Obesogenic Effects of Dietary Berry Fruits: A Review," *Food Research International* 147 (2021): 110539; M. J. Ko, R. H. Jayaramaiah, et al., "Evaluation of Bioactive Compounds in Strawberry Fruits by a Targeted Metabolomic Approach," *Horticulture Science and Technology* 35, no. 6 (2017): 805–819; I. Aragüez, E. Cruz-Rus, et al., "Proteomic Analysis of Strawberry Achenes Reveals Active Synthesis and Recycling of L-Ascorbic Acid," *Journal of Proteomics* 83 (2013): 160–179.

23. L. Wang, Y. Wei, et al., "Ellagic Acid Promotes Browning of White Adipose Tissues in High-Fat Diet-Induced Obesity in Rats Through Suppressing White Adipocyte Maintaining Genes," *Endocrine Journal* 66, no. 10 (2019): 923–936.

24. V. Baradaran Rahimi, M. Ghadiri, et al., "Antiinflammatory and Anti-Cancer Activities of Pomegranate and Its Constituent, Ellagic Acid: Evidence from Cellular,

Animal, and Clinical Studies," *Phytotherapy Research: PTR* 34, no. 4 (2020): 685–720; M. S. Ellulu, A. Rahmat, et al., "Effect of Vitamin C on Inflammation and Metabolic Markers in Hypertensive and/or Diabetic Obese Adults: A Randomized Controlled Trial," *Drug Design, Development and Therapy* 9 (2015): 3405–3412.

25. P. Aranaz, A. Romo-Hualde, et al., "Freeze-Dried Strawberry and Blueberry Attenuates Diet-Induced Obesity and Insulin Resistance in Rats by Inhibiting Adipogenesis and Lipogenesis," *Food and Function* 8, no. 11 (2017): 3999–4013.

26. I. Tlak Gajger and S. A. Dar, "Plant Allelochemicals as Sources of Insecticides," *Insects* 12, no. 189 (2021): 1–21.

27. F. Ibanez, W. Y. Bang, et al., "Solving the Controversy of Healthier Organic Fruit: Leaf Wounding Triggers Distant Gene Expression Response of Polyphenol Biosynthesis in Strawberry Fruit (Fragaria x ananassa)," *Scientific Reports* 9, no. 1 (2019): 1–11.

28. M. L. Bertoia, K. J. Mukamal, et al., "Changes in Intake of Fruits and Vegetables and Weight Change in United States Men and Women Followed for up to 24 Years: Analysis from Three Prospective Cohort Studies," *PLoS Medicine* 12, no. 9 (2015): 1–20.

29. A. Basu, K. Izuora, et al., "Dietary Strawberries Improve Cardiometabolic Risks in Adults with Obesity and Elevated Serum LDL Cholesterol in a Randomized Controlled Crossover Trial," *Nutrients* 13, no. 5 (2021): 1–14.

30. M.-C. Alessi, M. Poggi, et al., "Plasminogen Activator Inhibitor-1, Adipose Tissue and Insulin Resistance," *Current Opinion in Lipidology* 18, no. 3 (2007): 240–245.

31. S. J. Zunino, M. A. Parelman, et al., "Effects of Dietary Strawberry Powder on Blood Lipids and Inflammatory Markers in Obese Human Subjects," *British Journal of Nutrition* 108, no. 5 (2012): 900–909; A. Basu, M. Wilkinson, et al., "Freeze-Dried Strawberry Powder Improves Lipid Profile and Lipid Peroxidation in Women with Metabolic Syndrome: Baseline and Post Intervention Effects," *Nutrition Journal* 8, no. 43 (2009): 1–7.

32. J. Kowshik, H. Giri, et al., "Ellagic Acid Inhibits VEGF/VEGFR2, PI3K/Akt and MAPK Signaling Cascades in the Hamster Cheek Pouch Carcinogenesis Model," *Anti-Cancer Agents in Medicinal Chemistry* 14, no. 9 (2014): 1249–1260; Y. Ding, L. Wang, et al., "Protective Effects of Ellagic Acid Against Tetrachloride-Induced Cirrhosis in Mice Through the Inhibition of Reactive Oxygen Species Formation and Angiogenesis," *Experimental and Therapeutic Medicine* 14, no. 4 (2017): 3375–3380.

33. M. Kujawska and J. Jodynis-Liebert, "Potential of the Ellagic Acid-Derived Gut Microbiota Metabolite—Urolithin A in Gastrointestinal Protection," *World Journal of Gastroenterology* 26, no. 23 (2020): 3170–3181.

34. J. Schell, R. H. Scofield, et al., "Strawberries Improve Pain and Inflammation in Obese Adults with Radiographic Evidence of Knee Osteoarthritis," *Nutrients* 9, no. 949 (2017): 1–13.

35. R. Reifen, "Vitamin A as an Anti-Inflammatory Agent," *Proceedings of the Nutrition Society* 61, no. 3 (2002): 397–400; E. C. Lefferts, B. A. Hibner, et al., "Oral Vitamin C Restores Endothelial Function During Acute Inflammation in Young and Older Adults," *Physiological Reports* 9, no. 21 (2021): 1–13.

36. J. Fan, E. Park, et al., "Pharmacokinetic Parameters of Watermelon (Rind, Flesh, and Seeds) Bioactive Components in Human Plasma: A Pilot Study to Investigate the Relationship to Endothelial Function," *Journal of Agricultural and Food Chemistry* 68, no. 28 (2020): 7393–7403.

37. V. Otasevic, A. Korac, et al., "Nitric Oxide and Thermogenesis—Challenge in Molecular Cell Physiology," *Frontiers in Bioscience (Scholar Edition)* 3, no. 3 (2011): 1180–1195.

38. T. Lum, M. Connolly, et al., "Effects of Fresh Watermelon Consumption on the Acute Satiety Response and Cardiometabolic Risk Factors in Overweight and Obese Adults," *Nutrients* 11, no. 3 (2019): 1–13.

39. J. Xie, M. Liu, et al., "Zeaxanthin Ameliorates Obesity by Activating the β3-Adrenergic Receptor to Stimulate Inguinal Fat Thermogenesis and Modulating the Gut Microbiota," *Food and Function* 12, no. 24 (2021): 12734–12750; M. Liu, H. Liu, et al., "Anti-Obesity Effects of Zeaxanthin on 3T3-L1 Preadipocyte and High Fat Induced Obese Mice," *Food and Function* 8, no. 9 (2017): 3327–3338; N. Wang, D. Wang, et al., "Lutein Attenuates Excessive Lipid Accumulation in Differentiated 3T3-L1 Cells and Abdominal Adipose Tissue of Rats by the SIRT1-Mediated Pathway," *International Journal of Biochemistry and Cell Biology* 133 (2021): 1–11.

40. N. A. Khan, C. G. Edwards, et al., "Avocado Consumption, Abdominal Adiposity, and Oral Glucose Tolerance Among Persons with Overweight and Obesity," *Journal of Nutrition* 151, no. 9 (2021): 2513–2521.

41. L. Wang, L. Tao, et al., "A Moderate-Fat Diet with One Avocado per Day Increases Plasma Antioxidants and Decreases the Oxidation of Small, Dense LDL in Adults with Overweight and Obesity: A Randomized Controlled Trial," *Journal of Nutrition* 150, no. 2 (2020): 276–284.

42. N. Ahmed, M. Tcheng, et al., "Avocatin B Protects Against Lipotoxicity and Improves Insulin Sensitivity in Diet-Induced Obesity," *Molecular Nutrition and Food Research* 63, no. 24 (2019): 1–10.

43. S. Elgass, A. Cooper, et al., "Lycopene Inhibits Angiogenesis in Human Umbilical Vein Endothelial Cells and Rat Aortic Rings," *British Journal of Nutrition* 108, no. 3 (2012): 431–439; K. Zu, L. Mucci, et al., "Dietary Lycopene, Angiogenesis, and Prostate Cancer: A Prospective Study in the Prostate-Specific Antigen Era," *Journal of the National Cancer Institute* 106, no. 2 (2014): 1–10.

44. A. F. Vinha, S. V. P. Barreira, et. al., "Pre-Meal Tomato (Lycopersicon esculentum) Intake Can Have an Anti-Obesity Effect in Young Women?" *International Journal of Food Science and Nutrition* 65, no. 8 (2014): 1019–26.

45. H.-Y. Chung, A. L. A. Ferreira, et al., "Site-Specific Concentrations of Carotenoids in Adipose Tissue: Relations with Dietary and Serum Carotenoid Concentrations in Healthy Adults," *American Journal of Clinical Nutrition* 90 (2009): 533–539.

46. R. E. Graff, A. Pettersson, et al., "Dietary Lycopene Intake and Risk of Prostate Cancer Defined by ERG Protein Expression," *American Journal of Clinical Nutrition* 103, no. 3 (2016): 851–860; P. H. Gann, J. Ma, et al., "Lower Prostate Cancer Risk in Men with Elevated Plasma Lycopene Levels: Results of a Prospective Analysis," *Cancer Research* 59, no. 6 (1999): 1225–1230; E. Giovannucci, A. Ascherio, et al., "Intake of Carotenoids and Retinol in Relation to Risk of Prostate Cancer," *Journal of the National Cancer Institute* 87, no. 23 (1995): 1767–1776.

47. S. O. Antwi, S. E. Steck, et al., "Carotenoid Intake and Adipose Tissue Carotenoid Levels in Relation to Prostate Cancer Aggressiveness Among African-American and European-American Men in the North Carolina-Louisiana Prostate Cancer Project (PCaP)," *Prostate* 76, no. 12 (2016): 1053–1066.

48. Curiously, this benefit was only observed in white men in the study.

49. K. Takayanagi, S.-I. Morimoto, et al., "Mechanism of Visceral Fat Reduction in Tsumura Suzuki Obese, Diabetes (TSOD) Mice Orally Administered β-Cryptoxanthin from Satsuma Mandarin Oranges (Citrus unshiu Marc)," *Journal of Agricultural and Food Chemistry* 59, no. 23 (2011): 12342–12351.

50. L. Cheng, L. Shi, et al., "Rutin-Activated Adipose Tissue Thermogenesis Is Correlated with Increased Intestinal Short-Chain Fatty Acid Levels," *Phytotherapy Research: PTR* 36, no. 6 (2022): 2495–2510.

51. Y.-C. Zeng, L.-S. Pang, et al, "Protective Effect and Mechanism of Lycopene on Endothelial Progenitor Cells (EPCs) from Type 2 Diabetes Mellitus Rats," *Biomedicine and Pharmacotherapy = Biomedecine and Pharmacotherapie* 92 (2017): 86–94; J. Nones, A. P. Costa, et al., "The Flavonoids Hesperidin and Rutin Promote Neural Crest Cell Survival," *Cell and Tissue Research* 350, no. 2 (2012): 305–315.

52. J. F. Rinaldi de Alvarenga, P. Quifer-Rada, et al., "Mediterranean Sofrito Home-Cooking Technique Enhances Polyphenol Content in Tomato Sauce," *Journal of the Science of Food and Agriculture* 99, no. 14 (2019): 6535–6545.

53. B. Zhang, D. M. Tieman, et al., "Chilling-Induced Tomato Flavor Loss Is Associated with Altered Volatile Synthesis and Transient Changes in DNA Methylation," *Proceedings of the National Academy of Sciences of the United States of America* 113, no. 44 (2016): 12580–12585.

54. Y. Li, F. Yuan, et al., "Sulforaphane Protects Against Ethanol-Induced Apoptosis in Neural Crest Cells Through Restoring Epithelial-Mesenchymal Transition by Epigenetically Modulating the Expression of Snail1," *Biochimica et Biophysica Acta–Molecular Basis of Disease* 1865, no. 10 (2019): 2586–2594; L. M. Beaver, C. V. Löhr, et al., "Broccoli Sprouts Delay Prostate Cancer Formation and Decrease Prostate Cancer Severity with a Concurrent Decrease in HDAC3 Protein Expression in Transgenic Adenocarcinoma of the Mouse Prostate (TRAMP) Mice," *Current Developments in Nutrition* 2, no. 3 (2017): 1–12; S.-R. Jun, A. Cheema, et al., "Multi-omic Analysis Reveals Different Effects of Suforaphane on the Microbiome and Metabolome in Old Compared to Young Mice," *Microorganisms* 8, no. 10 (2020): 1–22; A. Mahn and A. Castillo, "Potential of Sulforaphane as a Natural Immune System Enhancer: A Review," *Molecules (Basel, Switzerland)* 26, no. 3 (2021): 1–14.

55. M. T. López-Chillón, C. Carazo-Diaz, et al., "Effects of Long-Term Consumption of Broccoli Sprouts on Inflammatory Markers in Overweight Subjects." *Clinical Nutrition* 38, no. 2 (2019): 745–752.

56. I. Çakır, P. L. Pan, et al., "Sulforaphane Reduces Obesity by Reversing Leptin Resistance," *eLife* 11 (2022): 1–28.

57. E. J. Llorent-Martínez, J. Ortega-Vidal, et al., "Comparative Study of the Phytochemical and Mineral Composition of Fresh and Cooked Broccolini," *Food Research International* 129 (2020): 1–8.

58. P. Felker, R. Bunch, et al., "Concentrations of Thiocyanate and Goitrin in Human Plasma, Their Precursor Concentrations in Brassica Vegetables, and Associated Potential Risk for Hypothyroidism," *Nutrition Reviews* 74, no. 4 (2016): 248–258.

59. X. Chen, J. Xie, et al., "Genistein Improves Systemic Metabolism and Enhances Cold Resistance by Promoting Adipose Tissue Beiging," *Biochemical and Biophysical Research Communications* 558 (2021): 154–160; B. Palacios-González, A. Vargas-Castillo, et al., "Genistein Increases the Thermogenic Program of Subcutaneous WAT and Increases Energy Expenditure in Mice," *Journal of Nutritional Biochemistry* 68 (2019): 59–68; A. Naaz, S. Yellayi, et al., "The Soy Isoflavone Genistein Decreases Adipose Deposition in Mice," *Endocrinology* 144, no. 8 (2003): 3315–3320.

60. X. O. Shu, Y. Zheng, et al., "Soy Food Intake and Breast Cancer Survival," *Journal of the American Medical Association* 302, no. 22 (2009): 2437–2443; Z. Yan, X. Zhang, et al., "Association Between Consumption of Soy and Risk of Cardiovascular Disease: A Meta-Analysis of Observational Studies," *European Journal of Preventive Cardiology* 24, no. 7 (2017): 735–747.

61. W. Li, W. Ruan, et al., "Soy and the Risk of Type 2 Diabetes Mellitus: A Systematic Review and Meta-Analysis of Observational Studies," *Diabetes Research and Clinical Practice* 137 (2018): 190–199.

62. A. Kurrat, T. Blei, et al., "Lifelong Exposure to Dietary Isoflavones Reduces Risk of Obesity in Ovariectomized Wistar Rats," *Molecular Nutrition and Food Research* 59, no. 12 (2015): 2407–2418.

63. N. Haghighat, D. Ashtary-Larky, et al., "Effects of 6 Months of Soy-Enriched High Protein Compared to Eucaloric Low Protein Snack Replacement on Appetite, Dietary Intake, and Body Composition in Normal-Weight Obese Women: A Randomized Controlled Trial," *Nutrients* 13, no. 7 (2021): 1–15.

64. M. Akhlaghi, M. Zare, et al., "Effect of Soy and Soy Isoflavones on Obesity-Related Anthropometric Measures: A Systematic Review and Meta-Analysis of Randomized Controlled Clinical Trials," *Advances in Nutrition* 8, no. 5 (2017): 705–717.

65. N. S. Chatterjee, P. K. Dara, et al., "Nanoencapsulation in Low-Molecular-Weight Chitosan Improves in Vivo Antioxidant Potential of Black Carrot Anthocyanin," *Journal of the Science of Food and Agriculture* 101, no. 12 (2021): 5264–5271.

66. T. Ahmad, M. Cawood, et al., "Phytochemicals in *Daucus carota* and Their Health Benefits—Review Article," *Foods* 8, no. 9 (2019): 1–22.

67. B. J. Burri, M. R. La Frano, et al., "Absorption, Metabolism, and Functions of β-Cryptoxanthin," *Nutrition Reviews* 74, no. 2 (2016): 69–82.

68. H. Hara, H. Takahashi, et al., "β-Cryptoxanthin Induces UCP-1 Expression via a RAR Pathway in Adipose Tissue," *Journal of Agricultural and Food Chemistry* 67, no. 38 (2019): 10595–10603.

69. K. Takayanagi, "Prevention of Adiposity by the Oral Administration of β-Cryptoxanthin," *Frontiers in Neurology* 2, no. 67 (2011): 1–6.

70. N. Yao, S. Yan, et al., "The Association Between Carotenoids and Subjects with Overweight or Obesity: A Systematic Review and Meta-Analysis," *Food and Function* 12 (2021): 4768–4782.

71. I. Sluijs, J. W. J. Beulens, et al., "Dietary Carotenoid Intake Is Associated with Lower Prevalence of Metabolic Syndrome in Middle-Aged and Elderly Men," *Journal of Nutrition* 139, no. 5 (2009): 987–992.

72. K. Fujihara, S. Nogawa, et al., "Carrot Consumption Frequency Associated with Reduced BMI and Obesity Through the SNP Intermediary rs4445711," *Nutrients* 13, no. 10 (2021): 1–11.

73. "Genome-Wide Association Studies Fact Sheet," National Human Genome Research Institute, last updated August 17, 2020, www.genome.gov/about-genomics/fact-sheets/Genome-Wide-Association-Studies-Fact-Sheet.

74. S. Dato, F. De Rango, et al., "Antioxidants and Quality of Aging: Further Evidences for a Major Role of TXNRD1 Gene Variability on Physical Performance at Old Age," *Oxidative Medicine and Cellular Longevity* 2015 (2015): 1–8.

75. H. Li, Y. Tian, et al., "Reviewing the World's Edible Mushroom Species: A New Evidence-Based Classification System," *Comprehensive Reviews in Food Science and Food Safety* 20, no. 2 (2021): 1982–2014.

76. B. V. McCleary and A. Draga, "Measurement of β-Glucan in Mushrooms and Mycelial Products," *Journal of AOAC International* 99, no. 2 (2016): 364–373.

77. V. Casieri, M. Matteucci, et al., "Long-Term Intake of Pasta Containing Barley (1-3) Beta-D-Glucan Increases Neovascularization-Mediated Cardioprotection Through Endothelial Upregulation of Vascular Endothelial Growth Factor and Parkin," *Scientific Reports* 7, no. 13424 (2017): 1–16; S. Agostini, E. Chiavacci, et al., "Barley Beta-Glucan Promotes MnSOD Expression and Enhances Angiogenesis Under Oxidative Microenvironment," *Journal of Cellular and Molecular Medicine* 19, no. 1 (2015): 227–238; K. Yamamoto, T. Kimura, et al., "Anti-Angiogenic and Anti-Metastatic Effects of Beta-1,3-D-Glucan Purified from Hanabiratake, Sparassis crispa," *Biological and Pharmaceutical Bulletin* 32, no. 2 (2009): 259–263.

78. D. Akramiene, A. Kondrotas, et al., "Effects of Beta-Glucans on the Immune System," *Medicina* 43, no. 8 (2007): 597–606; G. C.-F. Chan, W. K. Chan, et al., "The Effects of Beta-Glucan on Human Immune and Cancer Cells," *Journal of Hematology and Oncology* 2, no. 25 (2009): 1–11; L. Wu, J. Zhao, et al., "Antitumor Effect of Soluble β-Glucan as an Immune Stimulant," *International Journal of Biological Macromolecules* 179 (2021): 116–124.

79. K. H. Poddar, M. Ames, et al, "Positive Effect of Mushrooms Substituted for Meat on Body Weight, Body Composition, and Health Parameters. A 1-Year Randomized Clinical Trial," *Appetite* 71 (2013): 379–387.

80. L. Dicks, L. Jakobs, et al., "Fortifying a Meal with Oyster Mushroom Powder Beneficially Affects Postprandial Glucagon-Like Peptide-1, Non-Esterified Free Fatty Acids and Hunger Sensation in Adults with Impaired Glucose Tolerance: A Double-Blind Randomized Controlled Crossover Trial," *European Journal of Nutrition* 61, no. 2 (2022): 687–701.

81. S. Imai, N. Tsuge, "An Onion Enzyme That Makes the Eyes Water," *Nature* 419 (2002): 685.

82. C. Zhang, X. He, et al., "Allicin Regulates Energy Homeostasis Through Brown Adipose Tissue," *iScience* 23, no. 5 (2020): 101113.

83. M. Liu, P. Yang, et al., "Allicin Protects Against Myocardial I/R by Accelerating Angiogenesis via the miR-19a-3p/PI3K/AKT Axis," *Aging* 13, no. 19 (2021): 22843–22855; D. De Greef, E. M. Barton, et al., "Anticancer Potential of Garlic and Its Bioactive Constituents: A Systematic and Comprehensive Review," *Seminars in Cancer Biology* 73 (2021): 219–264.

84. V. M. Dirsch, A. K. Kiemer, et al., "Effect of Allicin and Ajoene, Two Compounds of Garlic, on Inducible Nitric Oxide Synthase," *Atherosclerosis* 139, no. 2 (1998): 333–339.

85. R. Bernini and F. Velotti, "Natural Polyphenols as Immunomodulators to Rescue Immune Response Homeostasis: Quercetin as a Research Model Against Severe COVID-19," *Molecules (Basel, Switzerland)* 26, no. 5803 (2021): 1–21; D. Xu, M.-J. Hu, et al., "Antioxidant Activities of Quercetin and Its Complexes for Medicinal Application," *Molecules* 24, no. 1123 (2019): 1–15; Y. Tan, C. C. Tam, et al., "Quercetin Ameliorates Insulin Resistance and Restores Gut Microbiome in Mice on High-Fat Diets," *Antioxidants* 10, no. 1251 (2021): 1–17; Y. Wang, M. Xiong, et al., "Quercetin Promotes Locomotor Function Recovery and Axonal Regeneration Through Induction of Autophagy After Spinal Cord Injury," *Clinical and Experimental Pharmacology and Physiology* 48, no. 12 (2021): 1642–1652; I. G. Osojnik Črnivec, M. Skrt, et al., "Waste Streams in Onion Production: Bioactive Compounds, Quercetin and Use of Antimicrobial and Antioxidative Properties," *Waste Management* 126 (2021):

476–486; D. J. Perdicaro, C. Rodriguez Lanzi, et al., "Quercetin Attenuates Adipose Hypertrophy, in Part Through Activation of Adipogenesis in Rats Fed a High-Fat Diet," *Journal of Nutritional Biochemistry* 79 (2020): 1–8.

86. Y. Pei, D. Otieno, et al., "Effect of Quercetin on Nonshivering Thermogenesis of Brown Adipose Tissue in High-Fat Diet-Induced Obese Mice," *Journal of Nutritional Biochemistry* 88 (2021): 1–8; L. A. Forney, N. A. Lenard, et al., "Dietary Quercetin Attenuates Adipose Tissue Expansion and Inflammation and Alters Adipocyte Morphology in a Tissue-Specific Manner," *International Journal of Molecular Sciences* 19, no. 895 (2018): 1–13.

87. M. Nishimura, T. Muro, et al., "Effect of Daily Ingestion of Quercetin-Rich Onion Powder for 12 Weeks on Visceral Fat: A Randomised, Double-Blind, Placebo-Controlled, Parallel-Group Study," *Nutrients* 12, no. 91 (2019): 1–12.

88. J. Kim and I. Jo, "Relationship Between Body Mass Index and Alanine Aminotransferase Concentration in Non-Diabetic Korean Adults," *European Journal of Clinical Nutrition* 64, no. 2 (2010): 169–175.

89. M. Kumar, M. D. Barbhai, et al., "Onion (Allium cepa L.) Peels: A Review on Bioactive Compounds and Biomedical Activities," *Biomedicine and Pharmacotherapy = Biomedicine and Pharmacotherapie* 146 (2022): 1–15.

90. J.-S. Lee, Y.-J. Cha, et al., "Onion Peel Extract Reduces the Percentage of Body Fat in Overweight and Obese Subjects: A 12-Week, Randomized, Double-Blind, Placebo-Controlled Study," *Nutrition Research and Practice* 10, no. 2 (2016): 175–181.

91. H. V. Beretta, F. Bannoud, et al., "Relationships Between Bioactive Compound Content and the Antiplatelet and Antioxidant Activities of Six *Allium* Vegetable Species," *Food Technology and Biotechnology* 55, no. 2 (2017): 266–275.

92. P. Arulselvan, C.-C. Wen, et al., "Dietary Administration of Scallion Extract Effectively Inhibits Colorectal Tumor Growth: Cellular and Molecular Mechanisms in Mice," *PloS One* 7, no. 9 (2012): 1–14.

93. B. B. Petrovska and S. Cekovska. "Extracts from the History and Medical Properties of Garlic," *Pharmacognosy Reviews* 4, no. 7 (2010): 106–110.

94. A. A. Sangouni, M. Alizadeh, et al., "Effects of Garlic Powder Supplementation on Metabolic Syndrome Components, Insulin Resistance, Fatty Liver Index, and Appetite in Subjects with Metabolic Syndrome: A Randomized Clinical Trial," *Phytotherapy Research: PTR* 35, no. 8 (2021): 4433–4441.

95. L. Perry, R. Dickau, et al., "Starch Fossils and the Domestication and Dispersal of Chili Peppers (Capsicum spp. L.) in the Americas," *Science* 315, no. 5814 (2007): 986–988.

96. S. Varghese, P. Kubatka, et al., "Chili Pepper as a Body Weight-Loss Food," *International Journal of Food Sciences and Nutrition* 68, no. 4 (2017): 392–401.

97. J.-S. Lee, S.-G. Kim, et al., "Acute Effects of Capsaicin on Proopioimelanocortin mRNA Levels in the Arcuate Nucleus of Sprague-Dawley Rats," *Psychiatry Investigation* 9, no. 2 (2012): 187–190.

98. S. Snitker, Y. Fujishima, et al., "Effects of Novel Capsinoid Treatment on Fatness and Energy Metabolism in Humans: Possible Pharmacogenetic Implications," *American Journal of Clinical Nutrition* 89, no. 1 (2009): 45–50.

Chapter 7: Treasure Hunt

1. Legumes are very common in Asian diets but tend to be fresh, such as snap peas or soybeans, or fermented, such as soybean paste.

2. S. Lösch, N. Moghaddam, et al., "Stable Isotope and Trace Element Studies on Gladiators and Contemporary Romans from Ephesus (Turkey, 2nd and 3rd Ct. AD)—Implications for Differences in Diet," *PloS One* 9, no. 10 (2014): 1–17.

3. F. Roy, J. I. Boye, et al., "Bioactive Proteins and Peptides in Pulse Crops: Pea, Chickpea and Lentil," *Food Research International* 43 (2010): 432–442.

4. M. T. Eng, "Chow: Navy Bean Soup," *Naval Historical Foundation*, www.navyhistory.org/2016/04/chow-navy-bean-soup/.

5. US Senate, "About Traditions and Symbols: Senate Bean Soup," Art and History, https://www.senate.gov/about/traditions-symbols/senate-bean-soup.htm.

6. V. Caracuta, O. Barzilai, et al., "The Onset of Faba Bean Farming in the Southern Levant," *Scientific Reports* 5 (2015): 1–9.

7. L. A. Bazzano, J. He, et al., "Legume Consumption and Risk of Coronary Heart Disease in US Men and Women: NHANES I Epidemiologic Follow-up Study," *Archives of Internal Medicine* 161, no. 21 (2001): 2573–2578; B. L. Luhovyy, R. C. Mollard, et al., "Canned Navy Bean Consumption Reduces Metabolic Risk Factors Associated with Obesity," *Canadian Journal of Dietetic Practice and Research* 76, no. 1 (2015): 33–37.

8. The beans were commercially available (H. J. Heinz) original beans in tomato sauce, original beans with pork in tomato sauce, deep-browned beans in tomato sauce, deep-browned beans with pork in tomato sauce, maple-style beans, and original beans with port and molasses.

9. S. Lemieux, D. Prud'homme, et al., "A Single Threshold Value of Waist Girth Identifies Normal-Weight and Overweight Subjects with Excess Visceral Adipose Tissue," *American Journal of Clinical Nutrition* 64, no. 5 (1996): 685–693.

10. E. L. de Hollander, W. J. Bemelmans, et al., "The Association Between Waist Circumference and Risk of Mortality Considering Body Mass Index in 65- to 74-Year-Olds: A Meta-Analysis of 29 Cohorts Involving More Than 58 000 Elderly Persons," *International Journal of Epidemiology* 41, no. 3 (2012): 805–817.

11. M. A. G. Hernández, E. E. Canfora, et al., "The Short-Chain Fatty Acid Acetate in Body Weight Control and Insulin Sensitivity," *Nutrients* 11, no. 8 (2019): 1–32.

12. N. Siva, C. R. Johnson, et al., "Lentil (Lens culinaris Medikus) Diet Affects the Gut Microbiome and Obesity Markers in Rat," *Journal of Agricultural and Food Chemistry* 66, no. 33 (2018): 8805–8813.

13. R. C. Mollard, B. L. Luhovyy, et al., "Regular Consumption of Pulses for 8 Weeks Reduces Metabolic Syndrome Risk Factors in Overweight and Obese Adults," *British Journal of Nutrition* 108 (2012): S111–S122.

14. S. J. Kim, R. J. de Souza, et al., "Effects of Dietary Pulse Consumption on Body Weight: A Systematic Review and Meta-Analysis of Randomized Controlled Trials," *American Journal of Clinical Nutrition* 103, no. 5 (2016): 1213–1223.

15. C. Papandreou, N. Becerra-Tomás, et al., "Legume Consumption and Risk of All-Cause, Cardiovascular, and Cancer Mortality in the PREDIMED Study," *Clinical Nutrition* 38, no. 1 (2019): 348–356.

16. D. El Khoury, C. Cuda, et al., "Beta Glucan: Health Benefits in Obesity and Metabolic Syndrome," *Journal of Nutrition and Metabolism* (2012): 1–28.

17. C. Shimizu, M. Kihara, et al., "Effect of High Beta-Glucan Barley on Serum Cholesterol Concentrations and Visceral Fat Area in Japanese Men—A Randomized, Double-Blinded, Placebo-Controlled Trial," *Plant Foods for Human Nutrition* 63, no. 1 (2008): 21–25.

18. D. Luna-Vital, I. Luzardo-Ocampo, et al., "Maize Extract Rich in Ferulic Acid and Anthocyanins Prevents High-Fat-Induced Obesity in Mice by Modulating SIRT1, AMPK and IL-6 Associated Metabolic and Inflammatory Pathways," *Journal of Nutritional Biochemistry* 79 (2020): 1–15; Q. Zhang, E. G. de Mejia, et al., "Relationship of Phenolic Composition of Selected Purple Maize (Zea mays L.) Genotypes with Their Anti-Inflammatory, Anti-Adipogenic and Anti-Diabetic Potential," *Food Chemistry* 289 (2019): 739–750.

19. H.-J. Kim, K. A. Koo, et al., "Anti-Obesity Activity of Anthocyanin and Carotenoid Extracts from Color-Fleshed Sweet Potatoes," *Journal of Food Biochemistry* (2020): e13438.

20. Y. Ding, Z. Gu, et al., "Clove Extract Functions as a Natural Fatty Acid Synthesis Inhibitor and Prevents Obesity in a Mouse Model," *Food and Function* 8, no. 8 (2017): 2847–2856.

21. X. Yuan, G. Wei, et al., "Rutin Ameliorates Obesity Through Brown Fat Activation," *FASEB* 31, no. 1 (2017): 333–345.

22. L. Cheng, L. Shi, et al., "Rutin-Activated Adipose Tissue Thermogenesis Is Correlated with Increased Intestinal Short-Chain Fatty Acid Levels," *Phytotherapy Research* 36, no. 6 (2022): 2495–2510.

23. S.-Y. Kim, M.-S. Lee, et al., "Tartary Buckwheat Extract Attenuated the Obesity-Induced Inflammation and Increased Muscle PGC-1a/SIRT1 Expression in High Fat Diet-Induced Obese Rats," *Nutrients* 11, no. 3 (2019): 1–14; H. Tomotake, N. Yamamoto, et al., "High Protein Buckwheat Flour Suppresses Hypercholesterolemia in Rats and Gallstone Formation in Mice by Hypercholesterolemic Diet and Body Fat in Rats Because of Its Low Protein Digestibility," *Nutrition* 22, no. 2 (2006): 166–173.

24. S. C. Chai, S. Hooshmand, et al., "Daily Apple versus Dried Plum: Impact on Cardiovascular Disease Risk Factors in Postmenopausal Women," *Journal of the Academy of Nutrition and Dietetics* 112, no. 8 (2012): 1158–1168.

25. E. Lever, S. M. Scott, et al., "The Effect of Prunes on Stool Output, Gut Transit Time and Gastrointestinal Microbiota: A Randomised Controlled Trial," *Clinical Nutrition* 38, no. 1 (2019): 165–173.

26. J. Bouayed, H. Rammal, et al., "Chlorogenic Acid, a Polyphenol from Prunus Domestica (Mirabelle), with Coupled Anxiolytic and Antioxidant Effects," *Journal of the Neurological Sciences* 262 (2007): 77–84.

27. M. L. Bertoia, K. J. Mukamal, et al., "Changes in Intake of Fruits and Vegetables and Weight Change in United States Men and Women Followed for up to 24 Years: Analysis from Three Prospective Cohort Studies," *PLoS Medicine* 12, no. 9 (2015): 1–20.

28. S. Bu, C. Yuan, et al., "Concentrated Extract of Prunus Mume Fruit Exerts Dual Effects in 3T3-L1 Adipocytes by Inhibiting Adipogenesis and Inducing Beiging/Browning," *Food and Nutrition Research* 65 (2021): 1–14.

29. K. H. Poddar, M. Ames, et al., "Positive Effect of Mushrooms Substituted for Meat on Body Weight, Body Composition, and Health Parameters. A 1-Year Randomized Clinical Trial," *Appetite* 71 (2013): 379–387; L. Dicks, L. Jakobs, et al., "Fortifying a Meal with Oyster Mushroom Powder Beneficially Affects Postprandial Glucagon-Like Peptide-1, Non-Esterified Free Fatty Acids and Hunger Sensation in Adults with Impaired Glucose Tolerance: A Double-Blind Randomized Controlled Crossover Trial," *European Journal of Nutrition* 61, no. 2 (2022): 687–701.

30. F. Galvão Cândido, F. X. Valente, et al., "Consumption of Extra Virgin Olive Oil Improves Body Composition and Blood Pressure in Women with Excess Body Fat: A

Randomized, Double-Blinded, Placebo-Controlled Clinical Trial," *European Journal of Nutrition* 57, no. 7 (2018): 2445–2455.

31. P. Royle and N. Waugh, "Literature Searching for Clinical and Cost-Effectiveness Studies Used in Health Technology Assessment Reports Carried Out for the National Institute for Clinical Excellence Appraisal System," *Health Technology Assessment* 7, no. 34 (2003): iii, ix–x, 1–51.

32. J. D. P. Ramírez-Anaya, C. Samaniego-Sánchez, et al., "Phenols and the Antioxidant Capacity of Mediterranean Vegetables Prepared with Extra Virgin Olive Oil Using Different Domestic Cooking Techniques," *Food Chemistry* 188 (2015): 430–438.

33. D. Yagnik, V. Serafin, et al., "Antimicrobial Activity of Apple Cider Vinegar Against Escherichia coli, Staphylococcus aureus and Candida albicans; Downregulating Cytokine and Microbial Protein Expression," *Scientific Reports* 8, no. 1 (2018): 1–12.

34. C. S. Johnston, C. M. Kim, et al., "Vinegar Improves Insulin Sensitivity to a High-Carbohydrate Meal in Subjects with Insulin Resistance or Type 2 Diabetes," *Diabetes Care* 27, no. 1 (2004): 281–282; F. Shishehbor, A. Mansoori, et al., "Vinegar Consumption Can Attenuate Postprandial Glucose and Insulin Responses; A Systematic Review and Meta-Analysis of Clinical Trials," *Diabetes Research and Clinical Practice* 127 (2017): 1–9.

35. H. Yamashita, K. Fujisawa, et al., "Improvement of Obesity and Glucose Tolerance by Acetate in Type 2 Diabetic Otsuka Long-Evans Tokushima Fatty (OLETF) Rats," *Bioscience, Biotechnology, and Biochemistry* 71, no. 5 (2007): 1236–1243.

36. T. Kondo, M. Kishi, et al., "Vinegar Intake Reduces Body Weight, Body Fat Mass, and Serum Triglyceride Levels in Obese Japanese Subjects," *Bioscience, Biotechnology, and Biochemistry* 73, no. 8 (2009): 1837–1843.

37. S.-J. Jang, Y.-J. Kim, et al., "Analysis of Microflora in Gochujang, Korean Traditional Fermented Food," *Food Science and Biotechnology* 20, no. 5 (2011): 1435–1440.

38. P. Mahoro, H.-J. Moon, et al., "Protective Effect of *Gochujang* on Inflammation in a DSS-Induced Colitis Rat Model," *Foods* 10, no. 5 (2021): 1–12; M. C. Dao, A. Everard, et al., "Akkermansia Muciniphila and Improved Metabolic Health During a Dietary Intervention in Obesity: Relationship with Gut Microbiome Richness and Ecology," *Gut* 65, no. 3 (2016): 426–436; B. Routy, E. Le Chatelier, et al., "Gut Microbiome Influences Efficacy of PD-1-Based Immunotherapy Against Epithelial Tumors," *Science* 359, no. 6371 (2018): 91–97.

39. Y.-S. Cha, S.-R. Kim, et al., "Kochujang, Fermented Soybean-Based Red Pepper Paste, Decreases Visceral Fat and Improves Blood Lipid Profiles in Overweight Adults," *Nutrition and Metabolism* 10, no. 1 (2013): 1–8.

40. J. E. Park, S.-H. Oh, et al., "*Lactobacillus Brevis* OPK-3 from Kimchi Prevents Obesity and Modulates the Expression of Adipogenic and Pro-Inflammatory Genes in Adipose Tissue of Diet-Induced Obese Mice," *Nutrients* 12, no. 3 (2020): 1–15; S. Y. Jo, E. A. Choi, et al., "Characterization of Starter Kimchi Fermented with Leuconostoc Kimchii GJ2 and Its Cholesterol-Lowering Effects in Rats Fed a High-Fat and High-Cholesterol Diet," *Journal of the Science of Food and Agriculture* 95, no. 13 (2015): 2750–2756.

41. S. Lim, J. H. Moon, et al., "Effect of Lactobacillus Sakei, a Probiotic Derived from Kimchi, on Body Fat in Koreans with Obesity: A Randomized Controlled Study," *Endocrinology and Metabolism* 35, no. 2 (2020): 425–434.

42. E. K. Kim, S.-Y. An, et al., "Fermented Kimchi Reduces Body Weight and Improves Metabolic Parameters in Overweight and Obese Patients," *Nutrition Research* 31, no. 6 (2011): 436–443.

43. C. Gärtner, W. Stahl, et al., "Lycopene Is More Bioavailable from Tomato Paste Than from Fresh Tomatoes," *American Journal of Clinical Nutrition* 66, no. 1 (1997): 116–122; N. Z. Unlu, T. Bohn, et al., "Lycopene from Heat-Induced Cis-Isomer-Rich Tomato Sauce Is More Bioavailable Than from All-Trans-Rich Tomato Sauce in Human Subjects," *British Journal of Nutrition* 98, no. 1 (2007): 140–146.

44. R. B. Toma, G. C. Frank, et al., "Lycopene Content in Raw Tomato Varieties and Tomato Products," *Journal of Food Service* 19, no. 2 (2008): 127–132.

45. X. Li, B. Xing, et al., "Network Pharmacology-Based Research Uncovers Cold Resistance and Thermogenesis Mechanism of Cinnamomum cassia," *Fitoterapia* 149 (2021): 1–15.

46. H. Y. Kwan, J. Wu, et al., "Cinnamon Induces Browning in Subcutaneous Adipocytes," *Scientific Reports* 7, no. 1 (2017): 1–12.

47. M. Rodrigues, C. Bertoncini-Silva, et al., "Beneficial Effects of Eugenol Supplementation on Gut Microbiota and Hepatic Steatosis in High-Fat-Fed Mice," *Food and Function* 13, no. 6 (2022): 3381–3390.

48. B. P. Lopes, T. G. Gaique, et al., "Cinnamon Extract Improves the Body Composition and Attenuates Lipogenic Processes in the Liver and Adipose Tissue of Rats," *Food and Function* 6, no. 10 (2015): 3257–3265.

49. S. G. Jain, S. Puri, et al., "Effect of Oral Cinnamon Intervention on Metabolic Profile and Body Composition of Asian Indians with Metabolic Syndrome: A Randomized Double-Blind Control Trial," *Lipids in Health and Disease* 16, no. 113 (2017): 1–11.

50. www.fao.org/nutrition/education/food-dietary-guidelines/regions/countries/india/en/.

51. X. Li, H.-Y. Lu, et al., "Cinnamomum Cassia Extract Promotes Thermogenesis During Exposure to Cold via Activation of Brown Adipose Tissue," *Journal of Ethnopharmacology* 266 (2021): 1–14; Y. Tamura, Y. Iwasaki, et al., "Ingestion of Cinnamaldehyde, a TRPA1 Agonist, Reduces Visceral Fats in Mice Fed a High-Fat and High-Sucrose Diet," *Journal of Nutritional Science and Vitaminology* 58, no. 1 (2012): 9–13.

52. Y.-H. Wang, B. Avula, et al., "Cassia Cinnamon as a Source of Coumarin in Cinnamon-Flavored Food and Food Supplements in the United States," *Journal of Agricultural and Food Chemistry* 61, no. 18 (2013): 4470–4476; F. Woehrlin, H. Fry, et al., "Quantification of Flavoring Constituents in Cinnamon: High Variation of Coumarin in Cassia Bark from the German Retail Market and in Authentic Samples from Indonesia," *Journal of Agricultural and Food Chemistry* 58, no. 19 (2010): 10568–10575.

53. J. Sharifi-Rad, Y. El Rayess, et al., "Turmeric and Its Major Compound Curcumin on Health: Bioactive Effects and Safety Profiles for Food, Pharmaceutical, Biotechnological and Medicinal Applications," *Frontiers in Pharmacology* 11 (2020): 1–23.

54. M. Okla, J. Kim, et al., "Dietary Factors Promoting Brown and Beige Fat Development and Thermogenesis," *Advances in Nutrition* 8, no. 3 (2017): 473–483; L.-Y. Wu, C.-W. Chen, et al., "Curcumin Attenuates Adipogenesis by Inducing Preadipocyte Apoptosis and Inhibiting Adipocyte Differentiation," *Nutrients* 11, no. 10 (2019): 1–22; S. Wang, X. Wang, et al., "Curcumin Promotes Browning of White Adipose Tissue in a Norepinephrine-Dependent Way," *Biochemical and Biophysical Research Communications* 466, no. 2 (2015): 247–253.

55. T. Islam, I. Koboziev, et al., "Curcumin Reduces Adipose Tissue Inflammation and Alters Gut Microbiota in Diet-Induced Obese Male Mice," *Molecular Nutrition and Food Research* 65, no. 22 (2021): 1–12.

56. T. Teich, J. A. Pivovarov, et al., "Curcumin Limits Weight Gain, Adipose Tissue Growth, and Glucose Intolerance Following the Cessation of Exercise and Caloric Restriction in Rats," *Journal of Applied Physiology* 123, no. 6 (2017): 1625–1634.

57. F. Di Pierro, A. Bressan, et al., "Potential Role of Bioavailable Curcumin in Weight Loss and Omental Adipose Tissue Decrease: Preliminary Data of a Randomized, Controlled Trial in Overweight People with Metabolic Syndrome. Preliminary Study," *European Review for Medical and Pharmacological Sciences* 19, no. 21 (2015): 4195–4202.

58. G. Shoba, D. Joy, et al., "Influence of Piperine on the Pharmacokinetics of Curcumin in Animals and Human Volunteers," *Planta Medica* 64, no. 4 (1998): 353–356.

59. S. M. Mousavi, A. Milajerdi, et al., "The Effects of Curcumin Supplementation on Body Weight, Body Mass Index and Waist Circumference: A Systematic Review and Dose-Response Meta-Analysis of Randomized Controlled Trials," *Critical Reviews in Food Science and Nutrition* 60, no. 1 (2020): 171–180.

60. J. Rogers, S. L. Urbina, et al., "Capsaicinoids Supplementation Decreases Percent Body Fat and Fat Mass: Adjustment Using Covariates in a Post Hoc Analysis," *BMC Obesity* 5 (2018): 1–10.

61. E. Lecumberri, L. Goya, et al., "A Diet Rich in Dietary Fiber from Cocoa Improves Lipid Profile and Reduces Malondialdehyde in Hypercholesterolemic Rats," *Nutrition* 23, no. 4 (2007): 332–341.

62. M. Wiese, Y. Bashmakov, et al., "Prebiotic Effect of Lycopene and Dark Chocolate on Gut Microbiome with Systemic Changes in Liver Metabolism, Skeletal Muscles and Skin in Moderately Obese Persons," *BioMed Research International* (2019): 1–15.

63. Y. Yamashita, M. Okabe, et al., "Prevention Mechanisms of Glucose Intolerance and Obesity by Cacao Liquor Procyanidin Extract in High-Fat Diet-Fed C57BL/6 Mice," *Archives of Biochemistry and Biophysics* 527, no. 2 (2012): 95–104.

64. Y. Gu, S. Yu, et al., "Dietary Cocoa Reduces Metabolic Endotoxemia and Adipose Tissue Inflammation in High-Fat Fed Mice," *Journal of Nutritional Biochemistry* 25, no. 4 (2014): 439–445.

65. T. Mitani, S. Watanabe, et al., "Theobromine Suppresses Adipogenesis Through Enhancement of CCAAT-Enhancer-Binding Protein β Degradation by Adenosine Receptor A1," *Biochimica et Biophysica Acta–Molecular Cell Research* 1864, no. 12 (2017): 2438–2448.

66. S. G. West, M. D. McIntyre, et al., "Effects of Dark Chocolate and Cocoa Consumption on Endothelial Function and Arterial Stiffness in Overweight Adults," *British Journal of Nutrition* 111, no. 4 (2014): 653–661.

67. M. Cuenca-García, J. R. Ruiz, et al., "Association Between Chocolate Consumption and Fatness in European Adolescents," *Nutrition* 30, no. 2 (2014): 236–239.

68. J. A. Greenberg and B. Buijsse, "Habitual Chocolate Consumption May Increase Body Weight in a Dose-Response Manner," *PloS One* 8, no. 8 (2013): e70271.

69. E. T. Massolt, P. M. van Haard, et al., "Appetite Suppression Through Smelling of Dark Chocolate Correlates with Changes in Ghrelin in Young Women," *Regulatory Peptides* 161, nos. 1–3 (2010): 81–86.

70. S. Naghshi, M. Sadeghian, et al., "Association of Total Nut, Tree Nut, Peanut, and Peanut Butter Consumption with Cancer Incidence and Mortality: A Comprehensive Systematic Review and Dose-Response Meta-Analysis of Observational Studies," *Advances in Nutrition* 12, no. 3 (2021): 793–808; M. Guasch-Ferré, X. Liu, et al., "Nut Consumption and Risk of Cardiovascular Disease," *Journal of the American College of Cardiology*

70, no. 20 (2017): 2519–2532; A. J. Ahola, C. M. Forsblom, et al., "Nut Consumption Is Associated with Lower Risk of Metabolic Syndrome and Its Components in Type 1 Diabetes," *Nutrients* 13, no. 11 (2021): 1–11; H. Li, X. Li, et al., "Nut Consumption and Risk of Metabolic Syndrome and Overweight/Obesity: A Meta-Analysis of Prospective Cohort Studies and Randomized Trials," *Nutrition and Metabolism* 15, no. 46 (2018): 1–10.

71. A. M. Tindall, C. J. McLimans, et al., "Walnuts and Vegetable Oils Containing Oleic Acid Differentially Affect the Gut Microbiota and Associations with Cardiovascular Risk Factors: Follow-up of a Randomized, Controlled, Feeding Trial in Adults at Risk for Cardiovascular Disease," *Journal of Nutrition* 150, no. 4 (2020): 806–817; S.-M. Ren, Q.-Z. Zhang, et al., "Anti-NAFLD Effect of Defatted Walnut Powder Extract in High Fat Diet-Induced C57BL/6 Mice by Modulating the Gut Microbiota," *Journal of Ethnopharmacology* 270 (2021): 1–10.

72. E. P. Neale, L. C. Tapsell, et al., "Impact of Providing Walnut Samples in a Lifestyle Intervention for Weight Loss: A Secondary Analysis of the Healthtrack Trial," *Food and Nutrition Research* 61, no. 1 (2017): 1–9.

73. L. C. Tapsell, M. Lonergan, et al., "Interdisciplinary Lifestyle Intervention for Weight Management in a Community Population (Healthtrack Study): Study Design and Baseline Sample Characteristics," *Contemporary Clinical Trials* 45, no. Pt B (2015): 394–403.

74. "Australian Guide to Healthy Eating," Eat for Health, January 5, 2017, www.eatfor health.gov.au/guidelines/australian-guide-healthy-eating.

75. M. Bes-Rastrollo, N. M. Wedick, et al., "Prospective Study of Nut Consumption, Long-Term Weight Change, and Obesity Risk in Women," *American Journal of Clinical Nutrition* 89, no. 6 (2009): 1913–1919.

76. M. Bes-Rastrollo, J. Sabaté, et al., "Nut Consumption and Weight Gain in a Mediterranean Cohort: The SUN Study," *Obesity* 15, no. 1 (2007): 107–116.

77. C. Franchi, I. Ardoino, et al., "Inverse Association Between Canned Fish Consumption and Colorectal Cancer Risk: Analysis of Two Large Case-Control Studies," *Nutrients* 14, no. 8 (2022): 1–9.

78. M. I. McBurney, N. L. Tintle, et al., "Using an Erythrocyte Fatty Acid Fingerprint to Predict Risk of All-Cause Mortality: The Framingham Offspring Cohort," *American Journal of Clinical Nutrition* 114, no. 4 (2021): 1447–1454.

79. T. B. Ahmad, D. Rudd, et al., "Correlation Between Fatty Acid Profile and Anti-Inflammatory Activity in Common Australian Seafood By-Products," *Marine Drugs* 17, no. 3 (2019): 1–20.

Chapter 8: The Daily Catch

1. S. H. Jónasdóttir, "Fatty Acid Profiles and Production in Marine Phytoplankton," *Marine Drugs* 17, no. 3 (2019): 151.

2. M. Fernández-Galilea, E. Félix-Soriano, et al., "Omega-3 Fatty Acids as Regulators of Brown/Beige Adipose Tissue: From Mechanisms to Therapeutic Potential," *Journal of Physiology and Biochemistry* 76, no. 2 (2020): 251–267; M. Pahlavani, F. Razafimanjato, et al., "Eicosapentaenoic Acid Regulates Brown Adipose Tissue Metabolism in High-Fat-Fed Mice and in Clonal Brown Adipocytes," *Journal of Nutritional Biochemistry* 39 (2017): 101–109.

3. N. S. Kalupahana, B. L. Goonapienuwala, et al., "Omega-3 Fatty Acids and Adipose Tissue: Inflammation and Browning," *Annual Review of Nutrition* 40 (2020): 25–49; E. Titos and J. Clària, "Omega-3-Derived Mediators Counteract Obesity-Induced Adipose Tissue Inflammation," *Prostaglandins and Other Lipid Mediators* 107 (2013): 77–84.

4. M. C. Basil and B. D. Levy, "Specialized Pro-Resolving Mediators: Endogenous Regulators of Infection and Inflammation," *Nature Reviews Immunology* 16 (2016): 51–67.

5. A. Ramel, J. A. Martinez, et al., "Effects of Weight Loss and Seafood Consumption on Inflammation Parameters in Young, Overweight and Obese European Men and Women During 8 Weeks of Energy Restriction," *European Journal of Clinical Nutrition* 64, no. 9 (2010): 987–993.

6. A. Ramel, M. T. Jonsdottir, et al., "Consumption of Cod and Weight Loss in Young Overweight and Obese Adults on an Energy Reduced Diet for 8 Weeks," *Nutrition, Metabolism, and Cardiovascular Diseases* 19, no. 10 (2009): 690–696.

7. Y. Sun, B. Liu, et al., "Association of Fried Food Consumption with All Cause, Cardiovascular, and Cancer Mortality: Prospective Cohort Study," *BMJ Clinical Research* 364 (2019): k5420.

8. www.sciencedirect.com/topics/agricultural-and-biological-sciences/fish-roe.

9. A. Nawaz, Y. Nishida, et al., "Astaxanthin, a Marine Carotenoid, Maintains the Tolerance and Integrity of Adipose Tissue and Contributes to Its Healthy Functions," *Nutrients* 13, no. 12 (2021): 4374.

10. M. Wang, H. Ma, et al., "Astaxanthin from *Haematococcus pluvialis* Alleviates Obesity by Modulating Lipid Metabolism and Gut Microbiota in Mice Fed a High-Fat Diet," *Food and Function* 12, no. 20 (2021): 9719–9738.

11. Y. Xu, W. Jiang, et al., "Astaxanthin Induces Angiogenesis Through Wnt/β-Catenin Signaling Pathway," *Phytomedicine* 22, no. 7–8 (2015): 744–751; J. Kowshik, A. B. Baba, et al., "Astaxanthin Inhibits JAK/STAT-3 Signaling to Abrogate Cell Proliferation, Invasion and Angiogenesis in a Hamster Model of Oral Cancer," *PloS One* 9, no. 10 (2014): e109114; S. Mohammadi, A. Barzegari, et al., "Astaxanthin Protects Mesenchymal Stem Cells from Oxidative Stress by Direct Scavenging of Free Radicals and Modulation of Cell Signaling," *Chemico-Biological Interactions* 333 (2021): 109324.

12. K. Marimuthu, P. Gunaselvam, et al., "Antibacterial Activity of Ovary Extract from Sea Urchin Diadema Setosum," *European Review for Medical and Pharmacological Sciences* 19, no. 10 (2015): 1895–1899.

13. D. Zhou, L. Qin, et al., "Optimisation of Hydrolysis of Purple Sea Urchin (Strongylocentrotus nudus) Gonad by Response Surface Methodology and Evaluation of in Vitro Antioxidant Activity of the Hydrolysate," *Journal of the Science of Food and Agriculture* 92, no. 8 (2012): 1694–1701; P. Cirino, C. Brunet, et al., "The Sea Urchin Arbacia lixula: A Novel Natural Source of Astaxanthin," *Marine Drugs* 15, no. 6 (2017): 187.

14. B. Lauby-Secretan, D. Loomis, et al., "Carcinogenicity of Polychlorinated Biphenyls and Polybrominated Biphenyls," *Lancet Oncology* 14, no. 4 (2013): 287–288. doi:10.1016/S1470-2045(13)70104-9.

15. P. F. Zagalsky, "A Study of the Astaxanthin-Lipovitellin, Ovoverdin, Isolated from the Ovaries of the Lobster, Homarus gammarus (L.)," *Comparative Biochemistry and Physiology Part B: Comparative Biochemistry* 80, no. 3 (1985): 589–597; N. M. Young and R. E. Williams, "The Circular Dichroism of Ovoverdin and Other Carotenoproteins from

the Lobster Homarus americanus," *Canadian Journal of Biochemistry and Cell Biology–Revue Canadienne de Biochimie et Biologie Cellulaire* 61, no. 9 (1983): 1018–1024. doi:10.1139/o83-130.

16. B. S. Beltz, M. E. Tlusty, et al., "Omega-3 Fatty Acids Upregulate Adult Neurogenesis," *Neuroscience Letters* 415, no. 2 (2007): 154–158.

17. T. T. Nguyen, W. Zheng, et al., "Significant Enrichment of Polyunsaturated Fatty Acids (PUFAs) in the Lipids Extracted by Supercritical CO_2 from the Livers of Australian Rock Lobsters (Jasus edwardsii)," *Journal of Agricultural and Food Chemistry* 63, no. 18 (2015): 4621–4628.

18. A. Albalat, L. E. Nadler, et al., "Lipid Composition of Oil Extracted from Wasted Norway Lobster (Nephrops norvegicus) Heads and Comparison with Oil Extracted from Antarctic Krill (Euphasia superba)," *Marine Drugs* 14, no. 12 (2016): 219.

19. Q. Wang, Z. Fan, et al., "Occurrence and Health Risk Assessment of Residual Heavy Metals in the Chinese Mitten Crab (Eriocheir sinensis)," *Journal of Food Composition and Analysis* 97 (2021): 103787.

20. Q. Wang, Z. Fan, et al., "Occurrence and Health Risk Assessment of Residual Heavy Metals in the Chinese Mitten Crab (Eriocheir sinensis)," *Journal of Food Composition and Analysis* 97 (2021): 103787.

21. Q. Wang, W. Wu, et al., "Nutritional Quality of Different Grades of Adult Male Chinese Mitten Crab, *Eriocheir sinensis*," *Journal of Food Science and Technology* 55, no. 3 (2018): 944–955.

22. T. Kleekayai, P. A. Harnedy, et al., "Extraction of Antioxidant and ACE Inhibitory Peptides from Thai Traditional Fermented Shrimp Pastes," *Food Chemistry* 176 (2015): 441–447.

23. L.-Y. Lee, N. A. Normaiyudin, et al., "First Description of Mantis Shrimp, Miyakella Nepa (Latreille, 1828), Feeding Preference Behaviour in Captive Conditions," *Aquaculture Reports* 22 (2022): 100969.

24. M. Balzano, D. Pacetti, et al., "Bioactive Fatty Acids in Mantis Shrimp, Crab and Caramote Prawn: Their Content and Distribution Among the Main Lipid Classes," *Journal of Food Composition and Analysis* 59 (2017): 88–94.

25. H.-J. Lee, P. S. Saravana, et al., "Extraction of Bioactive Compounds from Oyster (Crassostrea Gigas) by Pressurized Hot Water Extraction," *Journal of Supercritical Fluids* 141 (2018): 120–127.

26. A. F. Aldairi, R. A. Alyamani, et al., "Antioxidant and Antithrombotic Effects of Green Mussels (Perna canaliculus) in Rats," *Journal of Food Biochemistry* 45, no. 9 (2021): e13865; S. A. Cunha, R. de Castro, et al., "Hydrolysate from Mussel *Mytilus galloprovincialis* Meat: Enzymatic Hydrolysis, Optimization and Bioactive Properties," *Molecules* 26, no. 17 (2021): 5228.

27. A. G. Winter, R. L. H. Deits, and A. E. Hosoi, "Localized Fluidization Burrowing Mechanics of *Ensis Directus*," *Journal of Experimental Biology* 215, no. 12 (2012): 2072–2080.

28. S. Matsunaga, H. Ikeda, and R. Sakai, "Pectenovarin, a New Ovarian Carotenoprotein from Japanese Scallop *Mizuhopecten yessoensis*," *Molecules* 25, no. 13 (2020): 3042.

29. E. Prato, F. Biandolino, et al., "Bioactive Fatty Acids of Three Commercial Scallop Species," *International Journal of Food Properties* 21, no. 1 (2018): 519–532.

30. A protein from the black sea cucumber (*Holothuria leucospilota*) causes cancer cells to kill themselves when they are exposed to the substance in cell culture. Another sea

cucumber bioactive called nobiliside D (not a protein) kills cells from leukemia and lung, cervical, and breast cancer.

31. L. Guo, Z. Gao, et al., "Saponin-Enriched Sea Cucumber Extracts Exhibit an Antiobesity Effect Through Inhibition of Pancreatic Lipase Activity and Upregulation of LXR-β Signaling," *Pharmaceutical Biology* 54, no. 8 (2016): 1312–1325.

32. A. Ramalho, N. Leblanc, et al., "Characterization of a Coproduct from the Sea Cucumber *Cucumaria frondose* and Its Effects on Visceral Adipocyte Size in Male Wistar Rats," *Marine Drugs* 18, no. 11 (2020): 530.

33. S. K. Nadarajah, R. Vijayaraj, J. Mani, "Therapeutic Significance of *Loligo vulgaris* (Lamarck, 1798) Ink Extract: A Biomedical Approach," *Pharmacognosy Research* 9, Suppl. 1 (2017): S105–S109; S. Chen, J. Wang, et al., "Sulfation of a Squid Ink Polysaccharide and Its Inhibitory Effect on Tumor Cell Metastasis," *Carbohydrate Polymers* 81, no. 3 (2010): 560–566.

34. S. S. Shakthi, S. P. Archana, et al., "Biochemical Composition of Cuttle Fish Sepia Prabahari Ink and Its Bioactive Properties In-Vitro," *International Journal of Pharmaceutical Sciences and Research* 7, no. 7 (2016): 2966–2975.

35. University of Virginia, "Squid Ink from Jurassic Period Identical to Modern Cuttlefish Ink," *ScienceDaily*, May 21, 2012, www.sciencedaily.com/releases/2012/05/120521163 753.htm.

36. D. Ayas, Y. Ozogul, et al., "The Effects of Season and Sex on Fat, Fatty Acids and Protein Contents of Sepia Officinalis in the Northeastern Mediterranean Sea," *International Journal of Food Sciences and Nutrition* 63, no. 4 (2012): 440–445.

37. S.-H. Cha, E. J. Han, et al., "Taurine-Containing Hot Water Extract of Octopus Ocellatus Meat Prevents Methylglyoxal-Induced Vascular Damage," *Advances in Experimental Medicine and Biology* 1155 (2019): 471–482.

38. A. Torrinha, R. Cruz, et al., "Octopus Lipid and Vitamin E Composition: Interspecies, Interorigin, and Nutritional Variability," *Journal of Agricultural and Food Chemistry* 62, no. 33 (2014): 8508–8517; T. B. Ahmad, D. Rudd, et al., "Correlation Between Fatty Acid Profile and Anti-Inflammatory Activity in Common Australian Seafood By-Products," *Marine Drugs* 17, no. 3 (2019): 155; S. Ben-Youssef, S. Selmi, et al., "Total Lipids and Fatty Acids Composition of the Coastal and the Deep-Sea Common Octopus (Octopus vulgaris) Populations: A Comparative Study," *Nutrition and Health* 19, no. 3 (2008): 195–201.

39. Gareth Anthony Wilson, "The Lipid Composition of Patagonian Toothfish from the Macquarie Island Region: Ecological and Dietary Implications Within a Regional Food Web" (PhD thesis, University of Tasmania, 2004), https://eprints.utas.edu.au/22124/.

40. A. Cerrato, S. E. Aita, et al., "Comprehensive Identification of Native Medium-Sized and Short Bioactive Peptides in Sea Bass Muscle," *Food Chemistry* 343 (2021): 128443.

41. J. A. Vázquez, A. Meduíña, et al., "Production of Valuable Compounds and Bioactive Metabolites from By-Products of Fish Discards Using Chemical Processing, Enzymatic Hydrolysis, and Bacterial Fermentation," *Marine Drugs* 17, no. 3 (2019): 139.

42. F. P. Martínez-Antequera, J. A. Martos-Sitcha, et al., "Evaluation of the Inclusion of the Green Seaweed *Ulva ohnoi* as an Ingredient in Feeds for Gilthead Sea Bream (*Sparus aurata*) and European Sea Bass (*Dicentrarchus labrax*)," *Animals* 11, no. 6 (2021): 1684; E. Gisbert, K. B. Andree, et al., "Olive Oil Bioactive Compounds Increase Body Weight, and Improve Gut Health and Integrity in Gilthead Sea Bream (Sparus aurata)," *British Journal of Nutrition* 117, no. 3 (2017): 351–363.

43. Center for Food Safety and Applied Nutrition, "FDA/EPA 2004 Advice on What You Need to Know About Mercury in Fish and Shellfish," US Food and Drug Administration, July 2, 2019, www.fda.gov/food/metals-and-your-food/fdaepa-2004-advice-what-you-need-know-about-mercury-fish-and-shellfish.

44. K. M. I. Bashir, J. H. Sohn, et al., "Identification and Characterization of Novel Antioxidant Peptides from Mackerel (Scomber Japonicus) Muscle Protein Hydrolysates," *Food Chemistry* 323 (2020): 126809.

45. C. Offret, I. Fliss, et al., "Identification of a Novel Antibacterial Peptide from Atlantic Mackerel Belonging to the GAPDH-Related Antimicrobial Family and Its in Vitro Digestibility," *Marine Drugs* 17, no. 7 (2019): 413; N. Ennaas, R. Hammami, et al., "Purification and Characterization of Four Antibacterial Peptides from Protamex Hydrolysate of Atlantic Mackerel (Scomber scombrus) By-Products," *Biochemical and Biophysical Research Communications* 462, no. 3 (2015): 195–200.

46. F. Affane, S. Louala, et al., "Hypolipidemic, Antioxidant and Antiatherogenic Property of Sardine By-Products Proteins in High-Fat Diet Induced Obese Rats," *Life Sciences* 199 (2018): 16–22.

47. C. P. Rocha, D. Pacheco, et al., "Seaweeds as Valuable Sources of Essential Fatty Acids for Human Nutrition," *International Journal of Environmental Research and Public Health* 18, no. 9 (2021): 4968.

48. H. Maeda, M. Hosokawa, et al., "Fucoxanthin from Edible Seaweed, Undaria Pinnatifida, Shows Antiobesity Effect Through UCP1 Expression in White Adipose Tissues," *Biochemical and Biophysical Research Communications* 332, no. 2 (2005): 392–397; M. A. Gammone and N. D'Orazio, "Anti-Obesity Activity of the Marine Carotenoid Fucoxanthin," *Marine Drugs* 13, no. 4 (2015): 2196–2214.

49. L. Yang, L. Wang, et al., "Laminarin Counteracts Diet-Induced Obesity Associated with Glucagon-Like Peptide-1 Secretion," *Oncotarget* 8, no. 59 (2017): 99470–99481.

50. H. K. Maehre, M. K. Malde, et al., "Characterization of Protein, Lipid and Mineral Contents in Common Norwegian Seaweeds and Evaluation of Their Potential as Food and Feed," *Journal of the Science of Food and Agriculture* 94, no. 15 (2014): 3281–3290; P. A. Harnedy, M. B. O'Keeffe, et al., "Fractionation and Identification of Antioxidant Peptides from an Enzymatically Hydrolysed Palmaria Palmata Protein Isolate," *Food Research International* 100, part 1 (2017): 416–422; R. C. Robertson, F. Guihéneuf, et al., "The Anti-Inflammatory Effect of Algae-Derived Lipid Extracts on Lipopolysaccharide (LPS)-Stimulated Human THP-1 Macrophages," *Marine Drugs* 13, no. 8 (2015): 5402–5424.

51. N. Blouin, B. L. Calder, et al., "Sensory and Fatty Acid Analyses of Two Atlantic Species of Porphyra (Rhodophyta)," *Journal of Applied Phycology* 18, no. 1 (2006): 79–85.

Chapter 9: Liquid Gold

1. J. McNeil-Masuka and T. J. Boyer, "Insensible Fluid Loss," *StatPearls*, July 31, 2021.

2. P. Prinz, "The Role of Dietary Sugars in Health: Molecular Composition or Just Calories?" *European Journal of Clinical Nutrition* 73, no. 9 (2019): 1216–1223.

3. A. Choi, K. Ha, et al., "Frequency of Consumption of Whole Fruit, Not Fruit Juice, Is Associated with Reduced Prevalence of Obesity in Korean Adults," *Journal of the Academy of Nutrition and Dietetics* 119, no. 11 (2019): 1842–1851.

4. J. Suez, T. Korem, et al., "Artificial Sweeteners Induce Glucose Intolerance by Altering the Gut Microbiota," *Nature* 514, no. 7521 (2014): 181–186; W. Wang, J. E. Nettleton, et al., "A Metagenomics Investigation of Intergenerational Effects of Non-Nutritive Sweeteners on Gut Microbiome," *Frontiers in Nutrition* 8 (2022): 795848.

5. J. A. Nettleton, P. L. Lutsey, et al., "Diet Soda Intake and Risk of Incident Metabolic Syndrome and Type 2 Diabetes in the Multi-Ethnic Study of Atherosclerosis (MESA)," *Diabetes Care* 32, no. 4 (2009): 688–694.

6. B. Larsen, B. Klinedinst, et al., "Pick Your Poison Carefully: How Alcohol Consumption and Serum Biomarkers Influence Body Fat—A UK Biobank Study," *Innovation in Aging* 4, S1 (2020): 889.

7. J. D. Stookey, F. Constant, et al., "Drinking Water Is Associated with Weight Loss in Overweight Dieting Women Independent of Diet and Activity," *Obesity* 16, no. 11 (2008): 2481–2488.

8. M. Boschmann, J. Steiniger, et al., "Water-Induced Thermogenesis," *Journal of Clinical Endocrinology and Metabolism* 88, no. 12 (2003): 6015–6019.

9. K. Y. Chen, S. Smith, et al., "Room Indirect Calorimetry Operating and Reporting Standards (RICORS 1.0): A Guide to Conducting and Reporting Human Whole-Room Calorimeter Studies," *Obesity* 28, no. 9 (2020): 1613–1625.

10. V. A. Vij and A. S. Joshi, "Effect of 'Water Induced Thermogenesis' on Body Weight, Body Mass Index and Body Composition of Overweight Subjects," *Journal of Clinical and Diagnostic Research* 7, no. 9 (2013): 1894–1896.

11. M. Boschmann, J. Steiniger, et al., "Water Drinking Induces Thermogenesis Through Osmosensitive Mechanisms," *Journal of Clinical Endocrinology and Metabolism* 92, no. 8 (2007): 3334–3337.

12. "Plain Water, the Healthier Choice," Centers for Disease Control and Prevention, June 7, 2022, www.cdc.gov/nutrition/data-statistics/plain-water-the-healthier-choice .html.

13. IBWA, "Bottled Water Consumption Shift," October 14, 2021, bottledwater.org/ bottled-water-consumption-shift.

14. S. A. Mason, V. G. Welch, et al., "Synthetic Polymer Contamination in Bottled Water," *Frontiers in Chemistry* 6 (2018): 407.

15. "What a Bottled-Water Habit Means for Intake of 'Microplastics.'" *Nature* 570, no. 7761 (2019): 279.

16. R. Hursel and M. S. Westerterp-Plantenga, "Thermogenic Ingredients and Body Weight Regulation," *International Journal of Obesity* 34, no. 4 (2010): 659–669; F. Li, C. Gao, et al., "EGCG Reduces Obesity and White Adipose Tissue Gain Partly Through AMPK Activation in Mice," *Frontiers in Pharmacology* 9 (2018): 1366; X. He, S. Zheng, et al., "Chlorogenic Acid Ameliorates Obesity by Preventing Energy Balance Shift in High-Fat Diet-Induced Obese Mice," *Journal of the Science of Food and Agriculture* 101, no. 2 (2021): 631–637.

17. A. Mousavi, M. Vafa, et al., "The Effects of Green Tea Consumption on Metabolic and Anthropometric Indices in Patients with Type 2 Diabetes," *Journal of Research in Medical Sciences* 18, no. 12 (2013): 1080–1086.

18. W.-Q. Peng, G. Xiao, et al., "l-Theanine Activates the Browning of White Adipose Tissue Through the AMPK/α-Ketoglutarate/Prdm16 Axis and Ameliorates Diet-Induced Obesity in Mice," *Diabetes* 70, no. 7 (2021): 1458–1472.

19. D. J. Weiss and C. R. Anderton, "Determination of Catechins in Matcha Green Tea by Micellar Electrokinetic Chromatography," *Journal of Chromatography* A 1011, nos. 1–2 (2003): 173–180.

20. K. Jakubczyk, J. Kochman, et al., "Antioxidant Properties and Nutritional Composition of Matcha Green Tea," *Foods* 9, no. 4 (2020): 483.

21. M. E. T. Willems, M. A. Sahin, et al., "Matcha Green Tea Drinks Enhance Fat Oxidation During Brisk Walking in Females," *International Journal of Sport Nutrition and Exercise Metabolism* 28, no. 5 (2018): 536–541.

22. P. Xu, L. Ying, et al., "The Effects of the Aqueous Extract and Residue of Matcha on the Antioxidant Status and Lipid and Glucose Levels in Mice Fed a High-Fat Diet," *Food and Function* 7, no. 1 (2016): 294–300.

23. T. Wu, J. Xu, et al., "Oolong Tea Polysaccharide and Polyphenols Prevent Obesity Development in Sprague-Dawley Rats," *Food and Nutrition Research* 62 (2018): 10.29219/fnr.v62.1599.

24. K.-L. Kuo, M.-S. Weng, et al., "Comparative Studies on the Hypolipidemic and Growth Suppressive Effects of Oolong, Black, Pu-Erh, and Green Tea Leaves in Rats," *Journal of Agricultural and Food Chemistry* 53, no. 2 (2005): 480–489.

25. W. Rumpler, J. Seale, et al., "Oolong Tea Increases Metabolic Rate and Fat Oxidation in Men," *Journal of Nutrition* 131, no. 11 (2001): 2848–2852.

26. W.-J. Zhang, C. Liu, et al., "Comparison of Volatile Profiles and Bioactive Components of Sun-Dried Pu-Erh Tea Leaves from Ancient Tea Plants on Bulang Mountain Measured by GC-MS and HPLC," *Journal of Zhejiang University–SCIENCE B* 20, no. 7 (2019): 563–575; D. Wang, Y. Xiang, et al., "Pueribacillus theae gen. nov., sp. nov., Isolated from Pu'er Tea," *International Journal of Systematic and Evolutionary Microbiology* 68, no. 9 (2018): 2878–2882.

27. M.-H. Liao, X.-R. Wang, et al., "Pu'er Tea Rich in Strictinin and Catechins Prevents Biofilm Formation of Two Cariogenic Bacteria, *Streptococcus mutans* and *Streptococcus sobrinus*," *Journal of Dental Sciences* 16, no. 4 (2021): 1331–1334.

28. Y. Oi, I.-C. Hou, et al., "Antiobesity Effects of Chinese Black Tea (Pu-erh tea) Extract and Gallic Acid," *Phytotherapy Research* 26, no. 4 (2012): 475–481.

29. T.-Y. Yang, J. I. Chou, et al., "Weight Reduction Effect of Pu-Erh Tea in Male Patients with Metabolic Syndrome," *Phytotherapy Research* 28, no. 7 (2014): 1096–1101.

30. S.-L. Chu, H. Fu, et al., "A Randomized Double-Blind Placebo-Controlled Study of Pu'er Tea Extract on the Regulation of Metabolic Syndrome," *Chinese Journal of Integrative Medicine* 17, no. 7 (2011): 492–498.

31. H. F. L. Muhammad, D. C. Sulistyoningrum, et al., "The Interaction Between Coffee, Caffeine Consumption, UCP2 Gene Variation, and Adiposity in Adults—A Cross-Sectional Study," *Journal of Nutrition and Metabolism* (2019): 9606054.

32. A. Tagliabue, D. Terracina, et al., "Coffee-Induced Thermogenesis and Skin Temperature," *International Journal of Obesity and Related Metabolic Disorders* 18, no. 8 (1994): 537–541; D. E. Anderson and M. S. Hickey, "Effects of Caffeine on the Metabolic and Catecholamine Responses to Exercise in 5 and 28 Degrees C," *Medicine and Science in Sports and Exercise* 26, no. 4 (1994): 453–458.

33. D. Bracco, J. M. Ferrarra, et al., "Effects of Caffeine on Energy Metabolism, Heart Rate, and Methylxanthine Metabolism in Lean and Obese Women," *American Journal of Physiology* 269, no. 4, part 1 (1995): E671–E678.

34. S. C. Killer, A. K. Blannin, et al., "No Evidence of Dehydration with Moderate Daily Coffee Intake: A Counterbalanced Cross-Over Study in a Free-Living Population," *PloS One* 9, no. 1 (2014): e84154.

35. Josie Garthwaite, "What We Know About the Earliest History of Chocolate," *Smithsonian Magazine*, February 12, 2015, www.smithsonianmag.com/history/archaeology-chocolate-180954243.

36. L. Munguía, G. Gutiérrez-Salmeán, et al., "Beneficial Effects of a Flavanol-Enriched Cacao Beverage on Anthropometric and Cardiometabolic Risk Profile in Overweight Subjects," *Revista Mexicana de Cardiología* 26, no. 2 (2015): 78–86.

37. W. F. Chew, M. Masyita, et al., "Prevalence of Obesity and Its Associated Risk Factors Among Chinese Adults in a Malaysian Suburban Village," *Singapore Medical Journal* 55, no. 2 (2014): 84–91.

38. S. A. Keshavarz, Z. Nourieh, et al., "Effect of Soymilk Consumption on Waist Circumference and Cardiovascular Risks Among Overweight and Obese Female Adults," *International Journal of Preventive Medicine* 3, no. 11 (2012): 798–805.

39. S. Sethi, S. K. Tyagi, et al., "Plant-Based Milk Alternatives an Emerging Segment of Functional Beverages: A Review," *Journal of Food Science and Technology* 53, no. 9 (2016): 3408–3423.

40. Y.-F. Li, Y.-Y. Chang, et al., "Tomato Juice Supplementation in Young Women Reduces Inflammatory Adipokine Levels Independently of Body Fat Reduction," *Nutrition* 31, no. 5 (2015): 691–696.

41. A. J. Edwards, B. T. Vinyard, et al., "Consumption of Watermelon Juice Increases Plasma Concentrations of Lycopene and Beta-Carotene in Humans," *Journal of Nutrition* 133, no. 4 (2003): 1043–1050.

42. G. K. Dhamrait, K. Panchal, et al., "Characterising Nitric Oxide-Mediated Metabolic Benefits of Low-Dose Ultraviolet Radiation in the Mouse: A Focus on Brown Adipose Tissue," *Diabetologia* 63, no. 1 (2020): 179–193; C. M. Vincellette, J. Losso, et al., "Supplemental Watermelon Juice Attenuates Acute Hyperglycemia-Induced Macro- and Microvascular Dysfunction in Healthy Adults," *Journal of Nutrition* 151, no. 11 (2021): 3450–3458.

43. A. Hasani, S. Ebrahimzadeh, et al., "The Role of *Akkermansia muciniphila* in Obesity, Diabetes and Atherosclerosis," *Journal of Medical Microbiology* 70, no. 10 (2021): 10.1099/jmm.0.001435.

44. B. Routy, E. Le Chatelier, et al., "Gut Microbiome Influences Efficacy of PD-1-Based Immunotherapy Against Epithelial Tumors," *Science* 359, no. 6371 (2018): 91–97.

45. D. E. Roopchand, R. N. Carmody, et al., "Dietary Polyphenols Promote Growth of the Gut Bacterium Akkermansia Muciniphila and Attenuate High-Fat Diet-Induced Metabolic Syndrome," *Diabetes* 64, no. 8 (2015): 2847–2858. doi:10.2337/db14-1916; S. M. Henning, P. H. Summanen, et al., "Pomegranate ellagitannins Stimulate the Growth of Akkermansia muciniphila in Vivo," *Anaerobe* 43 (2017): 56–60; F. F. Anhê, D. Roy, et al., "A Polyphenol-Rich Cranberry Extract Protects from Diet-Induced Obesity, Insulin Resistance and Intestinal Inflammation in Association with Increased Akkermansia spp. population in the Gut Microbiota of Mice," *Gut* 64, no. 6 (2015): 872–883; F. F. Anhê, G. Pilon, et al., "Triggering Akkermansia with Dietary Polyphenols: A New Weapon to Combat the Metabolic Syndrome?" *Gut Microbes* 7, no. 2 (2016): 146–153.

46. H. Song, X. Shen, et al., "Pomegranate Fruit Pulp Polyphenols Reduce Diet-Induced Obesity with Modulation of Gut Microbiota in Mice," *Journal of the Science of Food and Agriculture* 102, no. 5 (2022): 1968–1977.

47. M. González-Ortiz, E. Martínez-Abundis, et al., "Effect of Pomegranate Juice on Insulin Secretion and Sensitivity in Patients with Obesity," *Annals of Nutrition and Metabolism* 58, no. 3 (2011): 220–223.

48. D. E. Roopchand, R. N. Carmody, et al., "Dietary Polyphenols Promote Growth of the Gut Bacterium Akkermansia muciniphila and Attenuate High-Fat Diet-Induced Metabolic Syndrome," *Diabetes* 64, no. 8 (2015): 2847–2858.

49. J. H. Hollis, J. A. Houchins, et al., "Effects of Concord Grape Juice on Appetite, Diet, Body Weight, Lipid Profile, and Antioxidant Status of Adults," *Journal of the American College of Nutrition* 28, no. 5 (2009): 574–582.

50. F. Zhou, J. Guo, et al., "Cranberry Polyphenolic Extract Exhibits an Antiobesity Effect on High-Fat Diet-Fed Mice Through Increased Thermogenesis," *Journal of Nutrition* 150, no. 8 (2020): 2131–2138.

51. T. N. C. Simão, M. A. B. Lozovoy, et al., "Reduced-Energy Cranberry Juice Increases Folic Acid and Adiponectin and Reduces Homocysteine and Oxidative Stress in Patients with the Metabolic Syndrome," *British Journal of Nutrition* 110, no. 10 (2013): 1885–1894.

52. A. S. Balcioğlu, M. E. Durakoglugil, et al., "Epicardial Adipose Tissue Thickness and Plasma Homocysteine in Patients with Metabolic Syndrome and Normal Coronary Arteries," *Diabetology and Metabolic Syndrome* 6 (2014): 62.

53. M. Tomás-Navarro, F. Vallejo, et al., "Encapsulation and Micronization Effectively Improve Orange Beverage Flavanone Bioavailability in Humans," *Journal of Agricultural and Food Chemistry* 62, no. 39 (2014): 9458–9462.

54. F. J. Martinez Noguera, P. E. Alcaraz, et al., "8 Weeks of 2S-Hesperidin Supplementation Improves Muscle Mass and Reduces Fat in Amateur Competitive Cyclists: Randomized Controlled Trial," *Food and Function* 12, no. 9 (2021): 3872–3882.

55. F. J. Martínez-Noguera, C. Marin-Pagán, et al., "Effects of 8 Weeks of 2S-Hesperidin Supplementation on Performance in Amateur Cyclists," *Nutrients* 12, no. 12 (2020): 3911.

56. J. J. Peterson, G. R. Beecher, et al., "Flavanones in Grapefruit, Lemons, and Limes: A Compilation and Review of the Data from the Analytical Literature," *Journal of Food Composition and Analysis* 19S (2006): S74–S80.

Chapter 10: Find Your Own Way

1. S. Degner, A. Papoutsis, and D. Romagnolo, "Health Benefits of Traditional Culinary and Medicinal Mediterranean Plants," *Complementary and Alternative Therapies and the Aging Population* (2009): 541–562, www.ncbi.nlm.nih.gov/pmc/articles/PMC7157932/.

2. Y. C. Yang, C. Boen, et al., "Social Relationships and Physiologial Determinants of Longevity Across the Human Life Span," *Proceedings of the National Academy of Sciences of the United States of America* 113, no. 3 (January 2016): 578–583, https://pubmed.ncbi.nlm.nih.gov/26729882/; S.-Q. Yuan, Y.-M. Liu, et al., "Association Between Eating Speed and Metabolic Syndrome: A Systematic Review and Meta-Analysis,"

Frontiers in Nutrition 20, no. 8 (October 2021): 700936, https://pubmed.ncbi.nlm.nih
.gov/34746200/.

3. M. L. Heiman and F. L. Greenway, "A Healthy Gastrointestinal Microbiome Is Depen-
dent on Dietary Diversity," *Molecular Metabolism* 5, no. 5 (May 2016): www.ncbi.nlm
.nih.gov/pmc/articles/PMC4837298/.

4. S. Lee, "#63 Research Your Own Experience," September 12, 2017, in *Bruce Lee Podcast*, https://brucelee.com/podcast-blog/2017/9/12/63-research-your-own-experience.

5. B. Lee and J. R. Little, *Striking Thoughts: Bruce Lee's Wisdom for Daily Living* (Tokyo:
Tuttle, 2016), 181.

6. Lee and Little, *Striking Thoughts*, 180.

7. E. Chamoun, D. M. Mutch, et al., "A Review of the Associations Between Single
Nucleotide Polymorphisms in Taste Receptors, Eating Behaviors, and Health," *Critical
Reviews in Food Science and Nutrition* 58, no. 2 (January 2018): 194–207, https://
pubmed.ncbi.nlm.nih.gov/27247080/.

8. N. Chaudhary, V. Kumar, et al., "Personalized Nutrition and -Omics," *Comprehensive
Foodomics* (2021): 495–507, www.ncbi.nlm.nih.gov/pmc/articles/PMC7217104/.

9. Editors of Blackbelt Magazine, *The Legendary Bruce Lee* (Santa Clarita, CA: Ohara
Publications, 1986), 46.

10. Lee and Little, *Striking Thoughts*, 105.

11. B. Lee, *Tao of Jeet Kune Do* (Oklahoma City: Black Belt Book, 1975).

12. S. Lee, "#20 Nutrition and Fitness," November 23, 2016, in *Bruce Lee Podcast*, https://
brucelee.com/podcast-blog/2016/11/23/20-nutrition-and-fitness.

13. S. Lee, "#102 The Intelligent Mind," June 13, 2018, in *Bruce Lee Podcast*, https://bru-
celee.com/podcast-blog/2018/6/13/102-the-intelligent-mind.

14. J. B. Nelson, "Mindful Eating: The Art of Presence While You Eat," *Diabetes Spectrum*
30, no. 3 (2017): 171–174.

15. A. Ruffault, S. Czernichow, et al., "The Effects of Mindfulness Training on Weight-
Loss and Health-Related Behaviours in Adults with Overweight and Obesity: A Systematic Review and Meta-Analysis," *Obesity Research and Clinical Practice* 11, no. 5,
suppl. 1 (2017): 90–111.

16. J. Daubenmier, P. J. Moran, et al., "Effects of a Mindfulness-Based Weight Loss Intervention in Adults with Obesity: A Randomized Clinical Trial," *Obesity* 24, no. 4
(2016): 794–804.

17. K. Hawton, D. Ferriday, et al., "Slow Down: Behavioural and Physiological Effects of
Reduced Eating Rate," *Nutrients* 11, no. 1 (2019): 50.

18. C. Cecchetto, M. Aiello, et al., "Increased Emotional Eating During COVID-19
Associated with Lockdown, Psychological, and Social Distress," *Appetite* 160 (2021):
105122.

Chapter 11: The Eat to Beat Protocol

1. V. D. Longo and S. Panda, "Fasting, Circadian Rhythms, and Time-Restricted Feeding
in Healthy Lifespan," *Cell Metabolism* 23, no. 6 (2016): 1048–1059; C. Patikorn, K.
Roubal, et al. "Intermittent Fasting and Obesity-Related Health Outcomes: An
Umbrella Review of Meta-Analyses of Randomized Clinical Trials," *JAMA Network
Open* 4, no. 12 (2021): 1–12; M. J. McAllister, A. E. Gonzalez, et al., "Time Restricted
Feeding Reduces Inflammation and Cortisol Response to a Firegrounds Test in

Professional Firefighters," *Journal of Occupational and Environmental Medicine* 63, no. 5 (2021): 441–447.

2. J. Rothschild, K. K. Hoddy, et al., "Time-Restricted Feeding and Risk of Metabolic Disease: A Review of Human and Animal Studies," *Nutrition Reviews* 72, no. 5 (2014): 308–318.

3. M. Bagherniya, A. E. Butler, et al., "The Effect of Fasting or Calorie Restriction on Autophagy Induction: A Review of the Literature," *Ageing Research Reviews* 47 (2018): 183–197.

4. M. M. Mihaylova, C.-W. Cheng, et al., "Fasting Activates Fatty Acid Oxidation to Enhance Intestinal Stem Cell Function During Homeostasis and Aging," *Cell Stem Cell* 22, no. 5 (2018): 769–778; C.-W. Cheng, G. B. Adams, et al., "Prolonged Fasting Reduces IGF-1/PKA to Promote Hematopoietic-Stem-Cell-Based Regeneration and Reverse Immunosuppression," *Cell Stem Cell* 14, no. 6 (2014): 810–823.

5. A. Maifeld, H. Bartolomaeus, et al., "Fasting Alters the Gut Microbiome Reducing Blood Pressure and Body Weight in Metabolic Syndrome Patients," *Nature Communications* 12, no. 1 (2021): 1–20; R. Mesnage, F. Grundler, et al., "Changes in Human Gut Microbiota Composition Are Linked to the Energy Metabolic Switch During 10 D of Buchinger Fasting," *Journal of Nutritional Science* 8 (2019): 1–14.

6. G. M. Tinsley, J. S. Forsse, et al., "Time-Restricted Feeding in Young Men Performing Resistance Training: A Randomized Controlled Trial," *European Journal of Sport Science* 17, no. 2 (2017): 200–207; S. Aoyama, H.-K. Kim, et al., "Distribution of Dietary Protein Intake in Daily Meals Influences Skeletal Muscle Hypertrophy via the Muscle Clock," *Cell Reports* 36, no. 1 (2021): 1–13.

7. M. P. Mattson, K. Moehl, et al., "Intermittent Metabolic Switching, Neuroplasticity and Brain Health," *Nature Reviews Neuroscience* 19, no. 2 (2018): 63–80.

8. X. Bian, L. Chi, et al., "The Artificial Sweetener Acesulfame Potassium Affects the Gut Microbiome and Body Weight Gain in CD-1 Mice," *PloS One* 12, no. 6 (2017): e0178426.

9. M. B. Abou-Donia, E. M. El-Masry, et al., "Splenda Alters Gut Microflora and Increases Intestinal p-Glycoprotein and Cytochrome p-450 in Male Rats," *Journal of Toxicology and Environmental Health Part A* 71, no. 21 (2008): 1415–1429; J. Suez, T. Korem, et al., "Artificial Sweeteners Induce Glucose Intolerance by Altering the Gut Microbiota," *Nature* 514, no. 7521 (2014): 181–186.

10. C. L. Frankenfeld, M. Sikaroodi, et al., "High-Intensity Sweetener Consumption and Gut Microbiome Content and Predicted Gene Function in a Cross-Sectional Study of Adults in the United States," *Annals of Epidemiology* 25, no. 10 (2015): 736–742.

11. S. Howell and R. Kones, "'Calories In, Calories Out' and Macronutrient Intake: The Hope, Hype, and Science of Calories," *American Journal of Physiology–Endocrinology and Metabolism* 313, no. 5 (2017): E608–E612.

12. N. B. Bueno, I. S. Vieira de Melo, et al., "Very-Low-Carbohydrate Ketogenic Diet v. Low-Fat Diet for Long-Term Weight Loss: A Meta-Analysis of Randomised Controlled Trials," *British Journal of Nutrition* 110, no. 7 (2013): 1178–1187; A. M. Bolla, A. Caretto, et al., "Low-Carb and Ketogenic Diets in Type 1 and Type 2 Diabetes," *Nutrients* 11, no. 5 (2019): 962; M. I. Friedman and S. Appel, "Energy Expenditure and Body Composition Changes After an Isocaloric Ketogenic Diet in Overweight and Obese Men: A Secondary Analysis of Energy Expenditure and Physical Activity," *PloS One* 14, no. 12 (2019): e0222971; P. Sumithran, L. A. Prendergast, et al., "Ketosis and

Appetite-Mediating Nutrients and Hormones After Weight Loss," *European Journal of Clinical Nutrition* 67, no. 7 (2013): 759–764.

13. C. D. Gardner, M. J. Landry, et al., "Effect of a Ketogenic Diet versus Mediterranean Diet on HbA1c in Individuals with Prediabetes and Type 2 Diabetes Mellitus: The Interventional Keto-Med Randomized Crossover Trial," *American Journal of Clinical Nutrition* 116, no. 3 (2022): nqac154.

14. Q. Y. Ang, M. Alexander, et al., "Ketogenic Diets Alter the Gut Microbiome Resulting in Decreased Intestinal Th17 Cells," *Cell* 181, no. 6 (2020): 1263–1275.

15. S. B. Eaton and M. Konner, "Paleolithic Nutrition. A Consideration of Its Nature and Current Implications," *New England Journal of Medicine* 312, no. 5 (1985): 283–289.

16. S. B. Eaton, M. Shostak, and M. Konner, *The Paleolithic Prescription: A Program of Diet and Exercise and a Design for Living* (New York: Perennial Library, 1989).

17. L. Cordain, *The Paleo Diet* (Hoboken, NJ: John Wiley & Sons, 2010).

18. E. V. A. de Menezes, H. A. C. Sampaio, et al., "Influence of Paleolithic Diet on Anthropometric Markers in Chronic Diseases: Systematic Review and Meta-Analysis," *Nutrition Journal* 18, no. 1 (2019): 41.

19. C. Mellberg, S. Sandberg, et al., "Long-Term Effects of a Palaeolithic-Type Diet in Obese Postmenopausal Women: A 2-Year Randomized Trial," *European Journal of Clinical Nutrition* 68, no. 3 (2014): 350–357.

20. W. Petroski and D. M. Minich, "Is There Such a Thing as 'Anti-Nutrients'? A Narrative Review of Perceived Problematic Plant Compounds," *Nutrients* 12, no. 10 (2020): 2929.

21. R.-Y. Huang, C. C. Huang, et al., "Vegetarian Diets and Weight Reduction: A Meta-Analysis of Randomized Controlled Trials," *Journal of General Internal Medicine* 31 (2016): 109–116.

22. H. Kahleova, E. Rembert, et al., "Effects of a Low-Fat Vegan Diet on Gut Microbiota in Overweight Individuals and Relationships with Body Weight, Body Composition, and Insulin Sensitivity. A Randomized Clinical Trial," *Nutrients* 12, no. 10 (2020): 2917.

23. G. M. Turner-McGrievy, N. D. Barnard, et al., "A Two-Year Randomized Weight Loss Trial Comparing a Vegan Diet to a More Moderate Low-Fat Diet," *Obesity* 15, no. 9 (2007): 2276–2281.

24. W. J. Moore, M. E. McGrievy, et al., "Dietary Adherence and Acceptability of Five Different Diets, Including Vegan and Vegetarian Diets, for Weight Loss: The New DIETs Study," *Eating Behaviors* 19 (2015): 33–38.

25. C. Weikert, I. Trefflich, et al., "Vitamin and Mineral Status in a Vegan Diet," *Deutsches Ärzteblatt International* 117, nos. 35–36 (2020): 575–582.

Chapter 13: Optimize Your Metabolism

1. E. N. C. Manoogian, L. S. Chow, et al., "Time-Restricted Eating for the Prevention and Management of Metabolic Diseases," *Endocrine Reviews* 43, no. 2 (2022): 405–436.

2. G. Kelsey, H. Kristin, et al., "Effects of 8-Hour Time Restricted Feeding on Body Weight and Metabolic Disease Risk Factors in Obese Adults: A Pilot Study," *Nutrition and Healthy Aging* 4, no. 4 (2018): 345–353; T. Moro, G. Tinsley, et al., "Effects of Eight Weeks of Time-Restricted Feeding (16/8) on Basal Metabolism, Maximal Strength,

Body Composition, Inflammation, and Cardiovascular Risk Factors in Resistance-Trained Males," *Journal of Translational Medicine* 14 (2016): 290.

3. M. Hatori, C. Vollmers, et al., "Time-Restricted Feeding Without Reducing Caloric Intake Prevents Metabolic Diseases in Mice Fed a High-Fat Diet," *Cell Metabolism* 15, no. 6 (2012): 848–860.

4. A. Huberman, producer, "Effect of Fasting and Time Restricted Eating on Fat Loss and Health," Huberman Lab Podcast, no. 41, October 11, 2021, www.youtube.com/watch?v=9tRohh0gErM&t=4s.

5. H. Jamshed, F. L. Steger, et al., "Effectiveness of Early Time-Restricted Eating for Weight Loss, Fat Loss, and Cardiometabolic Health in Adults with Obesity: A Randomized Clinical Trial," *JAMA Internal Medicine*, August 8, 2022. doi:10.1001/jamainternmed.2022.3050.

6. C. Andriessen, C. E. Fealy, et al., "Three Weeks of Time-Restricted Eating Improves Glucose Homeostasis in Adults with Type 2 Diabetes but Does Not Improve Insulin Sensitivity: A Randomised Crossover Trial," *Diabetologia* (2022). doi.org/10.1007/s00125-022-05752-z.

7. A. T. Hutchison, P. Regmi, et al., "Time-Restricted Feeding Improves Glucose Tolerance in Men at Risk for Type 2 Diabetes: A Randomized Crossover Trial," *Obesity* 27, no. 5 (2019): 724–732.

8. D. Liu, Y. Huang, et al., "Calorie Restriction with or Without Time-Restricted Eating in Weight Loss," *New England Journal of Medicine* 386 (2022): 1495–1504.

9. A. Leaf and J. Antonio, "The Effects of Overfeeding on Body Composition: The Role of Macronutrient Composition—A Narrative Review," *International Journal of Exercise Science* 10, no. 8 (2017): 1275–1296.

10. D. J. Morrison, G. M. Kowalski, et al., "Modest Changes to Glycemic Regulation Are Sufficient to Maintain Glucose Fluxes in Healthy Young Men Following Overfeeding with a Habitual Macronutrient Composition," *American Journal of Physiology–Endocrinology and Metabolism* 316, no. 6 (2019): E1061–E1070.

11. E. Robinson, P. Aveyard, et al., "Eating Attentively: A Systematic Review and Meta-Analysis of the Effect of Food Intake Memory and Awareness on Eating," *American Journal of Clinical Nutrition* 97, no. 4 (2013): 728–742.

12. A. Geliebter, C. L. Grillot, et al., "Effects of Oatmeal and Corn Flakes Cereal Breakfasts on Satiety, Gastric Emptying, Glucose, and Appetite-Related Hormones," *Annals of Nutrition and Metabolism* 66, nos. 2–3 (2015): 93–103; A. Warrilow, D. Mellor, et al., "Dietary Fat, Fibre, Satiation, and Satiety—A Systematic Review of Acute Studies," *European Journal of Clinical Nutrition* 73, no. 3 (2019): 333–344.

13. D. Jakubowicz, O. Froy, et al., "Meal Timing and Composition Influence Ghrelin Levels, Appetite Scores and Weight Loss Maintenance in Overweight and Obese Adults," *Steroids* 77, no. 4 (2012): 323–331.

14. B. Wansink, K. van Ittersum, et al., "Ice Cream Illusions Bowls, Spoons, and Self-Served Portion Sizes," *American Journal of Preventive Medicine* 31, no. 3 (2006): 240–243.

15. M. Hirshkowitz, K. Whiton, et al., "National Sleep Foundation's Sleep Time Duration Recommendations: Methodology and Results Summary," *Sleep Health* 1, no. 1 (2015): 40–43.

16. V. K. Chattu, M. D. Manzar, et al., "The Global Problem of Insufficient Sleep and Its Serious Public Health Implications," *Healthcare* 7, no. 1 (2018): 1–16.

17. J. M. Parish, "Sleep-Related Problems in Common Medical Conditions," *Chest* 135, no. 2 (2009): 563–572.

18. A.V. Nedeltcheva and F. A. J. L. Scheer, "Metabolic Effects of Sleep Disruption, Links to Obesity and Diabetes," *Current Opinion in Endocrinology, Diabetes, and Obesity* 21, no. 4 (2014): 293–298.

19. V. Bacaro, A. Blasio, et al., "Sleep Duration and Obesity in Adulthood: An Updated Systematic Review and Meta-Analysis," *Obesity Research and Clinical Practice* 14, no. 4 (2020): 301–309.

20. S. K. Sweet, B. A. Gower, et al., "Sleep Quality Is Differentially Related to Adiposity in Adults," *Psychoneuroendocrinology* 98 (2018): 46–51; V. Kunde, D. Leana, et al., "Measuring Visceral Adipose Tissue Metabolic Activity in Sleep Apnea Utilizing Hybrid 18F-FDG PET/MRI: A Pilot Study," *Nature and Science of Sleep* 13 (2021): 1943–1953.

21. J. Broussard and M. J. Brady, "The Impact of Sleep Disturbances on Adipocyte Function and Lipid Metabolism," *Best Practice and Research: Clinical Endocrinology and Metabolism* 24, no. 5 (2010): 763–773.

22. B. D. Wedger, C. Goblet, et al., "Systematic Analysis of Differential Rhythmic Liver Gene Expression Mediated by the Circadian Clock and Feeding Rhythms," *Proceedings of the National Academy of Sciences U.S.A.* 118, no. 3 (2021): 1–12.

23. R. B. Bazzite, L. G. Silva, et al., "Insulin Resistance in the Liver: Deficiency or Excess of Insulin?" *Cell Cycle* 13, no. 16 (2014): 2494–2500; R. F. D. Oliveira, T. M. da Costa Daniele, et al., "Adiponectin Levels and Sleep Deprivation in Patients with Endocrine Metabolic Disorders," *Revista da Associacao Medica Brasileira (1992)* 64, no. 12 (2018): 1122–1128.

24. O. A. Mullite-Gillman, Y. A. Kurnianingsih, et al., "Sleep Deprivation Alters Choice Strategy Without Altering Uncertainty or Loss Aversion Preferences," *Frontiers in Neuroscience* 9, no. 352 (2015): 1–12.

25. N. A. Jessen, A. S. F. Munk, et al., "The Glymphatic System: A Beginner's Guide," *Neurochemical Research* 40, no. 12 (2015): 2583–2599.

26. A.-M. Chang, D. Aeschbach, et al., "Evening Use of Light-Emitting Ereaders Negatively Affects Sleep, Circadian Timing, and Next-Morning Alertness," *Proceedings of the National Academy of Sciences of the U.S.A.* 112, no. 4 (2015): 1232–1237.

27. K. Yoda, M. Inaba, et al., "Association Between Poor Glycemic Control, Impaired Sleep Quality, and Increased Arterial Thickening in Type 2 Diabetic Patients," *PloS One* 10, no. 4 (2015): 1–12.

28. H. Dempsey-Jones, "The Surprising Science of Fidgeting," *The Conversation*, August 28, 2022, https://theconversation.com/the-surprising-science-of-fidgeting-77525.

29. J. A. Levine, S. J. Schleusner, et al., "Energy Expenditure of Nonexercise Activity," *American Journal of Clinical Nutrition* 72, no. 6 (2000): 1451–1454.

30. G. Hagger-Johnson, A. J. Gow, et al., "Sitting Time, Fidgeting, and All-Cause Mortality in the UK Women's Cohort Study," *American Journal of Preventive Medicine* 50, no. 2 (2016): 154–160.

31. "Calories Burned in 30 Minutes for People of Three Different Weights," *Harvard Health Publishing*, March 8, 2021, www.health.harvard.edu/diet-and-weight-loss/calories-burned-in-30-minutes-for-people-of-three-different-weights.

32. R. J. H. M. Verheggen, M. F. H. Maessen, et al., "A Systematic Review and Meta-Analysis on the Effects of Exercise Training versus Hypocaloric Diet: Distinct Effects

on Body Weight and Visceral Adipose Tissue," *Obesity Reviews* 17, no. 8 (2016): 664–690.

33. P. Aldiss, J. Betts, et al., "Exercise-Induced 'Browning' of Adipose Tissues," *Metabolism: Clinical and Experimental* 81 (2018): 63–70.

34. A. L. Hankinson, M. L. Daviglus, et al., "Maintaining a High Physical Activity Level Over 20 Years and Weight Gain," *Journal of the American Medical Association* 304, no. 23 (2010): 2603–2610; X. Tong, X. Chen, et al., "The Effect of Exercise on the Prevention of Osteoporosis and Bone Angiogenesis," *BioMed Research International* (2019): 1–8; J. Liang, X. Zhang, et al., "Promotion of Aerobic Exercise Induced Angiogenesis Is Associated with Decline in Blood Pressure in Hypertension: Result of EXCAVATION-CHN1," *Hypertension* 77, no. 4 (2021): 1141–1153; V. Frodermann, D. Rhode, et al., "Exercise Reduces Inflammatory Cell Production and Cardiovascular Inflammation via Instruction of Hematopoietic Progenitor Cells," *Nature Medicine* 25, no. 11 (2019): 1761–1771; M. U. Sohail, H. M. Yassine, et al., "Impact of Physical Exercise on Gut Microbiome, Inflammation, and the Pathobiology of Metabolic Disorders," *Review of Diabetic Studies* 15 (2019): 35–48; G. Wu, X. Zhang, et al., "The Epigenetic Landscape of Exercise in Cardiac Health and Disease," *Journal of Sport and Health Science* 10, no. 6 (2021): 648–659; J. Wang, S. Liu, et al., "Exercise Regulates the Immune System," *Advances in Experimental Medicine and Biology* 1228 (2020): 395–408.

35. D. J. Johns, J. Hartmann-Boyce, et al., "Diet or Exercise Interventions vs Combined Behavioral Weight Management Programs: A Systematic Review and Meta-Analysis of Direct Comparisons," *Journal of the Academy of Nutrition and Dietetics* 114, no. 10 (2014): 1557–1568; T. Wu, X. Gao, et al., "Long-Term Effectiveness of Diet-Plus-Exercise Interventions vs. Diet-Only Interventions for Weight Loss: A Meta-Analysis," *Obesity Reviews* 10, no. 3 (2009): 313–323.

36. E. D. Kirby, S. E. Muroy, et al., "Acute Stress Enhances Adult Rat Hippocampal Neurogenesis and Activation of Newborn Neurons via Secreted Astrocytic FGF2," *eLife* vol. 2 (2013): 1–23.

37. A. Mariotti, "The Effects of Chronic Stress on Health: New Insights into the Molecular Mechanisms of Brain-Body Communication," *Future Science OA* 1, no. 3 (2015): FSO23; P. H. Wirtz and R. von Känel, "Psychological Stress, Inflammation, and Coronary Heart Disease," *Current Cardiology Reports* 19, no. 11 (2017): 1–10; B. S. McEwen and R. M. Sapolsky, "Stress and Cognitive Function," *Current Opinion in Neurobiology* 5, no. 2 (1995): 205–216.

38. E. Epel, R. Lapidus, et al., "Stress May Add Bite to Appetite in Women: A Laboratory Study of Stress-Induced Cortisol and Eating Behavior," *Psychoneuroendocrinology* 26, no. 1 (2001): 37–49.

39. H. Herriot, C. Wrosch, et al., "Intra-Individual Cortisol Variability and Low-Grade Inflammation Over 10 Years in Older Adults," *Psychoneuroendocrinology* 77 (2017): 141–149.

40. K. Räikkönen, K. A. Matthews, et al., "Anger, Hostility, and Visceral Adipose Tissue in Healthy Postmenopausal Women," *Metabolism* 48, no. 9 (1999): 1146–1151.

41. P. Sun, S. Wei, et al., "Anger Emotional Stress Influences VEGF/VEGFR2 and Its Induced PI3K/AKT/mTOR Signaling Pathway," *Neural Plasticity* (2016): 1–12; J. Herold and J. Kalucka. "Angiogenesis in Adipose Tissue: The Interplay Between Adipose and Endothelial Cells," *Frontiers in Physiology* 11 (2021): 1–9.

42. V. K. Tsenkova, D. Carr, et al., "Anger, Adiposity, and Glucose Control in Nondiabetic Adults: Findings from MIDUS II," *Journal of Behavioral Medicine* 37, no. 1 (2014): 37–46.

43. K. Carrière, B. Khoury, et al., "Mindfulness-Based Interventions for Weight Loss: A Systematic Review and Meta-Analysis," *Obesity Reviews* 19, no. 2 (2018): 164–177.

44. H. Cramer, M. S. Thoms, et al., "Yoga in Women with Abdominal Obesity—A Randomized Controlled Trial," *Deutsches Ärzteblatt International* 113, no. 39 (2016): 645–652.

45. K. Unno, D. Furushima, et al., "Stress-Reducing Function of Matcha Green Tea in Animal Experiments and Clinical Trials," *Nutrients* 10, no. 10 (2018): 1–14; P. F. P. Chaves, P. A. S. Hocayen, et al., "Chamomile Tea: Source of a Glucuronoxylan with Antinociceptive, Sedative and Anxiolytic-Like Effects," *International Journal of Biological Macromolecules* 164 (2020): 1675–1682; J. L. Williams, J. M. Everett, et al., "The Effects of Green Tea Amino Acid L-Theanine Consumption on the Ability to Manage Stress and Anxiety Levels: A Systematic Review," *Plant Foods for Human Nutrition* 75, no. 1 (2020): 12–23; Y. Jia, J. Zou, et al., "Action Mechanism of Roman Chamomile in the Treatment of Anxiety Disorder Based on Network Pharmacology," *Journal of Food Biochemistry* 45, no. 1 (2021): 1–19.

46. P.-F. Tsai, S. Kitsch, et al., "Tai Chi for Posttraumatic Stress Disorder and Chronic Musculoskeletal Pain: A Pilot Study," *Journal of Holistic Nursing* 36, no. 2 (2018): 147–158.

47. V. Perciavalle, M. Blandini, et al., "The Role of Deep Breathing on Stress," *Neurological Sciences* 38, no. 3 (2017): 451–458; X. Ma, Z.-Q. Yue, et al., "The Effect of Diaphragmatic Breathing on Attention, Negative Affect and Stress in Healthy Adults," *Frontiers in Psychology* 8 (2017): 1–12.

48. M. A. H. Lentjes, "The Balance Between Food and Dietary Supplements in the General Population," *Proceedings of the Nutrition Society* 78, no. 1 (2019): 97–109.

49. M. E. Veatch-Blohm, I. Chicas, et al., "Screening for Consistency and Contamination Within and Between Bottles of 29 Herbal Supplements," *PloS One* 16, no. 11 (2021): 1–20.

50. C. M. White, "Dietary Supplements Pose Real Dangers to Patients," *Annals of Pharmacotherapy* 54, no. 8 (2020): 815–819.

51. K. Y. Z. Forrest and W. L. Stuhldreher, "Prevalence and Correlates of Vitamin D Deficiency in US adults," *Nutrition Research* 31, no. 1 (2011): 48–54; K. Amrein, M. Scherkl, et al., "Vitamin D Deficiency 2.0: An Update on the Current Status Worldwide," *European Journal of Clinical Nutrition* 74, no. 11 (2020): 1498–1513; P. D. Chandler, W. Y. Chen, et al., "Effect of Vitamin D3 Supplements on Development of Advanced Cancer: A Secondary Analysis of the VITAL Randomized Clinical Trial," *JAMA Network Open* 3, no. 11 (2020): 1–13.

52. C. Manyi-Loh, S. Mamphweli, et al., "Antibiotic Use in Agriculture and Its Consequential Resistance in Environmental Sources: Potential Public Health Implications," *Molecules* 23, no. 4 (2018): 795; D. Schar, E. Y. Klein, et al., "Global Trends in Antimicrobial Use in Aquaculture," *Scientific Reports* 10, no. 21878 (2020), https://doi.org/10.1038/s41598-020-78849-3.

53. V. H. Tournas, "Microbial Contamination of Select Dietary Supplements," *Journal of Food Safety* 29 (2009): 430–442.

54. "Public Notification: 'Libido Sexual Enhancer' Contains Hidden Drug Ingredient," U.S. Food and Drug Administration, October 23, 2015, https://www.fda.gov/drugs

/medication-health-fraud/public-notification-libido-sexual-enhancer-contains-hidden
-drug-ingredient.

55. A. Holborow, R. M. Purnell, et al., "Beware the Yellow Slimming Pill: Fatal 2,4-dini-
trophenol Overdose," *BMJ Case Reports* (2016): 1–3.

56. D. Yetman, "What to Know About DNP, the Weight-Loss Drug," *Healthline*, January
14, 2021, www.healthline.com/health/dnp-steroid.

57. R. L. Cosslett, "'I Thought It Was a Miracle. Then I Started Shaking': The Danger of
Buying Diet Pills Online," *Guardian*, November 3, 2018, www.theguardian.com/life
andstyle/2018/nov/03/diet-pills-danger-sweat-heart-attack-weight-loss-rhiannon-lucy
-cosslett.

58. "DMAA in Products Marketed as Dietary Supplements," US Food and Drug Administration, March 29, 2021, https://www.fda.gov/food/dietary-supplement-products-ingre
dients/dmaa-products-marketed-dietary-supplements; B. Venhuis, P. Keizers, et al., "A
Cocktail of Synthetic Stimulants Found in a Dietary Supplement Associated with
Serious Adverse Events," *Drug Testing and Analysis* 6, no. 6 (2014): 578–581; J. Grun-
dlingh, P. I. Dargan, et al., "2,4-dinitrophenol (DNP): A Weight Loss Agent with Significant Acute Toxicity and Risk of Death," *Journal of Medical* 7, no. 3 (2011):
205–212.

59. P. G. Shekelle, M. L. Hardy, et al., "Efficacy and Safety of Ephedra and Ephedrine for
Weight Loss and Athletic Performance: A Meta-Analysis," *Journal of the American
Medical Association* 289, no. 12 (2003): 1537–1545; "Small Entity Compliance Guide:
Final Rule Declaring Dietary Supplements Containing Ephedrine Alkaloids Adulter-
ated Because They Present an Unreasonable Risk," US Food and Drug Administration,
September 20, 2018, www.fda.gov/regulatory-information/search-fda-guidance-docu
ments/small-entity-compliance-guide-final-rule-declaring-dietary-supplements
-containing-ephedrine.

Index

Page numbers that appear in *italics* refer to illustrations. Page numbers followed by *n* refer to footnotes. Page numbers followed by *t* refer to tables.

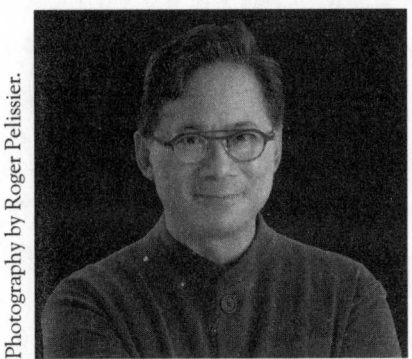

About the Author

Dr. William Li is a world-renowned physician, scientist, and *New York Times* bestselling author. Best known for his role as president and medical director of the Angiogenesis Foundation, Dr. Li began a crusade in 1994 to bring angiogenesis from the research laboratory to the patient's bedside. His work ultimately led to more than forty game-changing, FDA-approved interventions for cancer, cardiovascular disease, wound healing, and vision loss, which have impacted more than fifty million people worldwide. Today, Dr. Li's original vision to make angiogenesis part of mainstream medicine has been realized and his mission is expanding into new health frontiers that place health destiny under the power of individuals and not healthcare systems.

Dr. Li's pioneering approach to food as medicine involves using the rigorous tools of biology and biotechnology to understand not only the components of food but also how the body responds to what it is fed. His approach is leading to a deeper understanding of the cellular mechanisms responsible for the health benefits of food, and it is generating the scientific, clinical, and population-based evidence that paves the way toward disease prevention, better fitness, and faster recovery from illness.

A health futurist, Dr. Li has worked with top universities, leading companies, and scores of advocacy groups, governments, and institutions across five continents. He has forged collaborations with the National Institutes of Health, the World Health Organization, and the Food and Drug Administration. His accomplishments have been recognized by the Milken Institute, the Bill and Melinda Gates Foundation, Clinton Global Initiative, Virgin Unite, and the Richard Nixon Presidential Library, and the Vatican has thrice invited Dr. Li to present his work and vision for the future of health. He has advised King Charles III and Sir Richard Branson on diet and health. His wildly popular TED Talk "Can We Eat to Starve Cancer?" has garnered more than eleven million views. Bono, the lead singer of the band U2, writing in the *New York Times,* called Dr. Li one of the top ten people to watch in the coming decade "with the potential to change the world."

Dr. Li has authored more than one hundred scientific publications in leading journals, such as the *New England Journal of Medicine, Science, Nature Reviews, The Lancet,* and more. He has served on the faculties of Harvard, Tufts, and Dartmouth. A guest expert on CNN, ABC News, and MSNBC, Dr. Li has also been featured in *USA Today, TIME,* the *Wall Street Journal, The Atlantic,* and *NPR,* as well as numerous podcasts and radio shows. Dr. Li is a graduate of Harvard College and the University of Pittsburgh School of Medicine, and he completed his residency at Massachusetts General Hospital.

When he's not writing, disease fighting, or teaching, Dr. Li enjoys traveling, cooking, and listening to an eclectic music playlist.

 To learn more, visit:
www.drwilliamli.com
@drwilliamli